D1701296

THE CERVICAL SPINE SURGERY ATLAS

SECOND EDITION

THE CERVICAL SPINE SURGERY ATLAS

SECOND EDITION

HARRY N. HERKOWITZ, MD, EDITOR

Chairman, Department of Orthopedic Surgery
William Beaumont Hospital, Royal Oak, MI

The Cervical Spine Research Society
Editorial Committee

Charles R. Clark, Chair
Edward C. Benzel, MD
Bradford L. Currier, MD
John P. Dormans, MD
Jiri Dvorak, MD
Frank J. Eismont, MD
Steven R. Garfin, MD
Harry N. Herkowitz, MD
Christopher G. Ullrich, MD
Alexander R. Vaccaro, MD

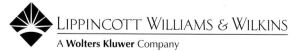

LIPPINCOTT WILLIAMS & WILKINS
A **Wolters Kluwer** Company
Philadelphia • Baltimore • New York • London
Buenos Aires • Hong Kong • Sydney • Tokyo

Acquisitions Editor: Robert Hurley
Developmental Editors: Lisa Consoli, Denise Martin
Supervising Editor: Steven P. Martin
Production Editor: Richard Rothschild, Print Matters, Inc.
Manufacturing Manager: Colin J. Warnock
Cover Designer: Patricia Gast
Compositor: Compset, Inc.
Printer: Edwards Brothers

© 2004 by LIPPINCOTT WILLIAMS & WILKINS
530 Walnut Street
Philadelphia, PA 19106 USA
LWW.com

All rights reserved. This book is protected by copyright. No part of this book may be
reproduced in any form or by any means, including photocopying, or utilized by any
information storage and retrieval system without written permission from the copyright
owner, except for brief quotations embodied in critical articles and reviews. Materials
appearing in this book prepared by individuals as part of their official duties as U.S.
government employees are not covered by the above-mentioned copyright.

Printed in the USA

Library of Congress Cataloging-in-Publication Data

The cervical spine surgery atlas / Harry N. Herkowitz, editor ; the Cervical Spine
  Research Society Editorial Committee, Charles R. Clark . . . [et al.].—2nd ed.
     p. ; cm.
  Rev. ed. of: The cervical spine / edited by Henry H. Sherk. c1994.
  Includes bibliographical references and index.
  ISBN 0-781-74435-0 (hc)
  1. Cervical vertebrae—Surgery—Atlases. I. Herkowitz, Harry N. II. Cervical Spine
Research Society. Editorial Committee. III. Cervical spine.
  [DNLM: 1. Cervical Vertebrae—surgery—Atlases. 2. Surgical Procedures,
Operative—methods—Atlases. WE 17 C4197 2003]
RD533.C455 2003
617.4'71—dc22

                                                                    2003058926

Care has been taken to confirm the accuracy of the information presented and to describe
generally accepted practices. However, the authors, editors, and publisher are not responsible
for errors or omissions or for any consequences from application of the information in
this book and make no warranty, expressed or implied, with respect to the currency,
completeness, or accuracy of the contents of the publication. Application of this information
in a particular situation remains the professional responsibility of the practitioner.

    The authors, editors, and publisher have exerted every effort to ensure that drug
selection and dosage set forth in this text are in accordance with current recommendations
and practice at the time of publication. However, in view of ongoing research, changes in
government regulations, and the constant flow of information relating to drug therapy and
drug reactions, the reader is urged to check the package insert for each drug for any change
in indications and dosage and for added warnings and precautions. This is particularly
important when the recommended agent is a new or infrequently employed drug.

    Some drugs and medical devices presented in this publication have Food and Drug
Administration (FDA) clearance for limited use in restricted research settings. It is the
responsibility of the health care provider to ascertain the FDA status of each drug or
device planned for use in their clinical practice.

10 9 8 7 6 5 4 3 2 1

This edition of the Cervical Spine Research Society Atlas is dedicated to our members who have passed on, many of whom were pioneers, innovators and educators. They formed the foundation upon which this society was founded. Their research, publications, lectures, and affinity for sharing knowledge with students, residents, fellows and colleagues set a fine example for those of us who followed.

Lewis D. Anderson, MD	1999
Claude Argenson, MD	2002
Elliott E. Blinderman, MD	2002
David W. Cahill, MD	2003
Ralph B. Cloward, MD	2001
J. William Fielding, MD	1998
Jacob J. Graham, MD	2000
Brian H. Huncke, MD	1995
Adolphe Jung, MD	1995
Joseph Ransohoff, MD	2002
Lee H. Riley Jr, MD	2001
Raymond Roy-Camille, MD	1997
E. Shannon Stauffer, MD	2002
Henk Verbiest, MD	1997
Josc Maria Vieira, MD	2003
Thomas S. Whitecloud, III, MD	2003

CONTENTS

CONTRIBUTORS

Jean Jacques Abitbol, MD, FRCSC California Spine Group, San Diego, CA

Kuniyoshi Abumi, MD Department of Orthopedic Surgery, Hokkaido University Hospital, Sapporo, Japan

Todd J. Albert, MD Rothman Institute, Philadelphia, PA

Howard S. An, MD Rush-Presbyterian-St. Luke's Medical Center, Chicago, IL

Paul A. Anderson, MD Associate Professor of Orthopedic Surgery and Rehabilitation, University of Wisconsin, Madison, WI

Ronald I. Apfelbaum, MD, FACS Professor, University of Utah, Department of Neurosurgery, Salt Lake City, UT

Hieu T. Ball, MD University of California, Davis, Bay Area Spine Institute, Walnut Creek, CA

Theodore A. Belanger, MD Miller Orthopedic Clinic, Charlotte, NC

Ashok Biyani, MD Medical College of Ohio, Department of Orthopedic Surgery, Toledo, OH

Christopher M. Bono, MD Boston University Medical Center, Department of Orthopedic Surgery, Boston, MA 02978

Jeffrey D. Coe, MD Medical Director of the Center for Spinal Deformity and Injury, Community Hospital of Los Gatos, Los Gatos, CA

Patrick J. Connolly, MD Institute for Spine Care, Syracuse, NY

Paul R. Cooper, MD New York University Medical Center, Department of Neurosurgery, New York, NY

Bradford L. Currier, MD Department of Orthopedics, Mayo Clinic, Rochester, MN

Rick B. Delamarter, MD The Spine Institute at Saint John's Health Center, Santa Monica, CA

Curtis A. Dickman, MD Associate Chief of Spinal Neurosurgery and Director of Spine Research, Barrow Neurological Institute, Division of Neurological Surgery, Phoenix, AZ

William F. Donaldson III, MD Department of Orthopedic Surgery and Neurological Surgery, University of Pittsburgh Medical Center, Pittsburgh, PA

Jason C. Eck, MS Center for Sports Medicine and Orthopedics, Chattanooga, TN

Frank Eismont, MD Department of Orthopedic Surgery, University of Miami, Miami, FL

Sanford E. Emery, MD Department of Orthopedics, University Orthopedic Associates, Cleveland, OH

Nancy E. Epstein, MD, FACS Division of Neurosurgery, Winthrop University Hospital, Mineola, NY, Professor, Albert Einstein College of Medicine, Bronx, NY

Michael G. Fehlings, MD, PhD, FRCSC Division of Neurosurgery, University of Toronto, Toronto, ON

Jeffrey S. Fischgrund, MD Department of Orthopedics, William Beaumont Hospital, Royal Oak, MI

Steven R. Garfin, MD Professor and Chair of Orthopedic Surgery, UCSD Medical Center, San Diego, CA

Alexander J. Ghanayem, MD Chief, Division of Spine Surgery, Loyola University Medical Center, Maywood, IL

L. Fernando Gonzalez, MD Division of Neurological Surgery, Barrow Neurological Institute, Phoenix, AZ

Eric J. Graham Department of Orthopedic Surgery, University of Pittsburgh Medical Center, Pittsburgh, PA

Dieter Grob, MD Chief, Spine Unit, Schultess Klinik, Zurich, Switzerland

John G. Heller, MD Emory Spine Center, Emory University, Department of Orthopedics, Atlanta, GA

Harry N. Herkowitz, MD Chairman, Department of Orthopedic Surgery, William Beaumont Hospital, Royal Oak, MI

Scott D. Hodges, DO Center for Sports Medicine and Orthopedics, Chattanooga, TN

Noboru Hosono, MD, PhD Department of Orthopedic Surgery, Osaka University Graduate School of Medicine, Osaka, Japan

Paul A. House, MD   Department of Neurosurgery, University of Utah Health Sciences Center, Salt Lake City, UT

Manabu Ito, MD, Dr Med Sci   Department of Orthopedic Surgery, Hokkaido University Graduate School of Medicine, Sapporo, Japan

James D. Kang, MD   Associate Professor of Orthopedic Surgery and Neurological Surgery, University of Pittsburgh Medical Center, Pittsburgh, PA

Christopher P. Kauffman, MD   Assistant Clinical Professor, UCSD, Dept of Orthopaedic Surgery, San Diego, CA

Choll W. Kim, MD, PhD   Assistant Professor Orthopedic Surgery, University of California, San Diego, CA

Yoshihisa Kotani, MD   Department of Orthopedic Surgery, Hokkaido University Graduate School of Medicine, Sapporo, Japan

Samir Kulkarni, MD   Research Institute International, Inc., Phoenix, AZ

Peter J. Lennarson, MD   Neurosurgical Service, Wright-Patterson AFB Medical Center, Wright-Patterson AFB, OH

Alan M. Levine, MD   Director of the Alvin and Lois Lapidus Cancer Institute, Sinai Hospital of Baltimore, University of Maryland, Baltimore, MD

Gary L. Lowery, MD, PhD   Chief of Spine Surgery, Phoenix Orthopedic Residency Program, Phoenix, AZ

Eric M. Massicotte, MD, MSc, FRCSC   University of Toronto, Division of Neurosurgery, Toronto, ON

Anthony J. Matan, MD   SUNY Upstate Medical University, Department of Orthopedic Surgery, Syracuse, NY

Randall R. McCafferty, MD   Chief, Neurosurgical Services, Wright-Patterson AFB Medical Center, Wright-Patterson AFB, OH

Robert A. McGuire Jr., MD   Professor and Chairman, Department of Orthopedics, University of Mississippi Medical Center, Jackson, MS

Howard Moses, MD, MS   Department of Neurology, Johns Hopkins School of Medicine, Lutherville, MD

Takenori Oda, MD, DMSc   Department of Orthopedics, National Osaka-Minami Hospital

Keiro Ono, MD   Osaka Graduate School of Medicine, Osaka Kosei-nenkin Hospital, Osaka, Japan

Chetan K. Patel, MD   William Beaumont Hospital, Department of Orthopedic Surgery, Royal Oak, MI

Marshal D. Peris, MD   Northern Westchester Hospital Center, Mount Kisco, NY

John K. Ratliff, MD   Rush-Presbyterian-St. Luke's Medical Center, Chicago, IL

Alok D. Sharan, MD   Albany Medical Center, Division of Orthopedic Surgery, Albany, NY

Kanwaldeep S. Sidhu, MD   St. John Hospital, The Hip and Knee Center, Detroit, MI

Jeff S. Silber, MD   Chief of Orthopedic Spine Surgery, Long Island Jewish Medical Center, New Hyde Park, NY

Vincent C. Traynelis, MD   University of Iowa Hospital, Division of Neurosurgery, Iowa City, IA

Eeric Truumees, MD   Department of Orthopedic Surgery, Willliam Beaumont Hospital, Royal Oak, MI

Alexander R. Vaccaro, MD   The Rothman Institute, Thomas Jefferson University, Philadelphia, PA

Kazuo Yonenobu, MD, PhD   Assistant Director, National Osaka-Minami Hospital, Kawachinagano-City, Japan

Thomas A. Zdeblick, MD   Professor and Chairman, Department of Orthopedic Surgery & Rehabilitation Medicine, University of Wisconsin, Madison, WI

PREFACE

Among the various missions of the Cervical Spine Research Society (CSRS), the most important is to educate those who have an interest in learning and mastering cervical spine disorders. This includes students, residents, fellows, and allied health personnel in addition to our medical and surgical members and colleagues. This is accomplished through our annual meeting, CSRS publications, CSRS instructional courses, and our CSRS website.

The second edition of the CSRS Atlas builds on the principles of the first edition in providing detailed information on surgical approaches and techniques. The second edition has been completely rewritten and updated to include the newest surgical techniques and instrumentation systems. The artwork in this edition is designed to give the reader a clear picture of approach and technique so that learning of these procedures will be made easier.

By combining the material contained in the Atlas with that of the 4th edition of the CSRS textbooks, students of cervical spine disorders will have a comprehensive study and learning guide to assist in mastering this most fascinating part of human anatomy.

The authors of this edition should be commended for their detailed and thorough chapters and for getting their work in under the deadline. On behalf of the members of the CSRS and the Editorial Board, we hope that you will find the CSRS Atlas enhances your understanding of cervical spine approaches and techniques.

Harry N. Herkowitz, MD

ACKNOWLEDGMENTS

Without the participation of the following people, this edition of the Cervical Spine Research Society Atlas would not be in print.

Christine Musich, my administrative assistant, whose organizational skills and ability to effectively communicate in a timely fashion with all the authors ensured that all of the chapters would be submitted on time.

Eeric Truumees, M.D., my former fellow, who assisted in organizing the chapters and subsections and whose ideas and comments contributed significantly to the Atlas.

Peggy Flaherty-Wlezien, our CSRS society manager, who is constantly "on top of all CSRS-related matters."

Robert Hurley of Lippincott Williams & Wilkins, who has continually supported CSRS publications and provided the editorial support to see these projects come to fruition.

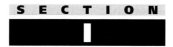

SURGICAL PREPARATION

1

CERVICAL TRACTION, POSITIONING, AND BRACES

EERIC TRUUMEES

Successful application of traction, operative positioning, and bracing techniques is critical in the successful operative management of cervical spine disorders. Patients with cervical trauma and deformity are often placed in traction for preoperative reduction and stabilization. Intraoperative traction provides stabilization and exposure. Appropriate patient positioning improves surgical exposure and decreases perioperative risk. Cervical braces are applied preoperatively and postoperatively for symptom relief and stabilization.

TRACTION

Cervical traction is indicated for the following:

- Temporary stabilization to preserve neurologic function in trauma patients
- Preoperative reduction in patients with deformity or displaced fractures
- Intraoperative stabilization and interspace distraction for anterior grafting
- Pain relief for patients with radiculopathy or muscle spasm

One of a variety of tong or pin devices may be used to apply skeletal traction. Cervical skin traction can be applied manually or via a head halter. The anesthetist may apply manual traction intraoperatively to distract the interspace for graft insertion. Interspace distraction may also be achieved with lamina spreaders, Caspar distractors, or other implanted devices.

A number of treatment parameters apply to the use of cervical traction. When traction is maintained preoperatively or postoperatively, prism glasses allow the alert patient to read or watch television. Turn off overhead lights when possible. Chewing and swallowing difficulties when recumbent present an aspiration risk. Pad and frequently check the occiput for signs of pressure sores.

Skin Traction

Cervical traction is quickly, easily, and noninvasively applied with a head halter. During surgery, such traction stabilizes the neck and improves access to the disc space. When used in the physical therapy department or as part of a "home traction kit," skin traction may decrease muscle spasm and radicular pain.

Halter traction is not useful in true cervical instability because of force and time limitations. Most patients will not tolerate more than 5 to 7 pounds or 2 to 3 hours of continuous traction. Some patients, particularly those with temporomandibular joint problems, complain of jaw pain with halter traction. A football mouthpiece may decrease jaw complaints.

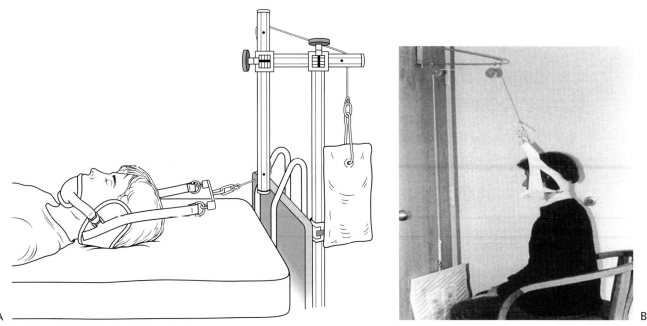

FIGURE 1.1. A: A spine patient in head halter traction. Note the spreader bar to keep the halter from pressing against the sides of the head. (From Zimmer, Inc. *Traction manual: a complete reference guide to the basics of traction.* Warsaw, IN: Zimmer, Inc., 1991, with permission.) **B:** This seated patient is undergoing skin traction as part of the treatment of cervical radiculopathy.

When the halter has been applied, inspect the chin piece and prevent throat constriction. Attach a wide spreader bar to prevent the halter straps from compressing the ears. Additional padding, felt, or cornstarch may reduce skin irritation (Fig. 1.1).

Gardner-Wells Tongs

Skeletal traction, through either tongs or a halo, has fewer force and temporal limitations. Of the wide variety of cervical tongs available, Gardner-Wells tongs are the most commonly used. These tongs are a quick and simple, but effective means by which a single operator can apply in-line cervical traction. Gardner-Wells tongs do not significantly limit voluntary rotation, flexion, or extension and must be used with caution in uncooperative patients. For further cervical control, apply a simple rigid collar or neck blocks in conjunction with tongs.

The indications for tongs traction are as follows:

- Reduction of cervical deformity, fracture, or dislocation in a patient likely to require surgical stabilization or nonhalo immobilization
- Temporary intraoperative stabilization and disc space access

Gardner-Wells tongs are composed of a U-shaped bar with two fixation pins. Typically, instructions for application of the tongs are welded to metal tongs. Newer graphite composite tongs are compatible with magnetic resonance imaging (Fig. 1.2). In both varieties, one of the fixation pins is solid and the other is spring-loaded. Tighten these pins simultaneously. When the indicator pin protrudes 1 mm, a pressure of 13.6 kg or 30 lb has been achieved. This pressure yields a pull-out strength of between 65 and 120 pounds. Some brands include a test bar to check the spring-loaded point and protect the tongs when not in use.

Apply Gardner-Wells tongs with the patient awake and minimally premedicated. No shave or Betadine prep is required. Inject the skin and the underlying galea with local

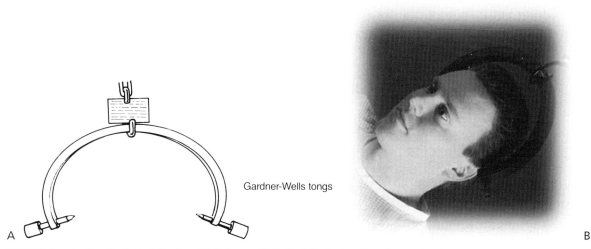

FIGURE 1.2. **A:** Standard steel Gardner-Wells tongs. Note that the instructions for application are welded to the traction hook. **B:** Graphite and titanium composite tongs are also available. These tongs are compatible with advanced imaging equipment, such as magnetic resonance imaging.

anesthetic over the intended entry sites. Plan pin sites below the equator (or widest portion) of the skull. For direct, in-line traction, place the pins below the temporal ridge and above the temporalis muscle immediately above and anterior to the pinnae (Fig. 1.3). In most patients, enter approximately 2 cm above the external auditory canal. Additional flexion requires a more posterior pin placement. Similarly, add an extension moment by moving the pin entry site slightly anterior to the pinna.

No skin incision is made. Bring the pins slowly against the anesthetized part of the scalp and tighten simultaneously until the marker pin protrudes 1 mm (Fig. 1.4). Rock the tongs to further seat the pins into the skull. Tighten the locking nuts. When traction is maintained longer than 24 hours, retighten the pins until the indicator pin is flush with the flat end of the screw. Do not tighten beyond this point.

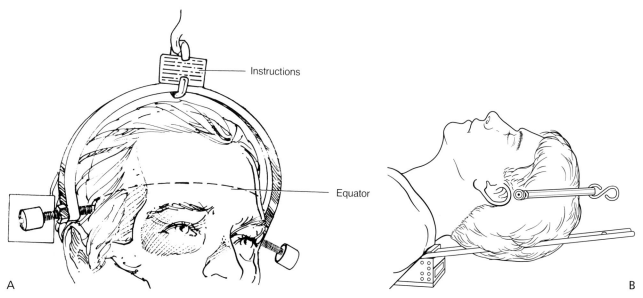

FIGURE 1.3. Correct positioning of Gardner-Wells tongs 1 to 2 cm above the external auditory meatus and below the temporal ridge. Tongs must be placed below the equator of the skull. (From Browner BD, Jupiter JB, Levine AM, et al., eds. *Skeletal trauma,* 2nd ed. Philadelphia: WB Saunders, 1998, p. 764, with permission.)

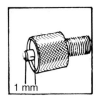

FIGURE 1.4. Tighten the screws simultaneously until the pressure pin on the spring-loaded screw protrudes 1 mm.

Mayfield Tongs

Mayfield tongs are not typically used for traction, but are included here as another important skeletal fixation device for cervical spine surgery. This device rigidly holds the head to the operating table and is particularly useful during complex posterior cervical reconstruction procedures. Mayfield tongs have a more elaborate **U**-shaped frame with width and rotational adjustability (Fig. 1.5). On one side, a hinged yoke holds two pins. The opposite side contains a single pin attachment.

To allow for facial swelling in long prone cases and for freedom of motion in patient positioning, ensure at least 2 cm between the Mayfield tongs and the bridge of the nose. Center the single Mayfield pin just above the ear as for Gardner-Wells tongs (see previous section). Span the opposite ear with the double pins at the same cranial-caudal level. The double pins may also span the temporal fossa. Place the anterior pins into the frontal bone approximately 1 cm above the eyebrow in the outer third of the orbit (see frontal halo pins).

After the pin sites have been selected, prepare the skin with Betadine. Select either pediatric or adult pins. Use sterile technique to insert the pins into their receptacles within the tongs. Open the tongs widely and align them with the skull. Bring the tongs together. Then, tension the pins on the skull with the calibrated tightening knob to 6 or 8 inch-pounds. Read the manufacturer's instructions for the calibration scale.

Halo Ring

A halo ring is useful for preoperative traction, to maintain head position during complex cervical spine operations, and as part of an orthotic device. However, halo ring application is more dangerous, more complex, and more time intensive than Gardner-Wells tongs application. Do not attempt placement without at least one assistant. Restrict halo traction to those patients presenting in a halo or requiring long-term halo brace immobilization. Halo skeletal traction has been described for chronic cervical spine deformities

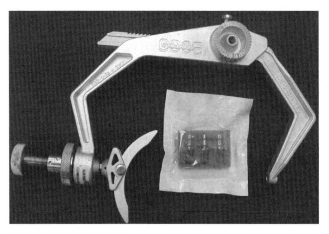

FIGURE 1.5. Mayfield tongs.

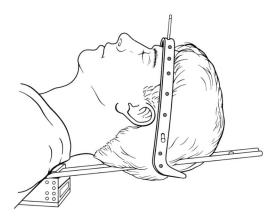

FIGURE 1.6. When a closed halo ring is employed, the halo head holder allows for proper positioning and access to the posterior ring. (From Browner BD, Jupiter JB, Levine AM, et al., eds. *Skeletal trauma,* 2nd ed. Philadelphia: WB Saunders, 1998, p. 762, with permission.)

prior to definitive operative stabilization. However, a high rate of infectious complications have been reported.

Position the patient on a spine board. Leave a semirigid collar in place until final halo tightening. For closed ring halo systems, move the patient to the end of the bed. Hang the head over the edge of the bed to access the posterior skull. Stabilize the head manually with axial distraction. If available, insert the special halo head support (Fig. 1.6). While one operator continues to stabilize the spine, slide the back panel under the patient's back between the scapulae. Attach the occipital support to the back panel and secure tightly. These special support systems are not needed with open-backed (horseshoe) halo rings (Fig. 1.7). As with any cervical spine positioning in children, beware of excess flexion due to the mismatch of head and body size. Use appropriate cut-outs or a split mattress.

A halo can be applied under general anesthesia, but, with spinal instability, apply the ring with the patient alert or under light sedation. Younger children may need deep sedation or general anesthesia.

Size the ring closely. At least 1 cm of clearance is needed between all points of the scalp and ring. If the ring touches the skin of the scalp, pressure sores develop. Position the ring below the equator of the skull no more than 1 cm above the ears or eyebrows (Fig. 1.8). Slippage occurs in rings placed too high on the convexity of the skull.

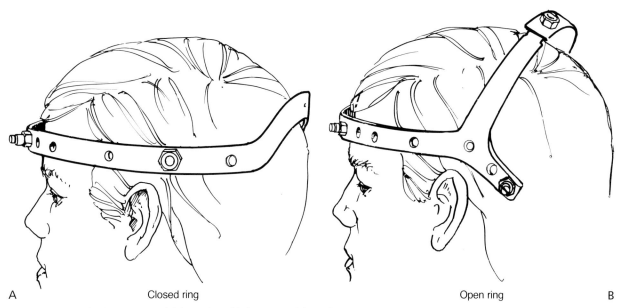

A   Closed ring   Open ring   B

FIGURE 1.7. Halo rings are available in closed (**A**) or open (**B**) configurations.

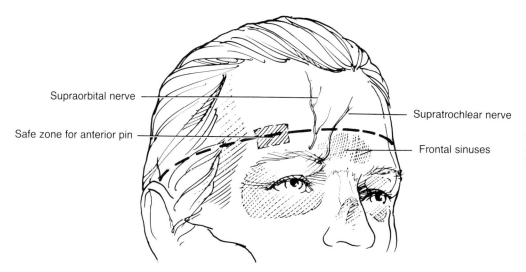

FIGURE 1.8. Anterior halo pins must be placed in the safe zone in the outer third of the orbital ridge. Medially, avoid the frontal sinuses and supraorbital and supratrochlear nerves. Laterally, avoid the thin temporal bone and temporal artery.

In adults, four pins fix the halo ring to the skull. One recent paper reported that, in force-deflection tests, six-pin halo constructs offer significantly higher loads to failure than four-pin constructs with no increase in pin site complications. Eight inch-pounds yields greater holding power and fewer pin site complications than lower torque settings for halo pins. The skulls of children or osteoporotic adults will not tolerate this much torque. In these individuals, a greater number of pins are placed with lower torque. Configurations utilizing 6 to 10 pins placed with finger tightening to 5 pounds of torque have been described. Tension all pins equally. Unequal tension will cause the halo to migrate in the direction of least force. Even in normal adults, halo pins may penetrate the inner table of the skull when torque exceeds 10 inch-pounds. If resistance to insertion suddenly decreases, stop inserting the pin. It is likely that the pin has penetrated the calvarium. If in doubt, obtain a postplacement skull computed tomographic (CT) scan. In some cases, use a preplacement CT scan to assess the following:

1. Skull thickness
2. Skull fractures
3. Lytic lesions
4. Location of suture lines in children

In small children, if the holding power of halo pins is in doubt, use tongs for reduction and apply a Minerva cast.

Temporarily hold the ring in position with plastic pods attached through the center forehead hole and two posterior holes (Fig. 1.9). A double-backed piece of adhesive tape helps to keep the pins from sliding. Place the two anterior pins in the supraorbital ridge "safe zone" between the middle to lateral thirds of the orbit. Over-medial pins may injure the supraorbital or supratrochlear nerves. Lateral pins may injure the temporal artery or zygomaticotemporal nerve, which supplies sensation to the temporal area. Lateral pins suffer from decreased strength in the thin temporal bone and may penetrate the temporalis muscle, affecting mandibular function. Stay within 1 cm of the orbit, to avoid the frontal sinus. Place the posterior pins immediately behind the pinnae.

Some authors recommend shaving the scalp over the posterior holes, but this is not necessary. Careful preparation of the skin, however, is essential. Inject a plain local anesthetic, such as 2% lidocaine, through the intended hole in the halo ring. First, create a bleb in the scalp. Then, track down to the galea. Avoid epinephrine to decrease the risk of skin necrosis. As with tongs, no skin incision is required (Fig. 1.10).

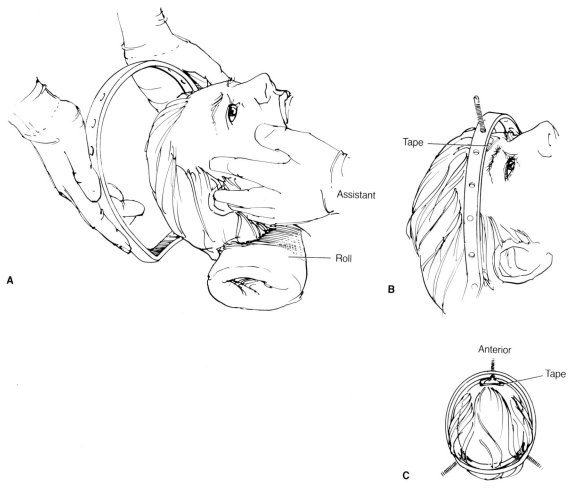

FIGURE 1.9. Application of the halo ring requires at least one assistant. **A:** Carefully position the head and size the ring. **B** and **C:** Temporarily maintain halo positioning using tape and plastic positioning pods.

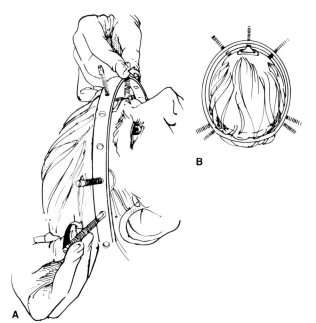

FIGURE 1.10. Recheck halo ring position from several vantage points. If the ring is optimally positioned, prepare the skin and inject local anesthetic. **A** and **B:** Insert diagonally opposite pins simultaneously until finger tight.

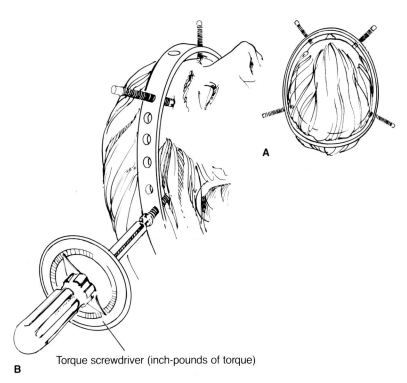

B

Torque screwdriver (inch-pounds of torque)

FIGURE 1.11. Once all pins are finger tight, complete the insertion using a torque wrench.

Prior to insertion of the anterior pins, ask the patient to close his or her eyes to avoid skin traction. Diagonally opposite pins are tightened simultaneously until all are finger tight (Fig. 1.11). Then, remove the baseplates and positioning pins. Finally, tension the pins with a torque wrench one inch-pound at a time. Finally, tighten the locking nuts (Fig. 1.12).

Once the ring is in place, apply a traction bar, or attach the halo to a vest or cast (Fig. 1.13). Surgery may be successfully performed either in the halo vest or with the halo ring attached to the operative table using a Mayfield halo holder (see below). At surgery, the posterior half of the shell may be temporarily removed, or the uprights may be left in place. If necessary, cut the vest back with a cast saw to allow adequate access to the neck.

Traction Assembly

Although wheelchair traction is used in certain cases of spinal deformity, most cervical traction is applied supine. A regular hospital bed or special spine frame can be employed.

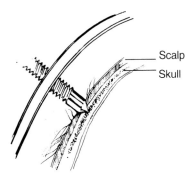

Scalp

Skull

FIGURE 1.12. Assess the maximal torque based on the quality of the patient's bone. In most adults, 6 to 8 inch-pounds of torque can be applied safely. Greater than 10 inch-pounds may cause the pins to protrude through the inner table of the skull.

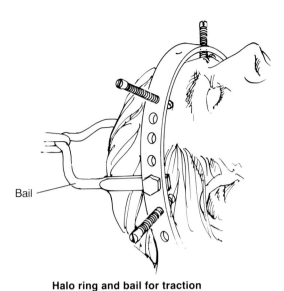

Halo ring and bail for traction

FIGURE 1.13. If the halo ring is to be used for in-line traction, attach a bail for the traction cord.

Excess friction between the bed and the patient's head, difficulty working around the size of the bed, and difficulty in obtaining radiographs limit the usefulness of a regular hospital bed. A Stryker turning frame improves patient and radiographic access and is appropriate for most preoperative traction. The patient can undergo either prone or supine surgery on this frame without removal of traction. Intraoperative cervical traction can be applied on a regular operating table through available head traction modules. Other operating tables, such as the Jackson frame, offer traction attachments as well.

With the exception of small amounts of force lost to friction, these in-line traction configurations deliver pound-for-pound force to the cervical spine. Use the patient's body weight and friction for countertraction. With higher tension, 20 degrees of reverse Trendelenburg positioning provides additional countertraction. A length of cord conveys traction force from the tongs through the frame to the attached weights. This material is subject to wear and bacterial contamination; it should not be reused. Tie special traction knots for safe, smooth maintenance of traction. The mnemonic for this knot is: Up and over, down and over, up and through (Fig. 1.14). Allow extra room at the end of the cord so that the knot may be adjusted without replacing the entire cord. Tape and check the knots to prevent slippage or entanglement in the pulley system. Prior to application of weight, spray the pulley apparatus with a silicone spray and secure the knot ends with adhesive tape.

When applying traction, the patient should be as awake and responsive as possible. Light IV sedation with short-acting agents is appropriate as long as it does not interfere

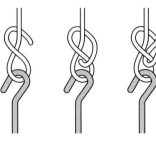

Up and over   Down and over   Up and through

FIGURE 1.14. The proper method to tie a traction knot. (From Zimmer, Inc. *Traction manual: a complete reference guide to the basics of traction.* Warsaw, IN: Zimmer, Inc., 1991, p. 8, with permission.)

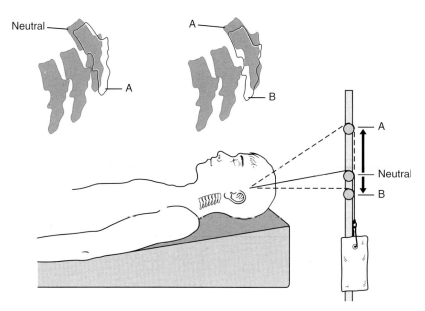

FIGURE 1.15. Changing the flexion moment of in-line traction will often assist with reduction. Flexion can be increased by raising the line of traction **(A)** or reduced by lowering the line of traction **(B)**. Often, the line of traction is raised to reduce perched facets. Once a reduction has been achieved, an extension moment and lower weights can be applied. (From Browner BD, Jupiter JB, Levine AM, et al., eds. *Skeletal trauma,* 2nd ed. Philadelphia: WB Saunders, 1998, p. 823, with permission.)

with neurologic examination. Gradually add weight to a hook at the end of the rope. Do not allow the weights to touch the floor, drag on bed parts, or become entangled with lines and monitoring devices.

Usually, pure axial traction is sufficient. In some trauma situations, increase flexion by adjusting the traction rope position or by placing a bolster between the patient's shoulder blades. This additional flexion moment helps unhook dislocated facets. An extension moment is preferred for many flexion unstable injuries, such as a flexion tear drop fracture (Fig. 1.15).

Optimal traction weight is controversial. Crutchfield's rule estimates the traction force needed to reduce cervical fractures or dislocations. Ten pounds distract the head, and 5 additional pounds are added for each interspace. Thus, a C4–5 fracture dislocation requires 30 pounds of traction, and a C5–6 requires 35 pounds. In reality, more distraction force is often needed. Some authors apply as much as 75% of body weight. If high weights are used, monitor the status of the skull pins. Manufacturer's labeling may limit applied weight to 50 pounds. Additional fixation may be required. A sharp increase in skull pain may predict impending pin failure.

Regardless of the ultimate traction force used, apply the force in a stepwise manner. *Always* start with 10 pounds to help exclude upper cervical instability and avoid overdistraction. Then gradually increase traction weight in 5- or 10-pound increments. Allow 15 minutes for ligamentous creep before applying additional weight. Repeat the radiographs and neurologic exams at each step (Fig. 1.16). Increase traction until the spine is in appropriate alignment. To reduce a facet dislocation, add weight until the facets are unlocked. Then, extend the neck slightly to allow the facets to slide into anatomic position. If the facets perch rather than reducing, change the traction angle to slight flexion. Once the spine is reduced, maintain 10 to 20 pounds of traction and apply a cervical collar. For flexion unstable injuries, maintain extension with a towel roll (Fig. 1.17).

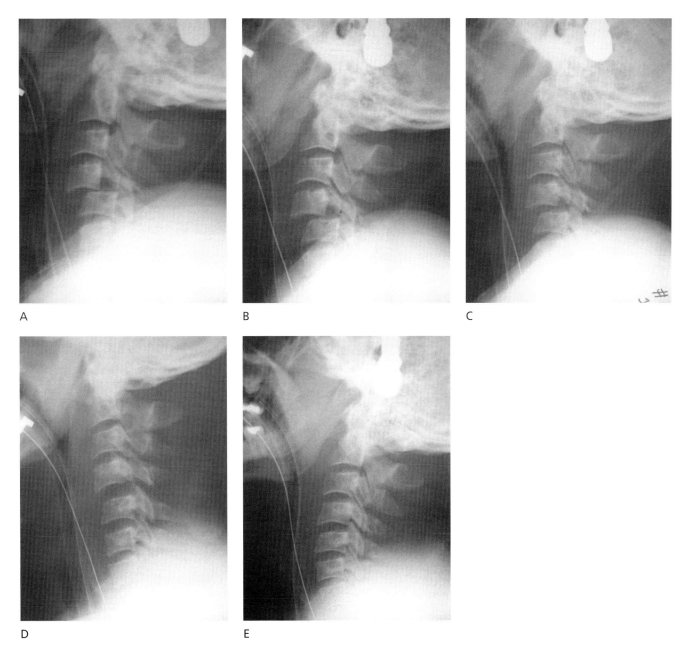

A   B   C

D   E

FIGURE 1.16. Radiographs demonstrating gradual reduction of bilateral dislocated cervical facets using Gardner-Wells tongs traction.

Patient Positioning

Supine and prone positioning are common during cervical spine operations. Seated and lateral positioning are also reported, but much less frequently employed. Safe positioning requires careful control of cervical alignment throughout the procedure. Neuro-muscular relaxation and general anesthesia leave the myelopathic patient susceptible to extreme spine positioning and subsequent spinal cord injury. Test the patient's ability to tolerate flexion and extension while alert and stay well within this range intraoperatively. Safe positioning relies on stable head control with tongs or head holders. Employ extra-long tubing and move anesthesia equipment further from the patient's head to allow access to the patient's head and rapid repositioning (Fig. 1.18). In select circumstances,

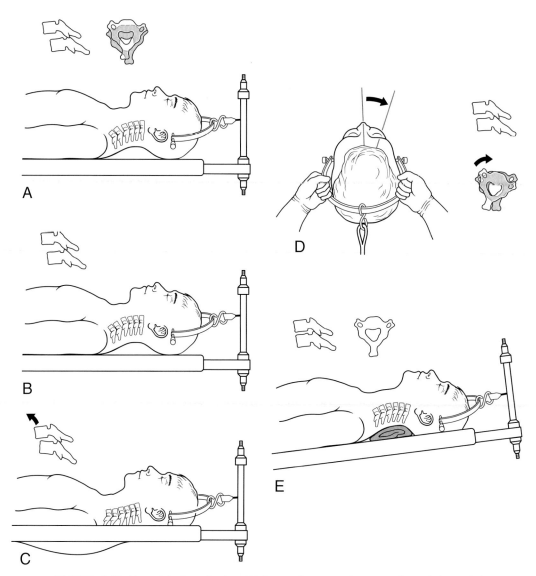

FIGURE 1.17. Use of in-line Gardner-Wells traction to reduce a unilateral facet dislocation. **A:** The patient is flat and supine on a Stryker turning frame with tongs in place. **B:** Weight is gradually increased, distracting the interspace. **C:** The bolster is removed from the shoulder blades to increase the flexion moment. **D:** Manually tilting the tongs away from the side of dislocation unlocks the dislocation. **E:** With the spine reduced, extension is added by placing a towel roll behind the neck. Weight may now be reduced. (From Browner BD, Jupiter JB, Levine AM, et al., eds. *Skeletal trauma,* 2nd ed. Philadelphia: WB Saunders, 1998, p. 824, with permission.)

fiberoptically intubate and transfer the patient while awake. Then perform a neurologic examination prior to anesthetization.

Lateral Decubitus Positioning

Lateral positioning will not be covered in detail here, but is used for a high thoracotomy approach used to address cervicothoracic junction pathology. Place the patient in the left decubitus position. The incision is made on the right because of the proximity of the heart on the left side. Employ an axillary roll and maintain position with a bean bag.

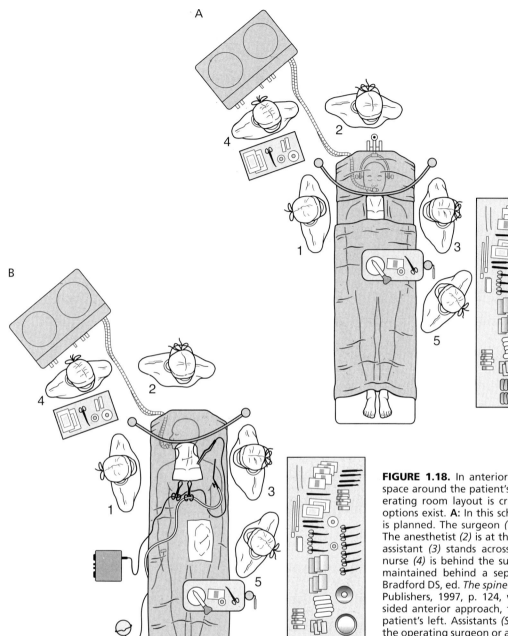

FIGURE 1.18. In anterior spine surgery, there is limited space around the patient's head and neck. Therefore, operating room layout is critical. A number of reasonable options exist. **A:** In this schematic, a right-sided approach is planned. The surgeon *(1)* stands on the patent's right. The anesthetist *(2)* is at the head of the bed. The surgical assistant *(3)* stands across from the surgeon, while the nurse *(4)* is behind the surgeon. Observers *(5 and 6)* are maintained behind a separate, sterile boundary. (From Bradford DS, ed. *The spine.* Philadelphia: Lippincott–Raven Publishers, 1997, p. 124, with permission.) **B:** For a left-sided anterior approach, the surgeon *(S1)* stands on the patient's left. Assistants *(S2 and S3)* may stand alongside the operating surgeon or across from him or her. The anesthesia team *(A1 and A2)* stands at the head of the bed behind a sterile boundary. (From Louis R. *Surgery of the spine: surgical anatomy and operative approaches.* Berlin: Springer-Verlag, 1982, p. 169, with permission.)

Supine Positioning

A majority of cervical spine procedures employ anterior approaches and are performed with the patient supine. These procedures include the Smith-Robinson anterior cervical discectomy with fusion and anterior approaches to tumors, fractures, infections, and deformities. Position the patient on a standard operating room (OR) bed. Occasionally, in trauma or complex circumferential spinal procedures, the Stryker turning frame or Jackson frame are used. These frames allow excellent access for intraoperative anteroposterior imaging (Fig. 1.19).

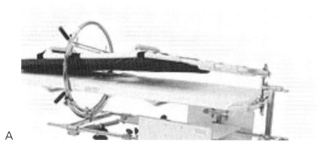

A

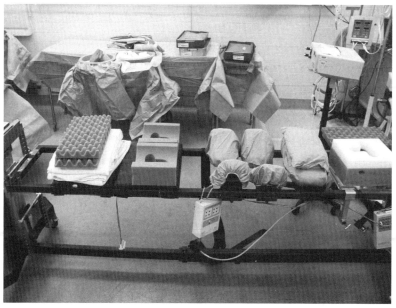

B

FIGURE 1.19. **A:** The Stryker turning frame is useful for both preoperative traction and intraoperative positioning. (Courtesy Stryker, Inc., Kalamazoo, MI.) **B:** The Jackson frame, like the Stryker turning frame, may be used to reposition the patient while maintaining in-line traction. Fluoroscopy and intraoperative radiographs are more easily obtained with these frames than with a standard operating room table.

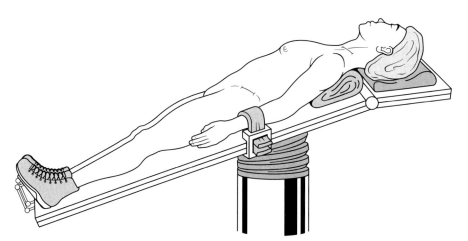

FIGURE 1.20. This patient is positioned supine for anterior cervical spine surgery. Slight reverse Trendelenburg position allows for better drainage. Occasionally, a footrest may be required to prevent distal migration of the patient. The neck is slightly extended using a blanket or towel roll between the shoulder blades. If iliac crest graft is to be obtained, the hip must be bumped up and draped. (From Louis R. *Surgery of the spine: surgical anatomy and operative approaches.* Berlin: Springer-Verlag, 1982, p. 169, with permission.)

Position the patient flat or in slight reverse Trendelenburg position. Reverse Trendelenburg improves visualization and venous drainage, and the body provides counterweight for traction. Place the neck in slight extension to increase exposure to the cervical spine using a small towel roll between the scapulae. Additional extension improves visualization of upper cervical levels. Rotate the head 15 degrees and tape the endotracheal tube to the side opposite that of the approach. In upper cervical cases, nasotracheal intubation allows the mandible to remain closed and improves exposure (Fig. 1.20).

Pad the occiput and stabilize the head. When using the standard OR head extension, concave pillows are suitable for this purpose. A Mayfield horseshoe headrest also controls head rotation and relieves posterior occipital pressure. Use 10 pounds of in-line skeletal traction in patients undergoing multilevel procedures or with unstable spines. A head halter may be acceptable for shorter procedures in the lower cervical spine. Continuous intraoperative traction may be avoided in favor of limited manual or instrument traction during decompression and bone graft insertion.

Tuck the patient's arms at the patient's sides. Pad the cubital tunnels and wrists. Position the shoulders such that they do not interfere with cross-table radiographs of lower cervical segments. Maintain shoulder position by *carefully* taping shoulders down with benzoin and 4-inch cloth tape. Overly aggressive shoulder retraction risks brachial plexus injury. To avoid continuous shoulder traction, pull on the arms during radiography only. Leave the hands accessible under the drapes or pass Kling rolls around the wrists and pass the roll from under the drapes (Fig. 1.21).

Flex the knees and hips with blanket rolls to keep the patent from migrating distally. Pad bony prominences and apply elastic stockings and sequential inflation devices. If

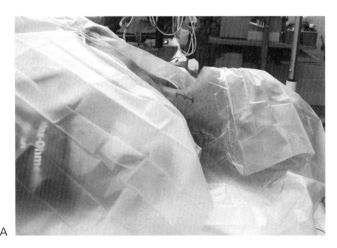
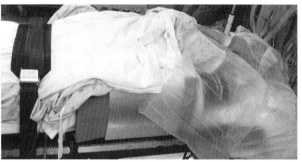

FIGURE 1.21. This patient has been positioned supine for anterior spinal surgery. **A:** The intended incision is marked out and the area is draped. **B:** The patient's arms are tucked. **C:** The neck is maintained in slight extension and rotated slightly to the right.

autologous fibula graft is to be harvested, bump one leg and apply a midthigh tourniquet. Similarly, if autologous iliac crest is to be harvested, place a blanket roll under the hip and maintain access to the area lateral to the anterior superior iliac spine.

Prone Positioning

Posterior approaches to the spine, including laminectomy, laminoplasty, laminoforaminotomy, and posterior stabilization procedures, require prone or seated positioning. Prone positioning, although less complex than seated positioning, requires careful attention to cervical alignment at all times (Fig. 1.22). A firm collar prevents excessive neck motion. Remove the collar once the patient's head has been rigidly fixed to the OR table. In some very unstable patients, even logrolling the patient prone may not be appropriate; use the wedge turning frame and continuous in-line skeletal traction to allow safer prone positioning.

For all prone spine surgery, ocular pressure and excessive hypotension must be fastidiously avoided because postoperative blindness continues to be reported. Posterior cervical spine procedures may be performed on a regular OR bed, Stryker turning frame, or Jackson frame. The Stryker and Jackson frames improve access for fluoroscopy as well as the option of patient rotation with continuous in-line traction. On a standard OR table, use a Wilson frame or towel rolls to decompress the abdomen (Fig. 1.23). Complete decompression decreases intraoperative bleeding and improves pulmonary compli-

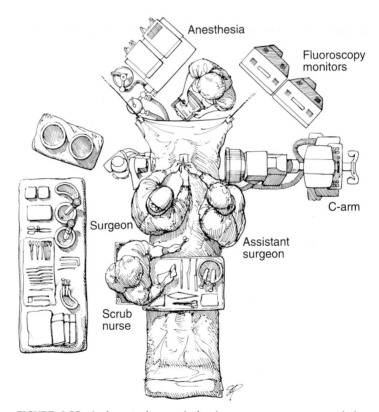

FIGURE 1.22. As in anterior cervical spine surgery, space around the patient's head and neck is limited. Therefore, the operating room layout must be preplanned. In this example of prone positioning for posterior cervical spine surgery, the surgeon stands on the patient's left side. The nurse stands behind the surgeon, and the assistant stands on the opposite side of the table. The anesthesia team remains at the head of the bed behind a sterile boundary. (From Dillin WH, Simeone FA, eds. *Posterior cervical spine surgery.* Philadelphia: Lippincott–Raven Publishers, 1998, p. 63, with permission.)

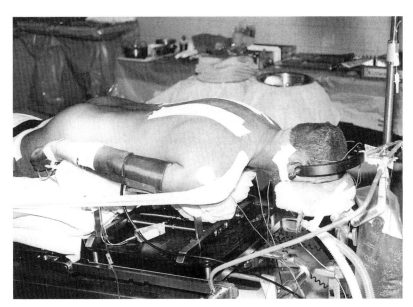

FIGURE 1.23. This patient is positioned prone for posterior cervical spine surgery on a regular operating room bed. In this case, blanket bolsters and a Wilson frame decompress the abdomen. A Mayfield horseshoe headrest is used to support the facet, and in-line traction is maintained through graphite Gardner-Wells tongs. The arms and dorsal skin have been taped down to increase exposure to the posterior cervical spine.

ance, but is difficult to achieve in larger or obese patients. The Jackson frame maintains the most favorable pulmonary compliance (Fig. 1.24).

A number of devices are available to maintain head position, but Mayfield tongs are preferred. A Mayfield horseshoe headrest with Gardner-Wells tongs may be applied in certain, shorter procedures (Fig. 1.25). Avoid horseshoe and other direct-contact facial supports in patients with short nasal bridges or exophthalmus. Further protect the eyes with lubricant and taping. Attach a mirror to the spinal frame and intermittently inspect the patient's face (Fig. 1.26). If a halo is to be used for postoperative immobilization, apply the ring preoperatively. Maintain head position intraoperatively in the vest or by fixing the ring to the OR table (Figs. 1.27–1.29).

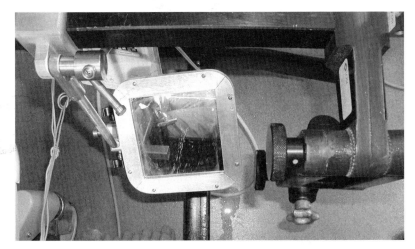

FIGURE 1.24. When patients are positioned prone, careful attention must be paid to ocular and facial pressure. Mirror attachments are available for the Stryker frame that allow intermittent assessment.

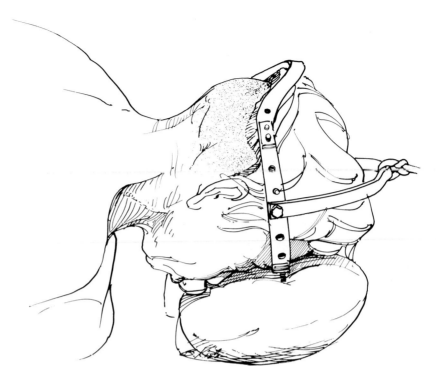

FIGURE 1.25. This patient is positioned for posterior cervical spine surgery using a Mayfield horseshoe headrest and halo traction.

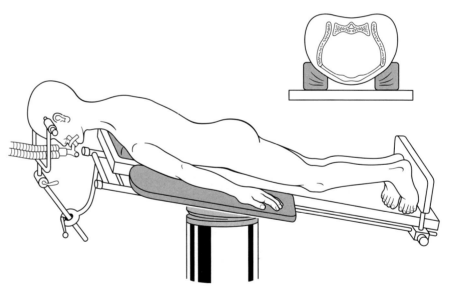

FIGURE 1.26. When patients are positioned prone, prevent pressure on the abdomen using blanket rolls, bolsters, or special prone surgery frames. (From Louis R. *Surgery of the spine: surgical anatomy and operative approaches.* Berlin: Springer-Verlag, 1982, p. 141, with permission.)

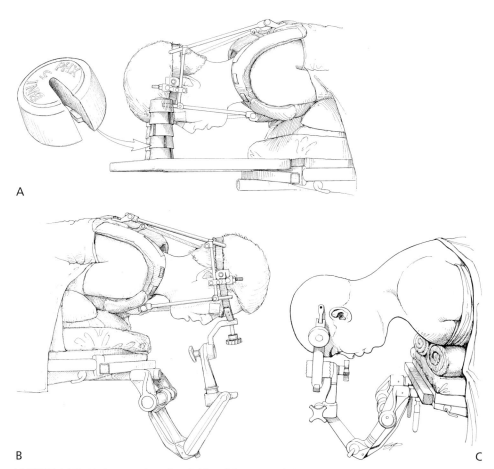

A

B   C

FIGURE 1.27. Various options for rigid stabilization of the cervical spine during prone surgery.
A: This patient is maintained in the halo. Traction weights are used as props to support the halo
uprights. **B:** Here, surgery also takes place in the halo. However, the ring is rigidly secured to the
table using a Mayfield halo attachment. **C:** In this patient, no halo has been applied. Mayfield
tongs hold the head rigidly to a regular operating room table. Bolsters decompress the abdomen.
(From Dillin WH, Simeone FA, eds. *Posterior cervical spine surgery.* Philadelphia: Lippincott–Raven
Publishers, 1998, p. 62, with permission.)

Adequate surgical access may require additional flexion or extension of the spine.
For example, C1–2 posterior stabilization procedures often require slight additional flexion. On the other hand, maintain spinal stability in facetal dislocations with slight extension. Do not overflex the neck merely to eliminate posterior skin folds. Benzoin and tape
can be used to retract excess skin.

Once the patient is positioned, recheck all leads, tubing, and bony prominences. Male
genitalia should hang freely, and pressure should be evenly distributed on the breasts.
Ensure appropriate spinal alignment with a lateral radiograph prior to draping. While the
radiograph is being developed, shave the patient's hair to the inion. Use benzoin and adhesive drapes to prevent prep solution from entering the eyes (Figs. 1.30 and 1.31).

Maintain the arms and shoulders at the patient's side. As with supine procedures,
caudal shoulder traction may improve intraoperative radiography, but avoid overtraction
and brachial plexus injury. Taping significantly delays emergent repositioning should resuscitation be required.

Seated Position

The seated position was introduced into neurosurgical practice for posterior fossa tumors
in 1913. More recently, the potential for serious complications has diminished imple-
mentation of this technique both in the United States and abroad. The seated position

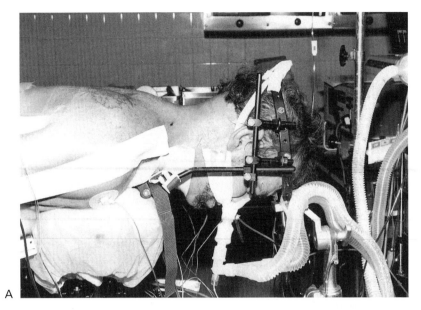

A

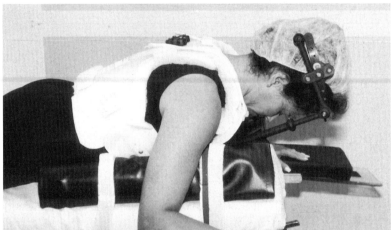

B

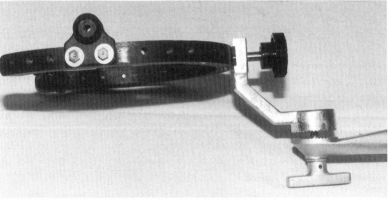

C

FIGURE 1.28. A and **B:** These patients are positioned for posterior cervical spine surgery while in a halo. The posterior vest and uprights have been removed, and addi-
tional stabilization of the ring has been achieved using a Mayfield halo attachment.
(Part B from Guanciale T. Positioning for posterior cervical spine surgery. In: Dillin
WH, Simeone FA, eds. *Posterior cervical spine surgery.* Philadelphia: Lippincott–Raven
Publishers, 1998:7–17, with permission.) **C:** A close-up view of the Mayfield halo at-
tachment. (From Guanciale T. Positioning for posterior cervical spine surgery. In: Dillin
WH, Simeone FA, eds. *Posterior cervical spine surgery.* Philadelphia: Lippincott–Raven
Publishers, 1998:7–17, with permission.)

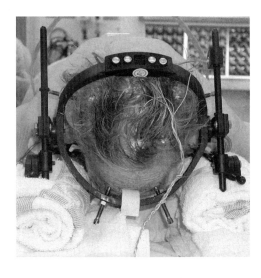

FIGURE 1.29. Axial view of a patient positioned prone for posterior cervical spine surgery while in a halo. The posterior vest and uprights have been removed. There is no pressure on the face.

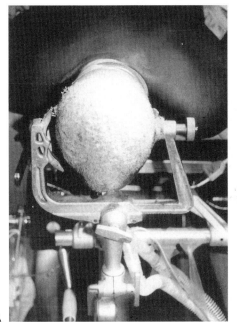

A

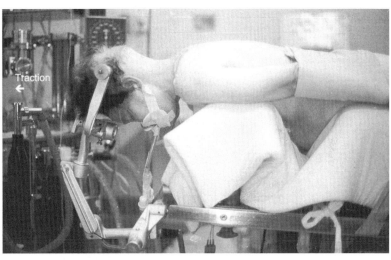

B

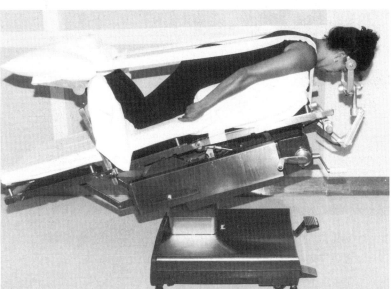

C

FIGURE 1.30. A: This axial view demonstrates proper prone positioning using Mayfield tongs. Note that the patient is rigidly fixed to the regular operating room table through the tongs attachment. There is no pressure on the face. **B:** This patient is positioned prone for posterior cervical spine surgery on a regular operating room table. Here, a Hall frame is used to support the trunk. Mayfield tongs maintain the head and neck in a slightly flexed position. (From Bradford DS, ed. *The spine*. Philadelphia: Lippincott–Raven Publishers, 1997, p. 141, with permission.) **C:** Another example of a patient positioned prone on a regular operating room table. In this case, blankets are used to decompress the chest and abdomen. A leg extension maintains knee flexion. The shoulders are retracted using 4-inch cloth tape. The Mayfield tongs maintain the neck in a slightly flexed position. (From Guanciale T. Positioning for posterior cervical spine surgery. In: Dillin WH, Simeone FA, eds. *Posterior cervical spine surgery*. Philadelphia: Lippincott–Raven Publishers, 1998:7–17, with permission.)

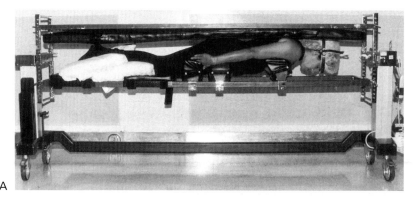

A

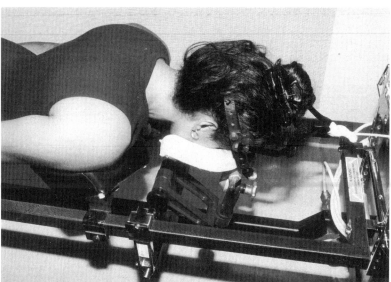

B

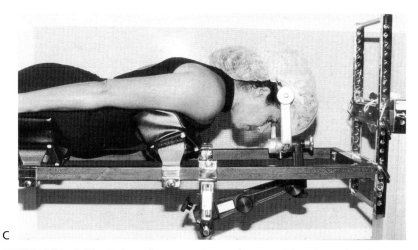

C

FIGURE 1.31. **A:** The Jackson frame may be used to reposition the patient in anterior and posterior cervical spine procedures while maintaining in-line cervical traction. **B:** This patient is positioned prone for posterior cervical spine surgery on a Jackson frame using a Mayfield horseshoe headrest and halo tong traction. **C:** These patients are positioned prone for posterior cervical spine surgery on a Jackson frame using Mayfield tongs. (All parts from Guanciale T. Positioning for posterior cervical spine surgery. In: Dillin WH, Simeone FA, eds. *Posterior cervical spine surgery.* Philadelphia: Lippincott–Raven Publishers, 1998:7–17, with permission.)

improves venous drainage and allows more rapid access to and control of bleeding points. A cleaner and more vertical surgical field improves visualization for foraminotomy and laminectomy procedures, especially in the upper cervical spine. On the other hand, positioning a microscope over the seated patient is more difficult. The seated position improves diaphragmatic excursion and ventilation. Access to the endotracheal tube and the anterior chest wall allows prompt resuscitative measures, when necessary. Ocular pressure is avoided, but sacral and sciatic nerve pressure injuries are reported. Avoid skin breakdown with extra padding or special gel seating.

Seated posterior spine surgery may be performed under local anesthesia, allowing cranial nerve assessment in cervicocranial procedures and spinal cord testing during cervical osteotomy.

These advantages of the seated position are offset by the potential for major vascular complications. As much as 1,500 mL of lower extremity venous pooling decreases cardiac preload. Compression dressings decrease such pooling, but must be carefully applied to prevent peroneal nerve injuries. Decrease postural hypotension by slowly moving the patient from the supine to the sitting position. Then, elevate the knees to the level of the heart.

Air embolism remains the most feared complication of seated cervical surgery and occurs in as many as 76% of cases. The majority of these events are subclinical and transesophageal echocardiographic findings only. Significant morbidity or mortality from venous embolism occurs in approximately 1% of cases. Clinically significant emboli are more common with suboccipital and widely decompressive procedures. Lower cervical procedures and foraminotomy procedures are rarely implicated.

Coagulate bleeding points immediately; maintain a moist tissue surface with regular irrigation; and wax exposed, cancellous bony surfaces to decrease the risk of air embolism. If embolism is detected, pack the wound and flood the tissue planes with fluid. A large intracardiac line may be used to aspirate the air from the heart. Then, search for the source of the embolus.

In the seated position, gravitational drainage of the cerebrospinal fluid allows air to accumulate in the subdural space if a durotomy has been inadvertently or intentionally created. Rarely, this volume of air may exert a mass effect with potentially lethal consequences, such as tonsillar herniation.

Obstruction of venous and lymphatic drainage from the tongue occurs when flexion of the head causes the chin to rest on the chest. The prolonged presence of an oral airway magnifies this obstruction, leading to macroglossia, airway obstruction, hypoxemia, and hypercapnia. Macroglossia is especially problematic in smaller and juvenile patients.

Thoroughly discuss the relative merits of seated positioning with the anesthesia team prior to surgery. The possibility of air embolism and serious sequelae restrict this technique in patients with the following conditions:

- Patent ventriculoatrial shunt
- Right atrial pressure in excess of left atrial pressure
- Patent foramen ovale
- Cerebral ischemia when upright and awake

Porter has described relative contraindications, including the following:

- Extremes of age
- Uncontrolled hypertension
- Chronic obstructive airways disease

If seated positioning has been selected, use a dental chair or a flexed OR table. A number of OR table configurations are described. The main differences surround the degree of flexion of the backrest. Move the backrest to 80 degrees to directly support the upper back, and use Mayfield tongs to secure the head (Fig. 1.32). Alternatively, slightly flex the backrest and maintain head position using a halo ring and pulley traction (Fig. 1.33).

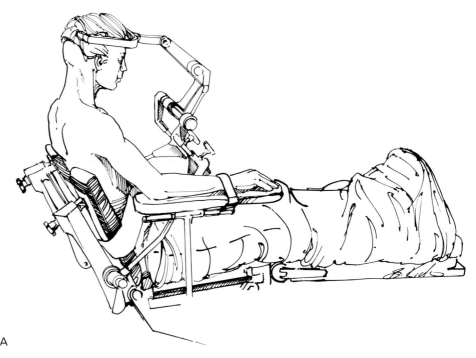

A

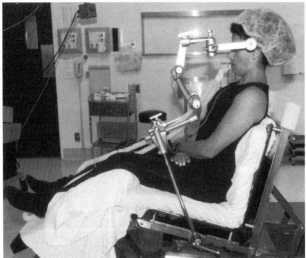

B

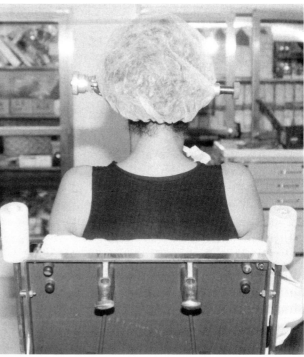

C

FIGURE 1.32. A: This patient is positioned for seated spine surgery using a regular operating room bed. The upper bed extension has been flexed to 80° to support the upper back. Head position is maintained with a Mayfield tongs attachment. The arms are supported with arm holders, and the patent has been belted into place. **B** and **C:** Similarly, this patient is seated on a regular operating room table. The table has been tilted back to help prevent distal migration of the patient. The backrest is flexed to 80°, and head position is maintained with Mayfield tongs. In this case, the arms are crossed in front of the patient. The posterior view demonstrates wide visualization of the posterior neck. (Parts B and C from Guanciale T. Positioning for posterior cervical spine surgery. In: Dillin WH, Simeone FA, eds. *Posterior cervical spine surgery.* Philadelphia: Lippincott–Raven Publishers, 1998:7–17, with permission.)

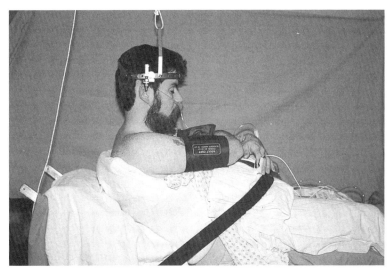

FIGURE 1.33. This patient has been positioned for posterior cervical spine surgery in the seated position. In this case, the upper operating room bed attachment is flexed to only 40°. Here, neck and head alignment is maintained through halo traction using a rope and pulley system. Note that the halo cast has already been applied. The patient is belted into position, and his arms are crossed in front of him. (From Bradford DS, ed. *The spine*. Philadelphia: Lippincott–Raven Publishers, 1997, p. 77, with permission.)

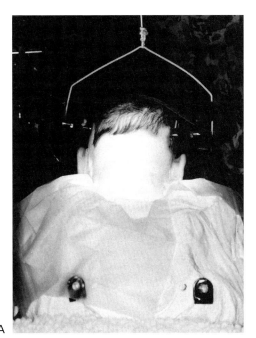

A

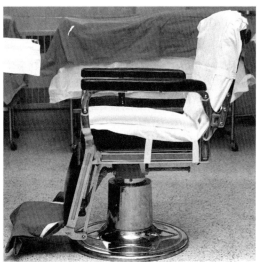

B

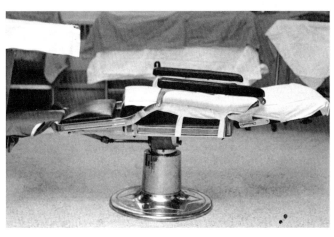

C

FIGURE 1.34. This patient has been positioned for posterior cervical spine surgery in the seated position. In this case, a dental chair is being used. Endotracheal intubation and vascular lines are secured while supine **(C)**. Then, the chair is flexed into the seated position **(B)**. Head and neck position in this case are being maintained using 9 pounds of halo traction using a cord and pulley system **(A)**. (From Dillin WH, Simeone FA, eds. *Posterior cervical spine surgery*. Philadelphia: Lippincott–Raven Publishers, 1998, p. 221, with permission.)

Intubate and secure an arterial line, precordial Doppler, and a right heart catheter while the patient is supine. Employ an esophageal stethoscope and transesophageal echocardiography. Avoid hypotensive anesthesia.

Then, flex the table and tilt it backward just enough to prevent the patient from sliding forward. In either case, make sure the patient is belted in to prevent distal migration. The hips and knees are flexed at the gatch in the table or with pillows. The arms are crossed in front of the patient, with cubital tunnel protectors in place. Once the head has been secured, remove the table extension to allow access to the back of the neck (Fig. 1.34).

NECK BRACES

Principles of Cervical Bracing

Cervical orthosis refers to an external brace applied to the neck to limit motion, correct deformity, decrease pain, and reduce axial loading. The earliest surviving documentation of cervical orthotics dates to the fifth Egyptian dynasty (2750–2625 BC). The biomechanical principles employed to relieve pain and control deformity have survived to the present. Today, a wide variety of cervical orthoses are named after their inventor (e.g., Benjamin-Taylor, Thomas, Guilford), the locality where they were designed (e.g., Philadelphia, Yale, Newport, Malibu, Miami), or by descriptions (e.g., four-poster, two-poster, sterno-occipital-mandibular immobilizer).

Important design characteristics when selecting a cervical orthosis include its weight, adjustability, functionality, cost, durability, and comfort. Adjustability is a critical factor. A poorly fitting brace gives little if any control over neck motion. A useful brace must be able to be fitted on a wide variety of patients. Functionality includes access to tracheostomy, wound, and drain sites as well as ease of application and removal. The material and comfort of the brace are important to avoid skin maceration from moisture and to improve compliance.

Cervical orthotics are indicated for

- Immobilization after surgery or trauma
- Pain relief
- Mechanical unloading
- Use as kinesthetic reminders

Proper brace selection relies on an understanding of cervical spine biomechanics as well as the vector of instability of the spine in question. Comparing maximal cervical range of motion in the brace versus native range of motion offers insights into the various braces and their effectiveness. The cervical spine is by far the most mobile segment of the spine. The normal cervical range of motion includes 140 to 150 degreesof sagittal plane flexion and extension, 150 to 180 degrees of rotation, and 90 degrees of lateral rotation. At all levels, flexion is greater than extension. However, the degree of motion in various planes varies with the level in question. The occiput to C1 articulation demonstrates significant flexion and extension, but limited side bending and rotation. The C1-C2 complex, on the other hand, accounts for half of the total cervical spine rotation. The region between C2 and C4 demonstrates the most side bending and rotation. C5 and C6 exhibit the greatest flexion and extension. This mobility as well as the inability to aggressively compress the soft tissues of the neck (trachea, carotid sheath, esophagus) limits the ability of an externally applied brace to restrict motion.

Cervical braces provide several functions. Most important, they restrict cervical motion to prevent further injury and to allow healing (Tables 1.1 and 1.2). The less rigid devices appear to function mainly as a kinesthetic reminder, preventing the patient from engaging in further injurious activity by using combinations of rigid and flexible materials to restrain cervical motion. Although a wide number of braces are available, they are divided into three categories. Category 1 includes braces that cover the neck alone. These

TABLE 1.1. MOTION ALLOWED IN VARIOUS TYPES OF CERVICAL BRACES

Test Situation	No. of Subjects (Male/Female)	Mean Age, Yrs (Range)	Mean Percentge of Normal Motion Allowed					
			Flexion-Extension	Significance*	Rotation	Significance*	Lateral Bending	Significance[a]
Normal unresticted (all subjects)	44 (19/25)	25.8 (20–36)	100		100		100	
Soft collar	20 (10/10)	26.2 (20–36)	74.2 ± 7.2	<.001	82.6 ± 4.6	<.001	92.3 ± 8.0	.057 (NS)
Philadelphia collar	17 (9/8)	25.8 (20–34)	28.9 ± 4.7	<.001	43.7 ± 6.7	<.001	66.4 ± 10.7	<.001
SOMI brace	22 (7/15)	25.0 (21–31)	27.7 ± 6.6	.772 (NS)	33.6 ± 6.4	<.05	65.6 ± 9.4	.899 (NS)
Four-poster brace	27 (11/16)	25.9 (21–36)	20.6 ± 5.4	<.05	27.1 ± 3.9	<.05	45.9 ± 7.5	<.001
Cervicothoracic brace	27 (11/16)	25.9 (21–36)	12.8 ± 3.0	<.05	18.2 ± 3.2	<.001	50.5 ± 7.1	.063 (NS)
Halo with plastic body vest	7 (6/1)	40.0 (20–48)	4		1		4	

SOMI, sterno-occipital-mandibular immobilizer; NS, not significant.
[a]Significance reported is the probability value of one brace or collar compared with the test situation directly above, using the paired *t* test. For example, flexion-extension in the soft collar was significantly different from normal unrestricted motion (*p* < .001), and the Philadelphia collar was significantly better in restricting flexion-extension than the soft collar (*p* < .001), whereas the SOMI brace was similar in effectiveness to the Philadelphia collar (*p* = .772).
From Browner BD, Jupiter JB, Levine AM, et al., eds. *Skeletal trauma,* 2nd ed. Philadelphia: WB Saunders, 1998, p. 811, with permission.

orthotics are subdivided into soft and rigid collars. Category 2 cervical braces extend further onto the patient's skull and thereby better control the upper cervical segments. Category 3 braces attach to the trunk to better control the lower cervical segments.

Drawbacks of bracing include the following:

- Brace pain and discomfort
- Skin breakdown
- Nerve compression
- Ingrown facial hair for men
- Muscle atrophy or contracture
- Increased segmental motion at ends of the orthosis
- Loss of reduction despite bracing
- Aspiration

TABLE 1.2. BRACES THAT PROVIDE THE BEST CONTROL OF FLEXION AND EXTENSION AT VARIOUS CERVICAL LEVELS

Segmental Levels	Flexion-Extension		Flexion		Extension	
	Brace	Mean Motion Allowed (Degrees)	Brace	Mean Motion Allowed (Degrees)	Brace	Mean Motion Allowed (Degrees)
C1-C2	Halo	3.4	SOMI	2.7	Cervicothoracic	2.5
C2-C3	Halo	2.4	SOMI	0.9	Four-poster	2.0
	Four-poster	3.7	Four-poster	1.6	Cervicothoracic	2.1
	Cervicothoracic	3.8	Cervicothoracic	1.8		
Middle (C3-C5)	Cervicothoracic	4.6	SOMI	1.7	Cervicothoracic	1.8
			Four-poster	2.0		
			Cervicothoracic	2.8		
Lower (C5-T1)	Cervicothoracic	4.0	Cervicothoracic	1.5	Cervicothoracic	2.5
			SOMI	2.9	Four-poster	2.5

From Browner BD, Jupiter JB, Levine AM, et al., eds. *Skeletal trauma,* 2nd ed. Philadelphia: WB Saunders, 1998, p. 811, with permission.

■ Decreased pulmonary capacity
■ Poor patient compliance
■ Psychological and physical dependency

Compliance falls with more restrictive braces. Even compliant patients often loosen their braces to the point of ineffectiveness. Neck size, body habitus, and shoulder and jaw motion also limit the effectiveness of cervical orthotics. Small children are difficult to effectively brace both because of patient size and lack of compliance. Patients with other injuries, particularly clavicular, scalp, facial, or thoracic trauma, have significant bracing limitations as well.

To maximize effectiveness, the least restrictive brace should be worn for the shortest effective interval. Close follow-up of braced patients will improve compliance and allow for orthotic changes, when necessary. To be effective, a cervical orthosis must be applied properly. Read and follow the manufacturer's guidelines. Fit changes with changing patient position. Typically, a snug fit requires 5 pounds of tension on the brace's elastic straps. Test the fit by attempting to place two fingers between the brace and the skin. Typically, when spinal instability is not an issue, orthosis is used until the patient can tolerate discomfort without the brace. After surgery or acute fractures, 6 to 12 weeks of bracing permits ligament and bone healing.

Simple Braces

The soft collar is a common orthotic fashioned from lightweight polyurethane foam covered with stockinette. These devices have Velcro closures and are easily applied and removed. Although they are comfortable, soft collars provide little true immobilization and allow up to 92% of normal motion in all planes. One study demonstrated the following limitations:

■ Flexion and extension by 5% to 15%
■ Lateral bending by 5% to 10%
■ Rotation by 10% to 17%

Soft collars do give a feeling of warmth, comfort, and security to patient. These soft braces are therefore indicated for minor cervical sprains and for temporary symptom relief in certain degenerative or postoperative cervical conditions. The average soft collar costs $50, but they are quickly soiled with long-term use (Fig. 1.35).

Hard cervical collars, such as the Thomas collar, are similar in shape to a soft collar but are made of Plastizote, a rigid polyethylene material. These collars are shaped like a ring with padding. In certain designs, height adjustability allows for better fit. Velcro

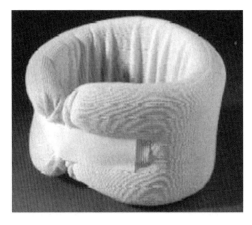

FIGURE 1.35. The soft cervical collar provides warmth and reassurance as well as a kinesthetic reminder, but little true control of cervical motion.

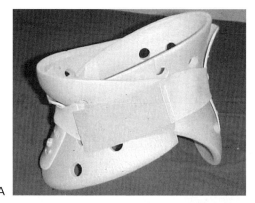

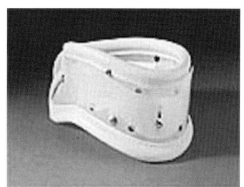

A

B

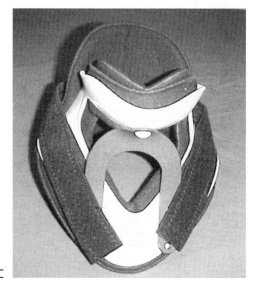

C

FIGURE 1.36. A: Close-up view of the Philadelphia collar. **B:** Close-up view of the Marlin collar. (Courtesy Rick Drazen, Progressive Orthotics.) **C:** Close-up view of the Thomas collar. The Thomas collar has relatively less cervical control due to its limited thoracic and cranial extension.

straps are used for easy donning and doffing. Although the average cost of these collars is $60, they are more durable than soft collars with long-term use. A hard collar restricts motion better than a soft collar, with full flexion and extension limited by 25%. These braces are less effective in restricting rotation and lateral bending. They are indicated to support the head during acute neck pain, relieve minor muscle spasm associated with spondylosis, provide psychological comfort, and for interim stability during halo application (Fig. 1.36).

Emergency collars such as the Stiffneck and Nec Loc are an important subgroup of category 1 orthotics (Fig. 1.37). These braces are compact and store easily in emergency vehicles. They are quickly transformed into sound cervical orthoses by twisting and snapping them into place. Various authors have found these braces to be as effective as Philadelphia collars. However, a short backboard and blocks remain a more effective form of emergency cervical spine immobilization than any collar device (Fig. 1.38).

Head cervical orthotics (HCOs) include the occiput and chin to decrease cervical range of motion. Unfortunately, the supported chin and clavicle are common places for skin breakdown and hair ingrowth. The classic HCO remains the Philadelphia collar, a semirigid two-piece Plastizote foam device. Plastic struts on the anterior and posterior sides lend additional support to the foam. The Philly collar is comfortable and available in various sizes. Further, Velcro straps allow easy removal and application, improving patient compliance. An anterior hole for tracheostomy patients and a thoracic extension for cervicothoracic junction injuries are available. A Philadelphia collar costs, on average, $125, but is difficult to clean and becomes soiled easily. The chin and clavicular extensions

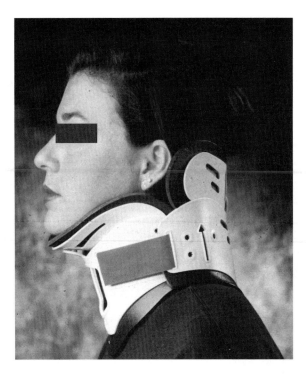

FIGURE 1.37. Examples of rigid collars commonly employed in emergency or extrication situations. **B:** The Nec Loc cervical extraction collar. (From Goldberg B, Hsu JD. *Atlas of orthoses and assistive devices,* 3rd ed. St. Louis: Mosby, 1997, p. 252, with permission.)

improve motion restrictions from simple soft and hard cervical collars and provide the following limitations:

- Flexion and extension by 65% to 70%
- Rotation by 60% to 65%
- Lateral bending by 30% to 35%

Philadelphia collars are indicated after anterior cervical fusion or halo removal. They are also commonly employed for suspected cervical trauma in unconscious patients and

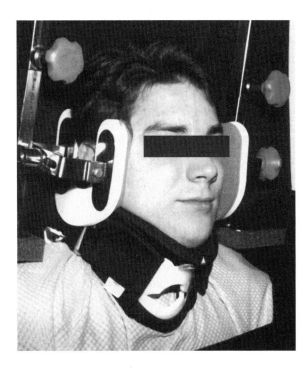

FIGURE 1.38. A backboard and blocks offer significantly more control of cervical motion than a collar alone.

after more significant cervical strains. Philadelphia collars break down over time and lose their effectiveness. Because they are not well vented, their use in a hot climate is associated with skin maceration. In supine patients, posterior scalp contact pressures routinely rise above capillary pressures, and pressure sores develop. A number of other rigid collar orthoses have therefore been devised, such as Newport, Marlin, Miami J, and Malibu collars.

The Miami J collar is another semirigid HCO comprising a two-piece polyethylene system with a soft washable lining (Fig. 1.39). Similar to the Philadelphia collar, an anterior opening for tracheostomy and a thoracic extension are available. The Miami J is available in various sizes and can also be heated and molded for a contoured fit. The average cost for a Miami J collar is $150. This collar limits

- Flexion and extension by 55% to 75%
- Rotation by 70%
- Lateral bending by 60%

The Miami J has similar indications to those of the Philadelphia collar.

The Malibu and Aspen collars are both two-piece semirigid HCOs similar to the Philadelphia collar. The Malibu is available in only one size but is adjustable in multiple planes for proper fit (Fig. 1.40). Straps around the chin, occiput, and lower cervical spine provide for tightening. The padding around the chin can be trimmed. The average cost for a Malibu collar is between $160 and $200. The Aspen collar is made of polyethylene with a soft foam liner and Velcro straps (Fig. 1.41). Both collars limit

- Flexion and extension by 55% to 60%
- Rotation by 60%
- Lateral bending by 60%

The indications for a Malibu or Aspen collar are similar to those for the Miami J and Philadelphia collars.

In one cadaver model, a 0.9-kg force resulted in a 58-degree arc of coronal motion in an unconstrained specimen. The Malibu, Miami J, Newport, and Philadelphia collars

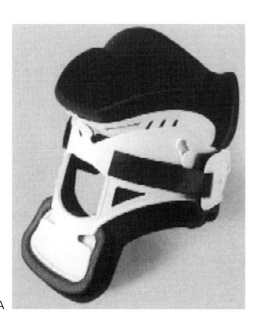
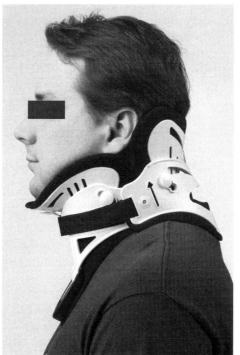

A   B

FIGURE 1.39. The Miami J collar is another popular category 1 orthosis.

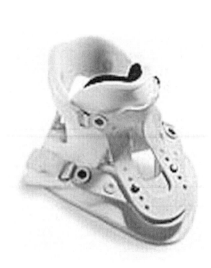

A

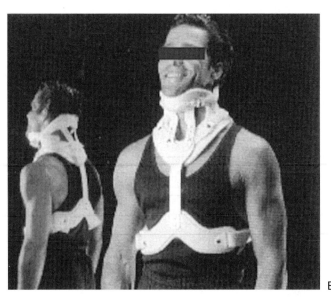

B

FIGURE 1.40. The Malibu collar offers significantly more cervical control than the Philadelphia collar. Control of the lower cervical segments is improved with a thoracic extension.

allowed 34.3, 37.8, 42.7, and 45.3 degrees of motion, respectively. Similarly, the unrestricted arc of sagittal flexion with 0.9 kg of applied force was nearly 70 degrees.In this plane, cervical orthoses fell into two groups. The Malibu and Miami J collars allowed 33 and 35.9 degrees. The Philadelphia and Newport collars allowed 40.5 and 43.9 degrees. An axial rotation arc of 63.1 degrees was recorded with the same 0.9 kg of applied force. The Philadelphia, Miami J, and Newport orthoses allowed just over 32 degrees of motion, a 51% restriction of normal motion. The Malibu brace further restricted rotation, allowing an average of 24.7 degrees.

The added pressure on the body obtained with cervical thoracic orthotics (CTOs) restricts middle to lower cervical spine motion better than head cervical orthoses. In models without significant head extensions, the upper cervical spine is less restricted. The sterno-occipital-mandibular immobilizer (SOMI) is a commonly employed, rigid three-poster CTO (Fig. 1.42). The average cost for a SOMI is $480. An anterior chest plate extends to the xiphoid process and has bars that curve over the shoulder. Straps from these bars go over the shoulder and cross to the opposite side of the anterior plate for fixation. The chin piece attaches to the chest plate and is removable during meals. The absence of posterior rods makes the SOMI ideal for bedridden patients. Proper adjustment is crucial to achieve any significant motion restriction. The lax connections between the occiput and mandibular pads make the SOMI more comfortable, but less effective than true two- or four-poster braces. The SOMI is most effective in controlling upper cervical flexion, but is less effective than other CTOs in controlling extension, limiting

- Flexion and extension by 70% to 75%
- Lateral bending by 35%
- Rotation by 60% to 65%

This upper cervical flexion control makes the SOMI ideal for stabilization of rheumatoid atlantoaxial instability. Other indications include immobilization of C2 neural arch fractures.

The Yale orthosis is a modified Philadelphia collar with a fiberglass thoracic extension. Typically, these braces cost $320. The Yale brace is easy to make and comfortable to wear. Midthoracic straps connect the two thoracic extensions. This thoracic extension improves control of injuries from C6 to T2. The occipital extension of the Yale brace rises higher on the skull posteriorly, increasing brace contact area and stability and limiting

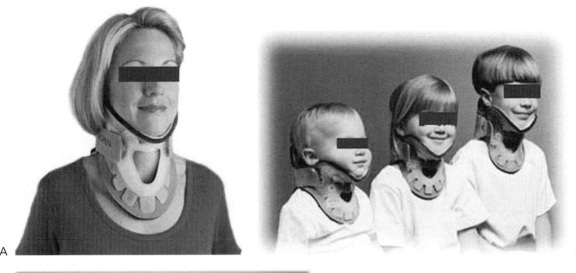

A

B

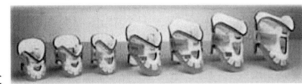

C

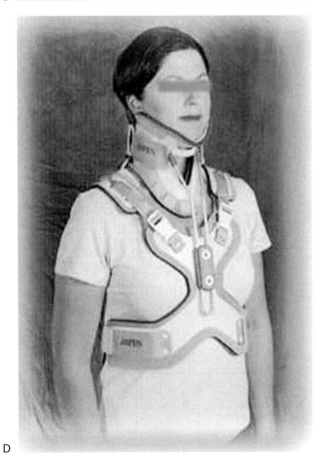

D

FIGURE 1.41. **A:** Aspen collars are also widely used category 1 cervical orthoses. **B** and **C:** They are available in a number of different sizes, which improves fit in smaller patients. **D:** As with Malibu collars, improved control of lower cervical segments is achieved with a thoracic extension.

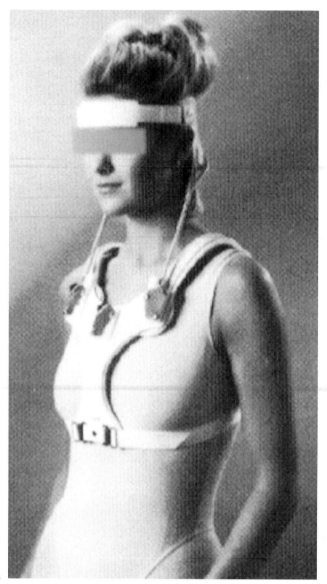

A

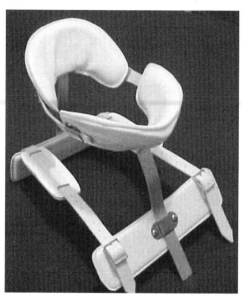

B

FIGURE 1.42. A: The sterno-occipital-mandibular immobilizer (SOMI) brace. **B:** The Dennison two-poster brace. (Courtesy of Rick Drazen, Progressive Orthotics.)

- Flexion and extension by 85%
- Rotation by 70% to 75%
- Lateral bending by 60%

These restriction of motion makes the Yale brace an appropriate choice for immobilization of minimally displaced or stabilized upper cervical fractures.

Other two- and four-poster braces are available. Most are rigid orthoses with anterior and posterior chest pads connected by straps. Molded occipital and mandibular support pieces connect to the chest pads with either two or four adjustable struts. These braces typically cost from $500 to $750. A four-poster design typically limits lateral bending and rotation better than a two-poster brace (Fig. 1.43). Additional straps often connect the occipital and mandibular support pieces. These posts leave the neck itself open, allowing heat to escape and assisting wound inspection. Two- and four-poster braces limit

- Flexion and extension by 80%
- Lateral bending by 55% to 80%
- Rotation by 50% to 70%

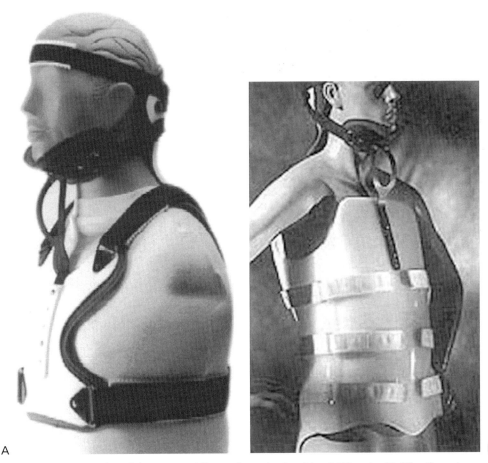

A

B

FIGURE 1.43. Examples of the Lerman Minerva brace both without **(A)** and with **(B)** a thoracic-lumbar-sacral orthosis (TLSO) attachment. These orthotics are effectively four-poster braces.

In Fisher and coworkers' roentgenographic study, the polyethylene collar, Philadelphia collar, four-poster, and SOMI brace were tested on normal subjects. The four-poster and SOMI restricted motion significantly more than the other braces.

The Halo Orthosis

The halo brace relies on skeletal fixation to the skull and a rigid four-poster design to offer significantly greater control of all three planes of cervical motion than other cervical orthotics (Fig. 1.44). Wolf and associates, studying halo vests and casts, found that sagittal flexion and extension were limited to 7.5 degrees. Lateral bending and rotation were limited to 4.1 and 2.2 degrees, respectively. The residual 4% to 31% of normal cervical range of motion that occurs at each level while in a halo relates most closely to the fit of the vest. Previously, casts were recommended to allow closer fit. More recently, the ease of vest application and the frequency of pressure sores has diminished enthusiasm for the halo cast. Patients with static spinal deformity (e.g., thoracic hyperkyphosis), small children, and others with an unusual body habitus remain well served by casts (Fig. 1.45).

The halo vest is available in several lengths. Use the half-vest for cervical spine pathologies above C4. The half-vest confers easy access to the chest wall in multitrauma patients with chest tubes. Pelvic extensions may increase control of cervicothoracic pathology. Most typically, apply a full-length vest. The average cost of the halo device with vest is $2,800.

The halo more completely controls upper cervical motion. "Snaking" decreases the control of lower cervical spine segments. Moreover, the halo does not shield the spine from significant compressive and distractive loads. For example, sitting subjects the

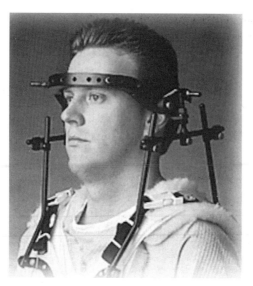

FIGURE 1.44. A patient wearing a standard halo vest.

cervical spine to 17 pounds of distractive force. Rising to walk converts this force to 4 pounds of compressive load.

Halo immobilization is commonly indicated for the following:

■ Unstable upper cervical spine trauma (such as a dens fracture)
■ After upper cervical spine reconstruction (such as a C1–2 Gallie fusion)
■ Control of certain longer subaxial surgical constructs (multilevel corpectomies)

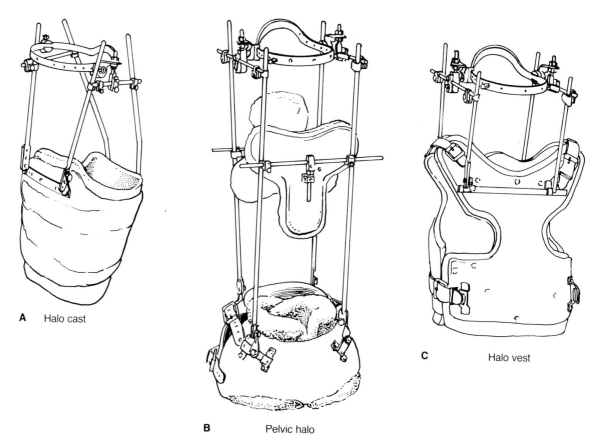

A   Halo cast

B   Pelvic halo

C   Halo vest

FIGURE 1.45. Halo rings may be attached to body casts **(A)**, a halo with pelvic extension **(B)**, or a standard halo vest **(C)**.

Halo vest immobilization is contraindicated in the following cases:

- Unstable skull fractures
- Lytic skull metastases
- Traumatized skin overlying pin sites
- Very young children (consider a Minerva cast)
- Very osteoporotic patients
- Patients with significant pulmonary problems

Application of the halo vest is relatively straightforward after the ring has been applied (see earlier in this chapter). To size the vest, measure the chest circumference at the xiphoid. Select the appropriate vest and logroll the patient up to 90 degrees. Slide the posterior vest underneath the patent and logroll the patient onto the vest (Fig. 1.46). Attach posterior uprights, followed by the anterior vest and uprights. Obtain a lateral radiograph to assess cervical alignment. Once the patient is standing,

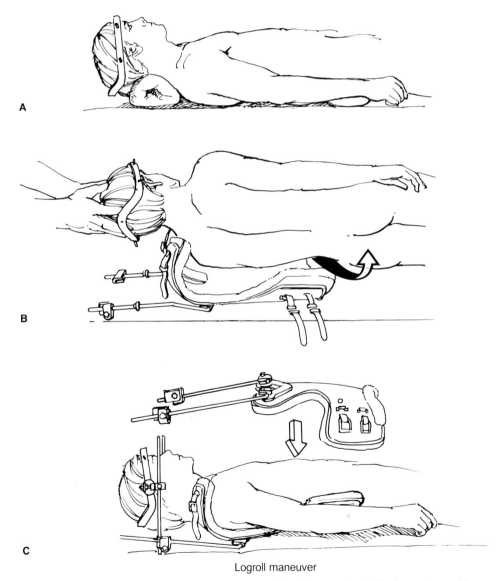

Logroll maneuver

FIGURE 1.46. A: Application of the halo vest is undertaken cautiously in the patient with an unstable cervical spine. **B:** Logroll the patient onto his or her side while maintaining in-line traction to the head. Then, place the posterior aspect of the vest, with uprights attached, under the patient. **C:** Roll the patient onto the posterior vest and attach the uprights to the halo ring. Next, apply the anterior vest and uprights.

check another x-ray to ensure maintenance of reduction. Overextension may lead to dysphagia.

Retighten the halo pins to the original torque at 48 hours. Thereafter, check the pins weekly to make sure they are finger tight. Infections usually occur in loose pins. Remove any loose pin that can be turned more than one full turn. Change this pin site and the diagonally opposite pin. Twice-daily hydrogen peroxide pin care may decrease the incidence of pin site infections. If an infection occurs before the brace can safely be removed, place a new pin into the adjacent, clean site. Also, inspect the skin under the vest, especially in paralyzed patients. Change the sheepskin lining as needed. Typically, after the expected period of healing (12 weeks for some injuries), the uprights of the halo are loosed. Flexion and extension radiographs are examined for evidence of continued instability. If the spine is stable, remove the halo and progress the patient into a CTO.

Complications associated with halo immobilization include long-term neck pain and stiffness. In one group of 83 patients treated in a halo from 10 to 12 weeks, 80% reported neck pain and limitation of motion long term. These patients returned to work, but demonstrated a statistically significant decrease of cervical rotation (18%) and side bending (18%). Sagittal plane flexion and extension remained normal. Halo placement may injure cranial nerve VI (abducens) or the supraorbital nerve. Twenty percent to 22% of patients sustain pin tract infections. In 1%, a brain abscess follows retightening of loose pins and penetration of the skull's inner table. Thirty-six percent to 60% report pin loosening, and 18% report severe pain. The anterior pins account for most complications. Pressure sores under the vest or cast and disfiguring scars are seen in approximately 10% to 30% of patients. Gastrointestinal and respiratory problems are reported. Obstructive pulmonary complications are particularly common, with a 10% loss of forced vital capacity in both a vest and a cast. Complications increase to up to 40% in children and thin-skulled patients.

Although halo braces are placed for a wide variety of disorders, brace failure with redislocation occurs in 10% of cases, while new neurologic injury is reported in 1% (Fig. 1.47).

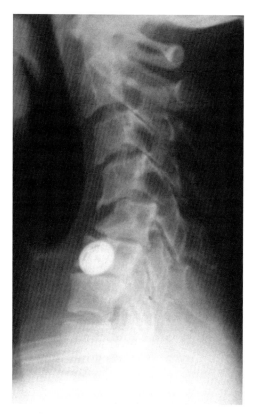

FIGURE 1.47. Loss of reduction of a halo brace applied for a flexion tear drop fracture.

BIBLIOGRAPHY

Botte MJ, Byrne TP, Abrams RA, et al. Halo skeletal fixation: techniques of application and prevention of complications. *J Am Acad Orthop Surg* 1996;4(1):44–53.

Bradford DS, ed. *The spine.* Philadelphia: Lippincott–Raven Publishers, 1997.

Browner BD, Jupiter JB, Levine AM, et al., eds. *Skeletal trauma,* 2nd ed. Philadelphia: WB Saunders, 1998.

Colachis SC, Strohm BR, Ganter EL. Cervical spine motion in normal women: radiographic study of effect of cervical collars. *Arch Phys Med Rehab* 1973;54:161–169.

Dormans JP, Criscitiello AA, Drummond DS, et al. Complications in children managed with immobilization in a halo vest. *J Bone Joint Surg Am* 1995;77(9):1370–1373.

Fisher SV. Proper fitting of the cervical orthosis. *Arch Phys Med Rehab* 1978;59:505–507.

Fisher SV, Bowar IF, Essam AA, et al. Cervical orthoses' effect on cervical spine motion: roentgenographic and goniometric method of study. *Arch Phys Med Rehab* 1977;58:109–115.

Fisher SV. Cervical orthotics. *Phys Med Rehab Clin North Am* 1992;3:29–43.

Fishman S, Berger N, Edelstein JE, et al. Spinal orthoses. In: Bunch WH et al., eds. *Atlas of orthotics.* St. Louis: Mosby, 1985:250–256.

Garfin SR, Botte MJ, Triggs KJ, et al. Subdural abscess associated with halo-pin traction. *J Bone Joint Surg Am* 1988;70(9):1338–1340.

Garfin SR, Botte MJ, Waters RL, et al. Complications in the use of the halo fixation device. *J Bone Joint Surg Am* 1986;68(3):320–325.

Graziano GP, Herzenberg JE, Hensinger RN. The halo-Ilizarov distraction cast for correction of cervical deformity. Report of six cases. *J Bone Joint Surg Am* 1993;75(7):996–1003.

Goldberg B, Hsu JD. *Atlas of orthoses and assistive devices,* 3rd ed. St. Louis: Mosby, 1997.

Guanciale T. Positioning for posterior cervical spine surgery. In: Dillin WH, Simeone FA, eds. *Posterior cervical spine surgery.* Philadelphia: Lippincott–Raven Publishers, 1998:7–17.

Hartman IT, Palumbo F, Hill BI. Cineradiography of the braced normal cervical spine. *Clin Orthop Related Res* 1975;109:97–102.

Johnson RM. Cervical orthoses. A study comparing their effectiveness in restricting cervical motion in normal subjects. *J Bone Joint Surg Am* 1957;39:111–139.

Kaufman WA, Lunsford TR, Lunsford BR, et al. Comparison of three prefabricated cervical collars. *Orthotics Prosthetics* 1986;39:4:21–28.

Kottke Fl, Mundale MO. Range of mobility of the cervical spine. *Arch Phys Med Rehab* 1959;379–82.

Lind B, Sihlbom H, Nordwall. A halo-vest treatment of unstable traumatic cervical spine injuries. *Spine* 1988;13(4):425–432.

Louis R. *Surgery of the spine: surgical anatomy and operative approaches.* Berlin: Springer-Verlag, 1982.

Lunsford TR, Davidson M, Lunsford BR. The effectiveness of four contemporary cervical orthoses in restricting cervical motion. *J Prosthetics Orthotics* 1994;6(4):93–99.

Manfredini M, Ferrante R, Gildone A, et al. Unilateral blindness as a complication of intraoperative positioning for cervical spinal surgery. *J Spinal Disord* 2000;13(3):271–272.

McGuire RA, Degnan G, Amundson GA. Evaluation of current extrication orthoses in immobilization of the unstable cervical spine. *Spine* 1990;15(10):1064–1067.

Nemeth JA. Six-pin halo fixation and the resulting prevalence of pin-site complications. *J Bone Joint Surg Am* 2001;83:377–382.

Palmon SC, Kirsch JR, Depper JA, et al. The effect of the prone position on pulmonary mechanics is frame-dependent. *Anesth Analg* 1998;87(5):1175–1180.

Podolsky S, Baraff LI, Simon RR, et al. Efficacy of cervical spine immobilization methods. *J Trauma* 1983;23(6):461–464.

Porter JM, Pidgeon C, Cunningham AJ. The sitting position in neurosurgery: a critical appraisal. *Br J Anaesth* 1999;82(1):117–128.

Sherk HH, ed. *The cervical spine: an atlas of surgical procedures.* Philadelphia: JB Lippincott Co., 1994.

Slabaugh RB, Nickel VL. Complications with use of the Stryker frame. *J Bone Joint Surg Am* 1978;60(8):1111–1112.

Smith GE. The most ancient splints. *Br Med J* 1980;1:732.

Sypert GW. External spinal orthotics. *Neurosurgery* 1987;20(4):642–649.

Wang GJ, Moskal JT, Albert T, et al. The effect of halo-vest length on stability of the cervical spine. A study in normal subjects. *J Bone Joint Surg Am* 1988;70(3):357–360.

Wolf LW, Johnson RM. *Cervical orthoses,* 2nd ed. Philadelphia: JB Lippincott, 1989.

Wolfe SW, Lospinuso MF, Burke SW. Unilateral blindness as a complication of patient positioning for spinal surgery. A case report. *Spine* 1992;17(5):600–605.

Zimmer, Inc. *Traction manual: a complete reference guide to the basics of traction.* Warsaw, IN: Zimmer, Inc., 1991.

PREOPERATIVE AND PERIANESTHETIC CONSIDERATIONS

KANWALDEEP S. SIDHU
J. J. ABITBOL

Careful preoperative planning for patients undergoing cervical spine surgery is essential to minimize complication rates. Elderly patients with rheumatoid arthritis, cervical stenosis, and myelopathic presentation may have significant associated comorbidities that may predispose them to life-threatening complications during and after reconstructive cervical surgery (1,2). In addition to obtaining the typical preoperative medical and cardiac clearance for elderly patients undergoing spinal procedures, specific precautions may be necessary to minimize risk of postoperative respiratory distress and neurologic deterioration.

Preoperative and perianesthetic considerations may involve the following:

- Assessing preoperative cervical instability and intubation techniques
- Timing of extubation
- Postoperative respiratory distress—edema or hematoma
- Immediate postoperative neurologic deterioration
- Neck and facial positioning

PREOPERATIVE CERVICAL INSTABILITY AND INTUBATION TECHNIQUES

Typical intubation techniques involve hyperextension of the cervical spine during insertion of the endotracheal tube (ETT). Excessive laryngoscope blade levering motion is undesirable in patients who have significant cord compression or instability secondary to trauma or rheumatoid arthritis. Alternatives to typical intubation techniques include manual in-line stabilization, fiberoptic intubation, and use of the intubating laryngeal mask airway (LMA) (3).

Trauma patients with demonstrated unstable cervical fractures on radiographs may be best intubated by manual in-line traction, use of the LMA, or awake fiberoptic intubation (3). The mechanism of injury (hyperflexion or extension) may be correlated with the fracture pattern visualized on the preoperative imaging studies.

Certain patients with flexion-compression cervical spine injuries with resulting spondylolisthesis may be relatively stable in extension and, as such, may be safely intubated using standard laryngoscope blade and manual in-line traction technique. Modified blades for safer intubation techniques have been described in the literature (4).

Mentzelopoulos et al. (5) reported on a technique using a modified blade facilitating glottic exposure by balloon inflation. They suggested that their device would reduce head extension during intubation. Seventeen elective surgery patients (in rigid cervical collars) underwent laryngoscopy using the standard curved blade and the modified blade. Head extension and levering motion angles were measured upon maximal glottic exposures.

Laryngoscopic view grade and oxygen saturation were also determined. They concluded that balloon laryngoscopy results in less head extension and less blade levering motion while facilitating similar laryngoscopic view and oxygen saturation.

Kihara et al. (6) reported on segmental cervical spine movement with the LMA during manual in-line cervical stabilization in patients with cervical pathology undergoing cervical spine surgery. In this study, 20 patients undergoing cervical spine surgery with neurologic symptoms preoperatively were intubated using the LMA. The LMA was inserted with the head and neck in neutral position. Intubation was facilitated by transillumination of the neck with a lightwand. Cervical motion was recorded with a single lateral cervical spine x-ray taken during various phases of intubation. The radiographs were digitized, and motion was measured from the occiput to C5. During insertion of the LMA and intubation, the average posterior displacement from C2–5 was 0.5 to 1 mm. During removal of the LMA there was no change. The authors concluded that the LMA produces segmental motion of the cervical spine despite manual in-line stabilization. However, this motion was in an opposite direction to direct laryngoscopy, suggesting that different approaches to airway management may be needed depending on the nature of cervical instability.

Cervical fractures involving disc space disruption and posterior ligamentous injury (anterior/posterior column) may be quite unstable in all planes. Clearly, this group of patients may be best intubated by awake fiberoptic intubation methods. Other options may include use of the lightwand device (Trachlight) and the LMA. Inoue et al. (7) compared the use of the lightwand versus the LMA in 148 prospectively randomized patients where clinical or radiographic evidence existed for cervical abnormality. In all patients, the head and neck were held in neutral position while intubation was accomplished via use of the above methods. Ninety-one percent of the first intubation attempts were successful in patients when the Trachlight was used, versus 73% in the LMA patients. The authors of this study concluded that the Trachlight may be more advantageous for orotracheal intubation in patients with cervical spine disorders than the LMA with respect to reliability, rapidity, and safety.

As opposed to trauma patients with cervical fractures where the degree of instability may be questionable, patients with rheumatoid arthritis undergoing elective reconstructive cervical procedures should have their instability quantified by preoperative flexion/extension radiographs (8). Rheumatoid cervical spines may have instability at the C0–1 level (cranial settling or basilar invagination), C1–2 level (atlantoaxial subluxation), or C2 to C7 levels (subaxial subluxations). Subtle signs of myelopathy may also be present in such patients. High-risk rheumatoid patients predisposed to neurologic deficits include those with atlantoaxial subluxation greater than 9 mm with vertical settling and posterior atlantodens interval less than 14 mm. Preoperative flexion/extension radiographs and magnetic resonance imaging (MRI) studies can define the extent of pathologic motion in addition to the presence of any cord compression. These factors are critical in determining the best intubation technique for a patient.

Kwek et al. (8) retrospectively reviewed 77 rheumatoid patients who underwent 132 operations under general or regional anesthesia. Most patients in this study had preoperative cervical spine flexion/extension x-rays for instability evaluation. Atlantoaxial subluxation was the most common defect encountered in this group. The authors concluded that detection of cervical spine instability was found to significantly affect anesthetic management, favoring techniques that avoided unprotected manipulations of the neck under anesthesia. Direct laryngoscopy may be difficult in such patients because of decreased range of motion of the cervical spine and mandibular joint leading to a reduced opening of the mouth and reduced dorsal extension of the cervical spine (9).

Some authors have suggested that routine preoperative cervical spine radiographs in rheumatoid patients undergoing elective orthopaedic surgery may not be necessary (10). Campbell et al. (10) retrospectively reviewed 128 patients with rheumatoid arthritis who had not had any preoperative symptoms of cervical cord compression. C1–2 subluxation was found in 5.5% of the patients. No significant differences in anesthetic management were found in patients with and without radiographic instability, and there were no adverse anesthesia-related outcomes.

Suderman et al. (3) reported on a 10-year review of 150 patients with traumatic cervical spine injuries with well-preserved neurologic function who underwent general anesthesia. Neurologic outcomes were compared with the mode of intubation. Preoperative neurologic deficits were identified in 33% of the patients, with most of them being single-level radiculopathies. Fifty-five percent of the patients had intubation performed after induction of general anesthesia, whereas 45% had awake fiberoptic intubation. Seventy-one percent of the patients had orotracheal intubation, with 29% undergoing nasotracheal intubation. Fifty-seven percent had cervical spine immobilization during intubation. Weighted traction or manual in-line stabilization were the most common methods employed for spinal stabilization. There were no differences in neurologic outcome between patients intubated after induction and those who received awake fiberoptic intubation. There were no differences between orotracheal and nasotracheal intubation. The authors of this study concluded that orotracheal intubation with in-line stabilization, either performed after induction of general anesthesia or with the patient awake, remains an excellent option for elective airway management in patients with cervical spine injuries.

The best intubation technique should be customized to the individual patient and to the skill level of the anesthesia personnel. Manual in-line intubation with the cervical collar on may be safer and more efficacious in certain instances where the anesthesia personnel are not comfortable with awake fiberoptic intubation methods. More often than not, a poorly executed awake fiberoptic intubation experience may not only be emotionally difficult for the patient, but can also seriously compromise the patient's neurologic status and mortality risk.

The positioning of the endotracheal tube (right versus left) is dependent on the preferred surgical approach. We prefer a left-sided approach (with the endotracheal tube taped to the right) in order to minimize risk of vocal cord paralysis secondary to injury to the recurrent laryngeal nerve. The path of the recurrent laryngeal nerve is more consistent and predictable on the left side, and thus there may be a decreased likelihood of nerve injury during surgical exposures from the left. Vocal cord paralysis has been reported in 5% of patients undergoing anterior cervical surgery (11). Not all vocal cord paralysis is secondary to surgical injury to the recurrent laryngeal nerve (12). Kriskovich et al. (12) reported on 900 consecutive patients undergoing anterior cervical spine surgery during which ETT cuff pressures were monitored. After the first 250 patients, a modified technique was employed in which ETT cuff pressures were released after retractor placement or repositioning was employed. In addition, intubated cadavers were studied with videofluoroscopy following retractor placement. Thirty cases of vocal cord paralysis consistent with recurrent laryngeal nerve palsy were identified, with three patients having permanent paralysis. With the modified technique, the incidence of temporary paralysis decreased from 6.4% to 1.69% (p = .0002). The cadaveric studies confirmed compromise of the intralaryngeal segment of the recurrent laryngeal nerve secondary to the retractor displacing the larynx against the shaft of the endotracheal tube. The authors concluded that the most common cause of vocal cord paralysis after anterior cervical surgery is compression of the recurrent laryngeal nerve within the endolarynx. They recommended ETT cuff pressure monitoring and release after retractor placement to help prevent injury to the nerve.

Do ETT cuff pressures affect the incidence of postoperative sore throat, hoarseness, and dysphagia after anterior cervical surgery? Ratnaraj et al. (13) reported prospectively on 51 patients scheduled for anterior cervical procedures. In all patients, the cuff pressure was adjusted to 20 mm Hg after intubation. The cuff pressures were measured following placement of retractors. Half the patients were randomized to a control group (no adjustment of ETT cuff pressures) or treatment group (cuff pressure 20 mm Hg). At 1 hour postoperative, there were no differences between the two groups. At 24 hours postoperative, 51% of the treatment group complained of a sore throat, compared with 74% of the control group. At 24 hours follow-up, the longer retractor times correlated with development of dysphagia ($p < .05$). Sixty-five percent of the female patients had sore throat versus 35% of the men ($p < .05$) The authors of this study concluded that there were three predictors of postoperative throat discomfort following anterior cervical surgery in which neck retraction is performed: increased endotracheal cuff pressure during neck retraction (sore throat), neck retraction time (dysphagia), and female sex (sore throat and hoarseness). They recommended decreasing the cuff pressures to 20 mm Hg uniformly in all patients to improve postoperative comfort.

Patients who are undergoing revision anterior cervical surgery should be carefully evaluated for previous partial vocal cord paralysis or recurrent laryngeal nerve injury. If previous compromise to the nerve or vocal cord function is confirmed, then the surgical approach must be from the same side of the neck as the previous scar. A contralateral surgical exposure is associated with the possibility of injury to the other recurrent laryngeal nerve. This may result in complete vocal cord paralysis with devastating life-threatening implications due to airway obstruction (14).

Exposure involving the upper cervical spine (C2 to C4) in obese patients may be quite difficult. Often, strong retraction may be needed to get the mandible out of the way. In this small subset of patients, consideration should be given to nasotracheal intubation versus an orotracheal airway. This would facilitate easier intraoperative retraction of the lower mandible and soft tissues.

TIMING OF EXTUBATION AND POSTOPERATIVE RESPIRATORY DISTRESS

Postoperative respiratory compromise and airway obstruction after anterior cervical surgery can be potentially lethal. Most patients undergoing routine anterior cervical procedures may be extubated safely immediately after the surgery. However, a small subset of patients undergoing major anterior reconstructive procedures involving long operating times, extensive upper cervical exposures, and high blood loss may need continued intubation for 24 to 48 hours in the intensive care setting (15). The two most common factors that can cause airway obstruction postoperatively are hematoma and pharyngeal edema (16). Hematoma is a compressive mechanical phenomenon that may need surgical evacuation. Treatment of pharyngeal edema is typically nonsurgical and involves the use of steroids to decrease edema plus airway management and possible reintubation.

Sagi et al. (15) performed a retrospective chart review of 311 anterior cervical procedures to look at the incidence of airway complications and the variables that predispose patients to these complications. Of the 311 patients studied, 19 (6.1%) had an airway complication and 6 (1.9%) required reintubation. One patient died. Symptoms developed an average of 36 hours postoperatively. Seventeen of 19 complications were caused by pharyngeal edema, not hematoma. The results are shown in Table 2.1. The authors of this study recommended that patients with prolonged procedures (>5 hours), with exposure of more than three vertebral bodies that include C2 to C4, or with more than 300 cc blood loss should be watched carefully for postoperative distress.

TABLE 2.1. INCIDENCE AND VARIABLES THAT PREDISPOSE PATIENTS TO AIRWAY COMPLICATIONS

Associated with airway compromise	No association with airway compromise
Exposure > 3 vertebral bodies	History of myelopathy or spinal cord injury
Blood loss > 300 cc	Smoking or pulmonary problems
Exposures involving C2, C3, C4	Anesthetic risk factors
Operative time > 5 hr	Absence of a drain

Data from Sagi HC, Beutler W, Carroll E, Connolly PJ. Airway complications associated with surgery on the anterior cervical spine. *Spine* 2002;27(9):949–953.

Epstein et al. (17) conducted a study to determine how to avoid postoperative reintubation and its associated morbidity in patients who have undergone extensive anterior posterior cervical surgery. The protocol described in this study involved continued intubation overnight and subsequent extubation on the first postoperative day or later, depending on an anesthesiologist's determination of reactive tracheal swelling based on direct fiberoptic visualization. Fifty-eight patients underwent multilevel anterior corpectomy with fusion, posterior wiring, and fusion and application of a halo. The average anterior fusion was three levels, whereas the posterior fusion and wiring was six levels. The average surgical time was 6 hours, with a blood loss requiring a transfusion of 2.6 units. Forty-eight patients where successfully extubated on the first postoperative day, 5 on the second, 3 on the third, 1 on the fourth, 2 on the fifth, and 3 on the seventh postoperative day. Three elective tracheostomies were done on the seventh postoperative day. Risk factors associated with delayed extubation or tracheostomy included the following:

- Operative time longer than 10 hours (12 patients)
- Weight greater than 220 lb (12 patients)
- Transfusion greater than 4 units (10 patients)
- Anterior cervical fusion reoperations (9 patients)
- Anterior cervical fusion including C2 (7 patients)
- Four-level anterior fusions (5 patients)
- Asthma (5 patients)

In the only case where emergent reintubation was needed, three of these risk factors were present. The authors of this study concluded that emergent reintubation following anterior posterior cervical surgery and fusion can be avoided by maintaining intubation overnight and subsequently having an anesthesiologist remove the tube after healing is fiberoptically confirmed.

Emery et al. (16) reviewed seven cases of upper airway obstruction that required reintubation immediately after anterior cervical surgery. All patients had moderate to severe myelopathy preoperatively. All underwent anterior cervical corpectomy and fusion. Five patients had no long-term sequelae, but two patients died. The airway obstruction was believed to be due to edema rather than hematoma. Risk factors common to all patients included moderate to severe myelopathy and multilevel corpectomy. Six patients were heavy smokers, and one had asthma.

Airway obstruction postoperatively may occur after isolated posterior cervical surgery. Wattenaker et al. (2) reported on 128 patients with rheumatoid arthritis who underwent a total of 128 consecutive posterior cervical spine operations. An upper airway obstruction developed after extubation postoperatively in 14% (8 of 58) of the patients who had been intubated without fiberoptic assistance versus 1% (1 of 70) who had been intubated fiberoptically ($p = .02$). The two groups were similarly matched for sex, age, severity of myelopathy, American Rheumatologic classification, use of preoperative traction, smoking history, duration of arthritis, size of ETT, duration of operation, anesthesia time, intraoperative fluid balance, and type of postoperative neck immobilization. The only statistically significant difference was the timing of extubation, which averaged 17.9 hours in the fiberoptic group and 10.6 hours in the nonfiberoptic group ($p = .02$) The authors concluded that nonfiberoptic intubation was a significant risk factor in this group of patients.

Appropriately chosen intubation techniques (fiberoptic, LMA, lightwand, etc.) combined with delayed extubation in select patients, once lack of pharyngeal edema has been confirmed visually, may decrease the rate of emergent reintubation after select cervical procedures.

The incidence of ENT complications due to anterior cervical approach was prospectively reported by Francois and colleagues (18). One hundred twenty-five anterior cervical surgery patients were placed in intensive care postoperatively, and an ENT examination with a fiberscope was employed in all patients preoperatively and postoperatively. Before surgery, two cases of vocal cord paralysis were found. Eighty-nine percent of the patients presented with subjective disorders preoperatively, such as sore throat, odynophagia, dysphagia, and hoarseness. Ninety-four percent of the patients had postoperative anomalies on the posterolateral pharyngeal wall, on the arytenoids, and on the vocal cords. Moderate to significant inflammatory or swollen lesions were found in 40% of the patients. Very significant circumferential swelling of the pharyngeal wall and the arytenoids was responsible for two patients requiring reintubation and return to the operating room. Severe inflammation correlated with the duration of surgery, numbers of levels fused, and the age of the patient ($p < .02$). Six patients had vocal cord paresis, which was permanent in three. All cases of vocal cord paralysis were associated with a right-sided approach.

Krnacik and Heggeness (19) reported airway obstruction due to severe angioedema after removal of a cervical osteophyte. Massive tongue swelling after spine surgery may compromise the airway also. Miura et al. (20) reported on four such cases related to fixation of the endotracheal tube and packing of surgical gauze around the tube resulting in compression of the base of the tongue. In their experience, the use of corticosteroids was effective in reducing swelling.

Prolonged hospitalization after reconstructive cervical surgery may be related to associated comorbidities. Harris et al. (1) studied preoperative and operative risk factors for prolonged hospitalization in 109 patients who underwent elective cervical surgery. They concluded that the following factors were related to the need for unanticipated postoperative critical care and prolonged hospitalization: multilevel decompression, preexisting myelopathy, pulmonary disease, cardiovascular disease, hypertension, and diabetes mellitus.

Airway compromise postoperatively may be the result of compressive hematoma at the surgical site. This can be a life-threatening complication and requires immediate intervention. Meticulous surgical exposure and hemostasis along with use of postoperative drainage can minimize this complication. The presence of hematoma underneath the platysma layer may not be totally obvious by inspection and palpation of the surgical site. A lateral cervical spine radiograph with a significant abnormality of the soft tissue shadow may indicate the presence of hematoma or pharyngeal edema. The presence of a drain at the surgical site, by itself, does not exclude the presence of a hematoma in a postoperative patient in respiratory distress. If the patient is complaining of shortness of breath (without frank respiratory distress) and the oxygen saturation is acceptable, then an MRI scan may help distinguish between soft tissue edema and hematoma.

In acute respiratory distress where hematoma is suspected, intubation may be extremely challenging unless the hematoma is first evacuated. Often, the compressive effect of the hematoma will cause a tracheal shift to the side opposite to the surgical exposure scar. During such an emergency, the incision suture line may need to be opened at bedside, and the hematoma should be manually removed. If possible, in a patient in respiratory distress with acceptable oxygen saturation and air exchange, this should be done under sterile conditions in the operating room. Intubation under such circumstances may be best accomplished by use of alternative techniques such as the LMA or awake fiberoptic. If all else fails, emergent tracheostomy may be needed to provide an airway.

Most patients with an expanding cervical hematoma at the surgical site will experience severe dysphagia as well as discomfort in a recumbent position. Patients who have severe dysphagia postoperatively, who are unable to swallow liquids, and who insist on sitting upright in bed should be carefully evaluated to rule out the presence of an expanding hematoma. The wall of the esophagus, which is soft and pliable compared with the trachea, is more susceptible to compressive forces. It would be highly unusual to have respiratory compromise due to hematoma in a patient who can tolerate a full liquid or regular diet. With high-risk patients, a tracheostomy kit or suture removal kit taped to the bedside may be a worthwhile precaution during the postoperative phase.

Burkey et al. (21) retrospectively reviewed 13,817 patients undergoing thyroidectomy and parathyroidectomy at the Mayo Clinic from 1976 to 2000. They identified 42 hematomas requiring reoperation. Symptoms of hematoma included respiratory distress in 21 patients (50%), pain or pressure in 11, dysphagia in 8, and drainage in 6 patients.

Eighteen hematomas presented within 6 hours, 16 between 7 and 24 hours, and 8 beyond 24 hours. The bleeding source was arterial in 11, venous in 8, thyroid or soft tissue in 13, and unknown in 10. No definite high-risk factors could be identified.

POSTOPERATIVE NEUROLOGIC DETERIORATION

Immediate postoperative neurologic deterioration is unusual after reconstructive cervical surgery. Several factors may be responsible for acute onset of postoperative neurologic deficit, including compressive hematoma adjacent to neural structures; cord compression due to strut grafts; cord syndrome due to surgical manipulation; edema; and intraoperative hypotension or positioning. An extensive discussion of all these factors is beyond the scope of this chapter; however, urgent reexploration may be needed in the immediate postoperative phase to minimize the risk of permanent neurologic injury.

Mechanical factors such as cord compression due to graft impingement and instrumentation may be ruled out by an immediate lateral cervical spine radiograph. Progressive quadriparesis in the immediate postoperative period is related to a hematoma until proven otherwise. An emergent MRI or reexploration of the surgical site should rule this out. The presence of anterior or central cord syndrome is typically associated with characteristic deficit rather than complete quadriplegia. Once obvious mechanical compressive factors are ruled out, cord syndrome may be treated medically with steroids, restoration of fluid balance, avoidance of hypotension, close observation, and appropriate medical support.

NECK AND FACIAL POSITIONING

Detailed discussion regarding neck and facial positioning has been covered in the previous chapter. A common feature of all congenital or inflammatory abnormalities of the cervical spine is a decrease in canal size, resulting in compromise of the neurologic structures. Hyperextension during intubation or positioning intraoperatively should be avoided because it may constrict an already compromised cervical cord, resulting in neurologic deficit. As discussed in the earlier section, no one method is the best for airway management; however, awake fiberoptic intubation may be the safest in patients where any hyperextension would risk neurologic injury. A preoperative clinical evaluation of the patient's active range of motion of the cervical spine may be a critical factor in deciding what a "tolerable" range of motion (in extension) may be for the individual patient prior to onset of radiculopathic or myelopathic symptoms.

Adequate spinal cord perfusion must be maintained in order to minimize risk of neurologic damage. Spinal cord flow seems to be regulated by the same factors as cerebral blood flow (11). Hypercapnia increases cord flow, whereas the reverse reduces it. Thus, normocapnia or mild hypocapnia is recommended. Intraoperative hypotension is often requested by surgeons in order to decrease the blood loss. However, in patients with a marginally perfused cord, reduction in blood flow may cause cord ischemia and therefore may be contraindicated.

When using prone positioning during posterior cervical procedures, care must be taken to avoid pressure on the eyes. Postoperative blindness is a rare but devastating complication after cervical surgery. Myers et al. (23) reported on 37 patients who experienced visual loss after spine surgery. Ninety-two percent of the cases involved posterior instrumented fusion with an average operative time of 410 minutes and blood loss of 3,500 cc. Most cases had significant intraoperative hypotension. Visual loss occurred secondary to ischemic optic neuropathy, retinal artery occlusion, or cerebral ischemia. Eleven of 30 cases were bilateral, and 15 patients had complete blindness in at least one eye. Most deficits were permanent. The use of a three-pin Mayfield head holder may be safest for avoidance of pressure on the facial structures. When a Mayfield horseshoe headrest is utilized, anesthesia personnel must frequently inspect the facial structures during the surgery to avoid pressure on the eyes. During such cases, exophthalmus or a flattened nasal ridge may allow transmission of pressure to the globe (24). Central retinal artery occlusion may also occur when a horseshoe headrest is utilized for patients in a prone position. This may be the result of excessive extraocular pressure and may be a cause of blindness after cervical surgery (25).

SUMMARY

Patients undergoing extensive reconstructive cervical surgery should be monitored closely for postoperative complications. The most dreaded complications include airway obstruction secondary to edema or hematoma. Poor outcomes may be minimized by anticipating patients who may be high risk and using careful preoperative planning and close perianesthetic monitoring. High-risk patients in whom airway problems may be anticipated include those with prolonged surgical times, high blood loss, three-level or greater corpectomy, and upper cervical spine exposures. Continued intubation for 24 to 48 hours postoperatively may be needed in select patients.

In addition, patients with preoperative cervical instability due to trauma, rheumatoid arthritis, or severe cord compression may need special consideration for intubation, including use of the laryngeal mask airway or awake fiberoptic laryngoscopy.

REFERENCES

1. Harris OA, Runnels JB, Matz PG. Clinical factors associated with unexpected critical care management and prolonged hospitalization after elective cervical spine surgery. *Crit Care Med* 2001; 29(10):1898–1902.
2. Wattenmaker T, Concepcion M, Hibberd P, et al. Upper-airway obstruction and perioperative management of the airway in patients managed with posterior operations on the cervical spine for rheumatoid arthritis. *J Bone Joint Surg Am* 1994;76(3):360–365.
3. Suderman VS, Crobsy ET, Lui A. Elective oral tracheal intubation in cervical spine injured adults. *Can J Anaesth* 1991;38(6):785–789.
4. MacIntyre PA, McLeod AD, Hurley R, et al. Cervical spine movements during laryngoscopy. Comparison of the Macintosh and McCoy laryngoscope blades. *Anaesthesia* 1999;54(5):413–418.
5. Mentzelopoulos SD, Romana CN, Corolanoglou DS, et al. Balloon versus conventional laryngoscopy: a comparison of laryngoscopic findings and intubation difficulty. *Anesth Analg* 2000;91 (6):1513–1519.
6. Kihara S, Watanabe S, Brimacombe J, et al. Segmental cervical spine movements with the intubating laryngeal mask during manual in-line stabilization in patients with cervical pathology undergoing cervical spine surgery. *Anesth Analg* 2000;91(1):195–200.
7. Inoue Y, Koga K, Shigematsu A. A comparison of two tracheal intubation techniques with Trachlight and Fastrach in patients with cervical spine disorders. *Anesth Analg* 2002;94(3):667–671.
8. Kwek TK, Lew TW, Thoo FI. The role of preoperative cervical spine x-rays in rheumatoid arthritis. *Anaesth Intensive Care* 1998;26(6):636–641.
9. Quoss A, Buurman C. Anesthesiological consideration in rheumatic diseases. *Anaesthesiol Reanim* 2000;26(5):116–121.
10. Campbell RS, Wou P, Watt I. A continuing role for preoperative cervical spine radiography in rheumatoid arthritis? *Clin Radiol* 1995;50(3):157–159.
11. Morpeth JF, Williams MF. Vocal cord paralysis after anterior cervical diskectomy and fusion. *Laryngoscope* 2000;110:43–46.
12. Kriskovich MD, Apfelbaum RI, Haller JR. Vocal fold paralysis after anterior cervical surgery: incidence, mechanism, and prevention of injury. *Laryngoscope* 2000;110(9):1467–1473.
13. Ratnaraj J, Todorov A, McHugh T, et al. Effects of decreasing endotracheal tube cuff pressures during neck retraction for anterior cervical surgery. *J Neurosurg* 2002;97(suppl 2):176–179.
14. Muzumdar DP, Deopujari CE, Bhojraj SY. Bilateral vocal cord paralysis after anterior cervical discoidectomy and fusion in a case of whiplash cervical spine injury. A case report. *Surg Neurol* 2000;53:586–588.

15. Sagi HC, Beutler W, Carroll E, et al. Airway complications associated with surgery on the anterior cervical spine. *Spine* 2002;27(9):949–953.
16. Emery SE, Smith MD, Bohlman HH. Upper airway obstruction after multilevel cervical corpectomy for myelopathy. *J Bone Joint Surg Am* 1991;73(4):544–551.
17. Epstein NE, Hollingsworth R, Nardi D, et al. Can airway complications following multilevel anterior cervical surgery be avoided? *J Neurosurg* 2001;94(suppl 2):185–188.
18. Francois JM, Castagnera L, Carrat X, et al. A prospective study of ENT complication following surgery of the cervical spine by the anterior approach (preliminary results). *Rev Laryngol Otol Rhinol (Bord)* 1998;119(2):95–100.
19. Krnacik MJ, Heggeness MH. Severe angioedema causing airway obstruction after anterior cervical surgery. *Spine* 1997;22(18):2188–2190.
20. Miura Y, Mimatsu K, Iwata H. Massive tongue swelling as a complication after spinal surgery. *J Spinal Disord* 1996;9(4):339–341.
21. Burkey SH, van Heerden JA, Thompson GB, et al. Reexploration for symptomatic hematomas after cervical exploration. *Surgery* 2001;130(6):914–920.
22. Beal JL, Lopin MC, Binnert M. Anesthesia for surgery of degenerative and abnormal cervical spine. *Ann Fr Anesth Reanim* 1993;12(4):385–392.
23. Myers MA, Hamilton SR, Bogosian AJ, et al. Visual loss as a complication of spine surgery. A review of 37 cases. *Spine* 1997;22(12):1325–1329.
24. Wolfe SW, Lospinuso MF, Burke SW. Unilateral blindness as a complication of patient positioning for spinal surgery. A case report. *Spine* 1992;17(5):600–605.
25. Bekar A, Tureyen K, Asksoy K. Unilateral blindness due to patient positioning during cervical syringomyelia surgery: unilateral blindness after prone position. *J Neurosurg Anesthesiol* 1996;8(3):227–229.

INTRAOPERATIVE NEUROMONITORING

HOWARD MOSES

BACKGROUND

Among the morbidities that can occur during spinal surgery, the most important is unintended injury to nervous structures. Intraoperative neuromonitoring (IONM) is the intraoperative evaluation of the nervous system to monitor nerve structures in an attempt to avoid injury to them during spinal surgery.

IONM can consist of continuous evaluation to identify neural dysfunction but also includes a number of discrete tests designed to address specific surgical questions as they arise. Although the discrete tests can be performed once or many times during a procedure, nevertheless they constitute "monitoring" in the strict sense. These forms of intraoperative neurologic evaluation provide critical information to the surgeon, allowing reversal or avoidance of neural insults.

Monitoring of the spinal cord by somatosensory evoked potentials was performed on animals in 1972 (1) and first applied to humans by McCallum and Bennett in 1975 (2).

IONM is available in almost all major surgical centers and in many community hospitals and is a recognized adjunct to spinal surgery as well as surgeries in other areas of the nervous system.

GOALS

The primary goal of IONM is the identification of intraoperative neural insults at a stage that allows intervention to eliminate or minimize resultant injury. To this end, evoked potentials can be monitored repeatedly throughout a procedure, with preservation or degradation of signal indicating the state of the corresponding neural pathways. Continuous electromyography can monitor nerve integrity. Multiple tests may be combined to best assess the complex neural structures that are at risk during any given case.

The use of IONM may assist a surgeon to proceed until signal changes are noted that suggest injury. Monitoring may pinpoint steps in surgery that lead to damage, allowing a surgeon to change his or her technique for subsequent surgeries.

Anatomic testing by IONM is used to determine that critical neural elements are not in the immediate surgical field prior to incision of that tissue, such as dissecting nerve roots from connective tissue and various spinal cord procedures.

IONM may help to predict postoperative outcome, identify intraoperative systemic changes, and reassure families that proper precautions are being taken.

GENERAL PRINCIPLES FOR MONITORING

Specific equipment and techniques for monitoring can be found in the references. Different institutions and hospitals prefer different equipment for the same procedure, depending on the surgeon, the equipment available, the engineers who are setting up the equipment, and the technicians performing the work.

Recordings from the anesthetized patient are obtained without pain in a relaxed condition that minimizes movement and muscle artifact. These advantages, however, are diminished by anesthetic suppression of some electrical signals, a noisy electrical environment, and at times limited access to electrodes that need to be adjusted or replaced.

Recordings over an extended time need allowance for varying conditions that may influence signal, such as blood anesthetic levels, blood pressure, temperature, medications, electrolytes, and blood loss.

In the operating room, decisions are made based on changes in the patient's own earlier baseline signals, for it is changes from the preoperative status that are of interest. Changes in the patient's own baseline data are the criteria for action; in particular, the amplitude of responses is a critically important parameter.

The initial steps of monitoring are performed during what is termed the *preoperative baseline period,* which is from the time of the patient's arrival in the preoperative area or operating room until exposure of the at-risk neural tissue. During this time, the patient is placed under anesthesia, electrodes are placed, and the patient is positioned for surgery. Preoperative baseline neurophysiologic data are acquired in the initial surgical exposure. At this time, initial evaluation of signals and multiple system checks are done to ensure their accuracy, and adjustments can be made to optimize signals and to equilibrate and adjust the anesthetic agents that will be used during the case. Elimination of the inducting anesthetic agents and establishment of a steady state in regard to other systemic variables are performed. As a result of the change in multiple variables, signals are likely to be more variable during the preoperative baseline period than during the bulk of the procedure (3). This preoperative baseline period is a low-risk period for neural injury, with the possible exception of positioning of the anesthetized patient. At this time, the patient is unconscious and the musculature is fully relaxed with a loss of normally protective painful feedback; thus, positioning may involve significant risk to the spinal cord. When this risk is high, such as with an unstable spine or severe spinal stenosis, testing is performed prior to and immediately after positioning.

Data collected during the baseline monitoring period form the basis of comparison for the remainder of the case and are collected after equilibration of systemic variables but before risk of surgical insult is present. During this time the quality and variability of signals are assessed and decisions are made as to which warning criteria will apply during the remainder of the procedure. If the signals are excellent, then warning criteria can be applied as outlined below, but if signals are of poor quality, a decision must be made as to whether a lower standard should be applied—for instance, simply the presence or absence of signals—or whether monitoring of that modality would be useful at all. Values for anesthetic doses, blood pressure, and body temperature are recorded at this time so that subsequent alterations can be identified and accounted for as they affect recorded signals.

After this, monitoring will continue, with comparisons made to baseline data through the remainder of the case. Specific action by the surgeon in response to degradation of signal by injury to nerve tissue will depend on the type of case monitored, the stage of the case, and the type of warning. The surgeon may reverse steps taken prior to the warning, stop the action that led to the warning, stop the surgery completely, or take no specific action at all. The anesthesiologist may cooperate by manipulating blood pressure, administering medication (for instance, steroids), or otherwise improving the patient's medical management. The surgeon may wish to partially wake the patient to assess motor function (Stagnara wake-up test) if signal degradation without persisting clinical deficit occurs.

IONM TESTING MODALITIES

Somatosensory Evoked Potentials

Somatosensory evoked potentials (SEPs) are well suited for IONM. Their amplitude and latency are defined and can be quantified for comparison throughout a procedure. They can asses neural function at all levels of the nervous system, from distal nerve to the somatosensory cortex. The level at which an electrical signal is interrupted due to neural insult can be localized to a peripheral nerve, spinal cord, or even brain. SEPs can be elicited from almost any nerve containing sensory fibers, with median, ulnar, and posterior tibial nerves used most frequently.

The most commonly used criterion for SEP is a drop in amplitude to below 50% of baseline. A less compelling but nevertheless warning standard is a latency prolongation of 10% over the baseline figure. These criteria are based on clinical experience, but exact cut-off values are arbitrary and standards will vary among IONM groups. These criteria are best used as an initial warning signal that a neurologic insult may be present; the actual relevance of such changes depends on many additional factors, such as the initial signal amplitude, initial signal variability, morphology of the signal, the presence of confounding system factors (e.g., alterations of anesthetic gases, low levels of neuromuscular blockage), the stage of the surgery, localization of the surgery, loss of the surgical level, and consistency of data degradation. All of these factors are critical in making decisions in the operating room, but no set formulas exist for their application and they are rarely discussed in the literature (Fig. 3.1).

Tibial Nerve Somatosensory Evoked Potentials

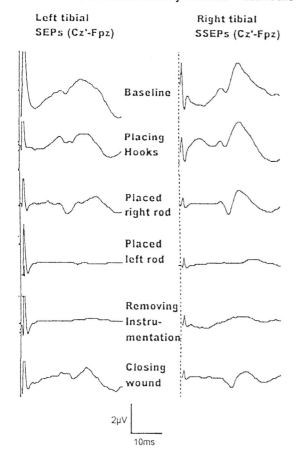

Left tibial
SEPs (Cz'-Fpz)

Right tibial
SSEPs (Cz'-Fpz)

Baseline

Placing
Hooks

Placed
right rod

Placed
left rod

Removing
Instru-
mentation

Closing
wound

2μV

10ms

FIGURE 3.1. Somatosensory evoked potential responses obtained during attempted correction of scoliotic deformity. Selected responses are displayed in a stacked format, with earlier responses at the top. Reproducible responses were present early in the procedure; these were abruptly lost bilaterally with attempts to correct the spinal curvature. Corrective forces on the spinal column were relaxed, and signals returned at the end of the procedure.

Appropriate surgeries for SEP monitoring are those that place the somatosensory pathways at significant risk, in which the SEP chosen is likely to have a reasonable sensitivity to an insult, and in which action by surgeons or anesthetists may be taken in response to a warning. Cervical and thoracic spinal surgeries as well as peripheral limb or joint surgeries are examples. SEP, however, has poor sensitivity at the spinal nerve root level since SEPs from peripheral nerves are typically mediated by multiple nerve roots and as such have poor sensitivity to monoradiculolopathies. Nevertheless, surgeries that place multiple nerve roots at risk simultaneously, for instance, the cauda equina, may still benefit from SEP monitoring. SEPs are now in widespread use during spinal deformity surgery and are considered by many to be a standard of care and have resulted in a 50% decline in major neurologic deficits associated with scoliosis surgery since their introduction. Experienced monitoring teams, however, have half the rate of neurologic deficits compared with the results of inexperienced teams.

SEP monitoring has eliminated the need for routine intraoperative wake-up tests, which have their own morbidities. SEPs also have a 98.9% specificity due to a high negative predicted value coupled with a low incidence of injury. False positive findings were actually common relative to true positive findings, with a predicted value of only 42% in 1995 scoliosis research studies. False negatives are less common but potentially more important since SEPs monitor only large fiber dorsal column–mediated sensory tracts, while postoperative motor function is typically the outcome of greatest interest. SEP as a proxy indicator of motor function is imperfect, and false negative results may occur with isolated motor injury, with delayed injury, or with only partial injury (4,5).

For arm somatosensory evoked potentials, the stimulus electrode placement for pure sensory nerve stimulation is as follows:

- Median nerve stimulation using ring electrodes on digits 2 or 3.
- Ulnar nerve stimulation using ring electrodes on digit 5.
- Radial nerve stimulation at the superficial sensory branch on the radial aspect of the dorsal side of the wrist. Musculocutaneous nerve stimulation at the cutaneous branch, 2 finger breadths below the lateral aspect of the cubital crease.

Although individual dermatomes can be stimulated, this is rarely done in routine clinical practice.

Scalp recordings use ipsilateral and contralateral electrodes, which may be referenced to each other or to a noncephalic reference.

Leg somatosensory evoked potentials can be performed with stimulation of the posterior tibial or peroneal nerves. The posterior tibial nerve is generally felt to be superior to the peroneal nerve for study because of the ease in identifying waveforms, particularly the lumbar potential. The posterior tibial nerve is stimulated at the ankle. The common peroneal nerve is stimulated at the knee. The stimulation parameters essentially are the same as those used for arm stimulation. Stimulation of the posterior tibial nerve is performed such that there is a small amount of plantar flexion of the toes in response to the stimulation. Stimulation of the peroneal nerve is performed such that there is a small amount of eversion of the foot. The stimulus rate is 4 to 7 per second; stimulus duration is usually 200 to 300 microseconds.

The posterior tibial nerve is exposed at the medial malleolus. The cathode (negative stimulating electrode) is placed midway between the medial border of the achilles tendon and the posterior border of the medial malleolus. The anode (positive stimulating electrode) is placed 3 cm distal to the cathode. The ground electrode is attached to the skin of the calf proximal to the stimulating electrodes.

The peroneal nerve is exposed in the popliteal fossa and over the fibular head. The cathode is placed over the lateral part of the popliteal fossa just medial to the tendon of the biceps femoris and below the leg crease. The tendon of the biceps femoris stands out when the patient flexes the knee against resistance while the knee is at approximately a 90-degree angle. The anode is placed 3 cm distal to the cathode. A ground electrode is placed on the leg proximal to the stimulating electrodes.

For tibial nerve stimulation at the ankle, recording electrodes are placed in the following locations for cervical spine surgery: midline between CZ and PZ, and ipsilateral cortex between C3/4 and P3/4. Recording time normally is set at 60 msec, although if good cerebral potentials are not seen, increasing the recording time to 100 msec is warranted to ensure that a delayed response is detected. Between 1,000 and 4,000 responses are averaged to produce a good response with peroneal or tibial nerve stimulation. Smaller nerves may require more averaged responses. A sweep length of at least 60 msec is used, although longer lengths may be used for delayed cerebral responses.

Motor Evoked Potentials

The most reliable method to assess central motor pathways is through transcranial motor evoked potentials (TcMEP). These are a relatively new addition to the IONM suite. They are now in routine use by some services but may still be inhibited due to persisting problems. Responses are elicited with high-intensity, high-rate trains of transcranial electrical or magnetic pulses (3 to 7 pulses at 300–500 Hz). The resulting descending volley is then recorded from the spinal cord surface by epidural or subdural electrodes or from limb muscles.

Motor evoked potentials (MEPs) are an important addition to SEPs because motor tracts and the large fiber dorsal column sensory tracts assessed by SEPs may be injured individually within the nervous system (6,7). This potential disassociation is very significant within the spinal cord because motor tracts lie within the distribution of the anterior spinal artery, making them selectively vulnerable to ischemic injury. Motor function preservation is the most critical concern of the patient and involved surgeons in most cases.

MEPs should not be confused with spinally elicited peripheral nerve responses (SEPNRs). SEPNRs use spinal cord stimulation to produce a descending volley that can be recorded (average response) over peripheral nerves. This test was originally developed as a test for motor function and was initially called "neurogenic motor evoked potentials"(8), but it is actually primarily a sensory response with little or no motor information (5,9,10). A variant of this test using a train of stimuli and muscle recording has been recorded to assess motor pathways (11). Cases with the strongest indication for MEPs are those in which there is a high likelihood of isolated motor tract injury without associated somatosensory tract injury, such as spinal cord tumors, thoracic aorta aneurysm repair, vascular spinal cord procedures, and high-risk spinal deformity surgeries. Uses for MEP monitoring continue to evolve, and further uses are still to be delineated. MEP testing is typically done in conjunction with SEP testing.

The type of MEP performed determines the warning criteria. TcMEP data recorded from muscles is more variable than spinal cord potentials recorded from epidural or subdermal electrodes. For muscle recording, the only agreed-upon criterion for significance of MEP degradation is complete loss of previously reliable signals (Fig. 3.2). Some groups report use of stricter criteria as a percentage of amplitude loss relative to baseline (12). An alternate method is to record signals at their threshold for acquisition, with an increase in threshold as an indicator of probable injury (13). Even more stringent amplitude criteria may be used when direct spinal cord monitoring is employed, with a 50% loss of amplitude considered significant (14). MEP latency measures are poor indicators of motor injury (12).

MEPs are highly predictive of postoperative motor function (12,15) and are superior to SEPs for this purpose (16,17). This is especially important during spinal deformity surgery and thoracic aneurysm surgery, where the sensitivity of SEP is poor (16,18) whereas initial reports of MEP sensitivity are excellent (12).

MEP testing however, is highly sensitive to most commonly used anesthetic agents (17,18) other than narcotics and ketamine (18,19). This sensitivity is even more pronounced when MEPs are elicited with magnetic stimulation (20). As a result, anesthetic agents optimized for MEPs may be more difficult to manage, may not allow timely

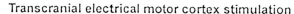

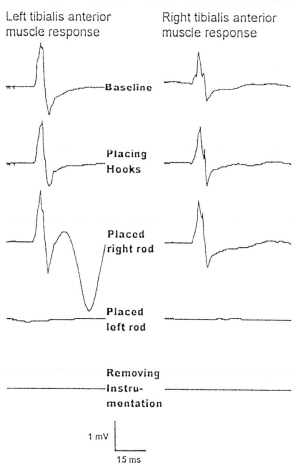

Transcranial electrical motor cortex stimulation

Left tibialis anterior
muscle response

Right tibialis anterior
muscle response

Baseline

Placing
Hooks

Placed
right rod

Placed
left rod

Removing
Instru-
mentation

1 mV

15 ms

FIGURE 3.2. Motor evoked potential responses obtained during correction of scoliotic deformity. Selected responses are displayed in a stacked format, with earlier responses at the top. Initial signals were robust but then were abruptly lost bilaterally after attempts to reverse the spinal curvature. Signals subsequently returned (not shown). In a follow-up procedure, these signals were lost each time spinal derotation was attempted and were regained on subsequent relaxation.

wake-up tests, and are often more expensive than standard regimens. Effective TcMEP presents a problem in the United States, where there are no FDA-approved transcranial stimulators and, as a result, approved electrical stimulators are used off-label and non-FDA-approved devices are used under research conditions. Furthermore, FDA stimulators do not provide an ideal stimulus when used alone.

Electric stimulation is anodal rather than cathodal as is used for peripheral nerve stimulation. A flat anode is placed on the scalp over the motor strip, and a long beltlike cathode goes around the head. Recording electrodes are placed over the muscle to be studied, often the abductor digiti minimi. The patient is asked to make a mild voluntary contraction of the studied muscle. This facilitates the response so that a lower stimulus intensity is required, which prevents the stimulation from involving more extensive muscle contraction.

Magnetic stimulation is delivered by a manufactured induction coil held in the hand, placed over the motor cortex; direct contact with the skin is not necessary.

Recordings of the MEPs are usually made from the arm, although the leg can be used. In the arm, the most commonly examined muscles are the abductor digiti minimi, abductor pollicis brevis, first dorsal interosseous, biceps, and triceps. In the leg, the tibialis anterior is the most often studied. The active recording electrode is placed over the belly of the muscle. The reference electrode is placed distally over the tendon or a distal joint.

Band pass usually is set at 3 to 3,000 Hz. Gain is determined by the amplitude of the response. Analysis time initially is set to 50 msec.

Electromyography

Electromyographic (EMG) activity can be monitored in any muscle accessible to a needle, wire, or surface electrode. Muscle activity can be continuously monitored (free-running EMG) or can be evaluated under electrical stimulation of associated nerves (motor nerve conduction studies, "trigger EMG"). Free-running EMG and motor nerve conduction studies are often complementary and used in conjunction. Only irritation of peripheral nerves reliably evokes EMG activity, and free-running EMG is not used for evaluation of central pathways. EMG monitoring is most effective in cases where nerve injury results from repetitive mechanical irritation of the nerve. It may be used in spinal surgery to monitor lumbosacral nerve roots during spinal surgeries at that level. EMG monitoring can be applied in any case that puts a nerve root at risk during skull base surgery, cervical spine surgery with risk of radicular injury, lumbosacral spine surgery, and any surgery placing peripheral nerve at risk, for instance, joint, pelvic, and plexus surgeries. Thoracic myotomes may be monitored primarily to prevent postoperative pain, but this is uncommon given the lesser impact of motor dysfunction in the thoracic myotomes.

Motor Nerve Conduction Studies

Motor nerve conduction studies (MNCS) are commonly performed in association with free-running EMG monitoring. MNCS can assess the continuity of nerves from the point of stimulation to the muscle, especially when the nerve in question is at high risk of injury, and under certain conditions may predict degree of injury (21). MNCS can indicate whether neural structures are in or near an area of proposed resection or cautery. This is important because motor nerves may be obscured by tumor or may be difficult to distinguish from connective tissue or scar, for instance, arachnoiditis. In these instances, a searching stimulus can be used to ensure that nerves are not within a target area of tissue.

MNCS are useful in the placement of pedicle screws used alone or to anchor spinal instrumentation. Holes drilled in the vertebral pedicle so that screws can be inserted may perforate the cortical rim of the pedicle, and a screw placed in it may impinge upon exiting nerve roots, with a resultant radiculopathy or pain. However, any hole that perforates a pedicle bicortically creates a low-impedance pathway for electrical current outflow to the adjacent nerve roots. The intensity of current needed to depolarize these roots (the threshold) is lower when a perforation results (22).

Warning criteria for identification of malpositioned pedicle screws are based on the electrical threshold for activation of nearby nerve roots. The threshold levels indicating pedicle screw malpositioning vary from center to center depending on stimulation methods and individual preferences. Hole thresholds of less than 5 mA and screw thresholds of less than 7 mA are likely to represent pedicle wall perforations. Hole thresholds of 5 to 7 mA and screw thresholds of 7 to 10 mA may or may not reflect pedicle perforation, and the surgeon may choose to use, redirect, or abandon the hole based on other factors such as probing of the pedicle wall for defect and the viability of redirection in alternative fixation sites. Hole thresholds over 7 mA and screw thresholds over 10 mA suggest the screw is placed entirely within the pedicle.

Computed tomographic studies of pedicle screw placement found that screws with an electrical threshold above critical level can be stated as being within the pedicle with 93% to 98% confidence (23,24), whereas intraoperative radiographic guidance only provides 63% to 83% accuracy (25,26). Accurate identification of malpositioned screws using MNCS reduces neurologic injury in appropriate surgeries (27). Preexisting nerve root compression (28) or high levels of neuromuscular blockage (29) may elevate measured thresholds, leading to false negative results.

MNCS may be used in the same types of cases as listed previously for free-running EMG and are often used in conjunction with EMG. Any case where nerve muscle pairs are accessible may be tested with MNCS for identification of function or anatomy.

OTHER TYPES OF TESTING USED IN INTRAOPERATIVE NEUROMONITORING

Other types of tests include the following:

- *Reflex and f-wave monitoring:* H-reflex and f-wave evaluation can assess the involved neural pathway. More rostral neural mediation of these responses may result in signal loss due to spinal cord injury, resulting in the electrophysiologic equivalent of "spinal shock."
- *Repetitive nerve stimulation:* Used to test for a neuromuscular blockade (29–31) and for selective dorsal rhizotomy (32,33).
- *Stagnara wake-up test:* The neurologic examination can be directly assessed during surgeries by the Stagnara wake-up test (34). Anesthetic agents are withdrawn and allowed to wane until the patient is able to follow commands, at which time gross motor function can be directly assessed in the at-risk limbs. This was used routinely in some cases of spinal surgery prior to widespread utilization of IONM. It has been largely replaced by other tests because of its ability to access function at only one point during a surgery as well as because of the potential delay in surgery, the patient recall, and risk of unintentional extubation or hemodynamic instability. It is still used by many surgeons, but usually only as an adjunct to assess the extent of insults detected by other IONM tests.

ANESTHETIC AGENTS AND OTHER SYSTEMIC VARIABLES

Anesthetic and other systemic variables affect IONM signals in qualitative but not quantitative ways. Detailed reviews of this topic can be found elsewhere (35). Generally, effects are global for similar types of signals. An increase in the inhaled concentration of nitrous oxide will reduce the amplitude of both upper and lower limb cortical SEP responses and will do so bilaterally. Typically, the changes seen are of similar magnitude, although it is not uncommon for one or more signals to be affected more dramatically in terms of percentage decline. This may make interpretation of anesthetic-related changes uncertain, and therefore stability of both anesthetic and systemic parameters is of great importance.

The best anesthetic regimen for monitoring is one in which excellent signals are obtained after full equilibration of the routine and in which this routine remains stable. There is, however, considerable individual variation in how patients' electrical potentials respond to the many possible anesthetic regimens, and thus flexibility and cooperation between the anesthesia and IONM teams will best meet the shared goals of anesthesia, amnesia, analgesia, and adequate insight into the integrity of the patient's nervous system.

CONCLUSION

IONM has become an important component of many types of spinal surgery, and for some of these procedures there is strong evidence of a reduced complication rate.

A surgery with a high risk of neural injury and definite steps that might be taken if an insult is identified will benefit from IONM-provided insight into the pathways at risk. A surgery with low risk of morbidity and little that can be done upon identification of an insult will almost certainly not benefit from IONM, but even low-risk surgeries with effective intervention options may benefit from IONM (e.g., scoliosis). Cost-benefit analyses will tend to favor IONM even if a reduced complication rate can be demonstrated, because of the severe nature of most neurologic injuries. The cost- benefit balance will shift, however, with lower complication rates, less severe injuries, and if the sensitivity of IONM tests is poor.

REFERENCES

1. Croft TJ, Brodkey JS, Nulsen FE. Reversible spinal cord trauma: a model for electric monitoring of spinal cord function. *J Neurosurg* 1972;36:402–406.
2. McCallum JE, Bennett MH. Electrophysiologic monitoring of spinal cord function during intraspinal surgery. *Surg Forum* 1975;26:469–471.
3. Luk KD, Hu Y, Wong YW, et al. Variability of somatosensory-evoked potentials in different stages of scoliosis surgery. *Spine* 1999;24:1799–1804.
4. Lesser RP, Raudzens P, Luders H, et al. Postoperative neurological deficits may occur despite unchanged intraoperative somatosensory evoked potentials. *Ann Neurol* 1986;19:22–25.
5. Minahan RE, Sepkuty JP, Lesser RP, et al. Anterior spinal cord injury with preserved neurogenic "motor" evoked potentials. *Clin Neurophysiol* 2001;112:1442–1450.
6. Ben-David B, Haller G, Taylor P. Anterior spinal fusion complicated by paraplegia. A case report of a false-negative somatosensory-evoked potential. *Spine* 1987;12:536–539.
7. Ben-David B, Taylor PD, Haller GS. Posterior spinal fusion complicated by posterior column injury. A case report of a false-negative wake-up test. *Spine* 1987;12:540–543.
8. Owen JH. Intraoperative stimulation of the spinal cord for prevention of spinal cord injury. *Adv Neurol* 1993;63:271–288.
9. Su CF, Haghighi SS, Oro JJ, et al. "Backfiring" in spinal cord monitoring. High thoracic spinal cord stimulation evokes sciatic response by antidromic sensory pathway conduction, not motor tract conduction. *Spine* 1992;17:504–508.
10. Toleikis JR, Skelly JP, Carlvin AO, et al. Spinally elicited peripheral nerve responses are sensory rather than motor. *Clin Neurophysiol* 2000;111:736–742.
11. Mochida K, Shinomiya K, Komori H, et al. A new method of multisegment motor pathway monitoring using muscle potentials after train spinal stimulation. *Spine* 1995;20:2240–2246.
12. de Haan P, Kalkman CJ, De Mol BA, et al. Efficacy of transcranial motor-evoked myogenic potentials to detect spinal cord ischemia during operations for thoracoabdominal aneurysm. *J Thorac Cardiovasc Surg* 1997;113:87–100.
13. Calancie B, Harris W, Broton JG, et al. "Threshold-level" multipulse transcranial electrical stimulation of motor cortex for intraoperative monitoring of spinal motor tracts: description of method and comparison to somatosensory evoked potential monitoring. *J Neurosurg* 1998;88:457–470.
14. Morota N, Deletis V, Constantini S, et al. The role of motor evoked potentials during surgery for intramedullary spinal cord tumors. *Neurosurgery* 1997;41:1327–1336.
15. Yang LH, Lin SM, Lee WY, et al. Intraoperative transcranial electrical motor evoked potential monitoring during spinal surgery under intravenous ketamine or etomidate anesthesia. *Acta Neurochir* 1994;127:191–198.
16. Meylaerts SA, Jacobs MJ, Iterson van V, et al. Comparison of transcranial motor evoked potentials and somatosensory evoked potentials during thoracolumbar aortic aneurysm repair. *Ann Surg* 1999;230:742–749.
17. Pechstein U, Nadstawek J, Zentner J, et al. Isoflurane plus nitrous oxide versus propofol for recording of motor evoked potentials after high frequency repetitive electrical stimulation. *Electroencephalog Clin Neurophysiol* 1998;108:175–181.
18. Galla JD, Ergin MA, Lansman SL, et al. Use of somatosensory evoked potentials for thoracic and thoracoabdominal aortic resections. *Ann Thorac Surg* 1999;67:1947–1952.
19. Kalkman CJ, Drummond JC, Ribberink AA, et al. Effects of propofol, etomidate, midazolam and fentanyl on motor evoked responses to transcranial electrical or magnetic stimulation in humans. *Anesthesiology* 1992;76:502–509.
20. Ubags LH, Kalkman CJ, Been HD, et al. The use of ketamine or etomidate to supplement sufentanil/N20 anesthesia does not disrupt monitoring of the myogenic transcranial motor evoked responses. *J Neurosurg Anesthesiol* 1997;9:228–233.
21. Ubags LH, Kalkman CJ, Been HD, et al. A comparison of myogenic motor evoked responses to electrical and magnetic transcranial stimulation during nitrous oxide/opioid anesthesia. *Anesth Analg* 1999;88:568–572.
22. Goldbrunner RH, Schlake HP, Milewski C, et al. Quantitative parameters of intraoperative electromyography predict facial nerve outcomes for vestibular schwannoma surgery. *Neurosurgery* 2000;46:1140–1146.
23. Calancie B, Madsen P, Lebwohl N. Stimulus-evoked EMG monitoring during transpedicular lumbosacral spine instrumentation. Initial clinical results. *Spine* 1994;19:2780–2786.

24. Glassman SD, Dimar JR, Puno RM, et al. A prospective analysis of intraoperative electromyographic monitoring of pedicle screw placement with computed tomographic scan confirmation. *Spine* 1995;20:1375–1379.
25. Maguire J, Wallace S, Madiga R, et al. Evaluation of intrapedicular screw position using intraoperative evoked electromyography. *Spine* 1995;20:1068–1074.
26. Ferrick MR, Kowalski JM, Simmons ED. Reliability of roentgenogram evaluation of pedicle screw position. *Spine* 1998;22:1249–1253.
27. Darden DV, Wood KE, Hatley MK, et al. Evaluation of pedicle screw insertion monitored by intraoperative evoked electromyography. *J Spinal Disord* 1996;9:8–16.
28. Holland NR, Lukaczyk TA, Riley LH, et al. Higher electrical stimulus intensities are required to activate chronically compressed nerve roots. Implications for intraoperative electromyographic pedicle screw testing. *Spine* 1998;23:224–227.
29. Minahan RE, Riley L, Lukaczyk TA, et al. The effect of neuromuscular blockage on pedicle screw stimulation thresholds. *Spine* 2000;25:2526–2530.
30. Ali HH, Savarese JJ. Monitoring of neuromuscular function. *Anesthesiology* 1976;45:216–249.
31. Minahan RE, Riley L, Lukaczyk TA, et al. Measures of partial neuromuscular blockage for lumbosacral spinal surgeries. American Academy of Neurology Meeting, poster presentation P02.135, 1999.
32. Logigian EL, Shefner JM, Goumnerova L, et al. The critical importance of stimulus intensity in intraoperative monitoring for partial dorsal rhizotomy. *Muscle Nerve* 1996;19:415–422.
33. Mittal S, Farmer JP, Poulin C, et al. Reliability of intraoperative electrophysiological monitoring in selective posterior rhizotomy. *J Neurosurg* 2001;95:67–75.
34. Vauzelle C, Stagnara P, Jouvinroux P. Functional monitoring of spinal cord activity during spinal surgery. *Clin Orthop* 1973;93:173–178.
35. Sloan TB. Anesthetic effect on electrophysiologic records. *J Clin Neurophysiol* 1998;15:217–226.

APPROACHES TO THE CERVICAL SPINE

APPROACHES TO THE CERVICAL SPINE: OVERVIEW, EXPOSURE, INDICATIONS, AND CONTRAINDICATIONS

ALEXANDER J. GHANAYEM

Reconstructive, corrective, and functional restorative procedures of the cervical spine can usually all be demonstrated in their outcome by radiographic imaging. The simple, yet satisfying, successful one-level anterior cervical discectomy and fusion (ACDF) or corrective osteotomy for cervical kyphosis can readily be demonstrated by plain radiographs. A sagittal magnetic resonance imaging (MRI) scan will demonstrate how effective a transoral resection of the odontoid can be to relieve spinal cord and brainstem compression in a rheumatoid patient with cranial settling and atlantoaxial subluxation. The "before and after" pictures do not reveal all of the events that took place during surgery but rather the end result. Technical aspects of decompressive, corrective, and stabilization procedures have evolved since Robinson and Smith's first report of the ACDF (1)

The keys to any successful surgical procedure lie in the details. Of course, proper indications must also be present. A well-thought-out surgical exposure of the cervical spine is vital because it provides the surgeon safe and proper access to perform the necessary technical portions of a procedure. Inadequate exposure or visualization can be the downfall of a perfectly planned surgical procedure. For example, anterior odontoid screw insertion through an incision placed too cephalad or caudal will adversely affect the proper screw insertion angle (2). Overzealous retraction during an ACDF can leave a patient dissatisfied with his or her residual swallowing or with phonation dysfunction, even though the procedure achieved technical success for the radiculopathy. Without proper preoperative planning and attention to detail with respect to the surgical approach, the approach can become half the battle. Conversely, proper surgical planning and a detailed understanding of the relevant surgical anatomy will result in adequate exposure while minimizing complications. In this scenario, getting there can be half the fun.

INDICATIONS

The indication for a particular approach depends on the anatomic level or levels to be addressed and the techniques employed. Usually, these two considerations are one and the same. There are, however, two exceptions:

1. Anterior odontoid screw insertion. The operative level is C2, but the surgical approach is performed at about the C5 level. This allows for the proper insertion angle of the odontoid screw.
2. Posterior C1–2 transarticular screw insertion. While C1–2 is exposed posteriorly at the level, additional small paramedian incisions, usually at the lower cervical or upper thoracic level, are needed for proper screw insertion angle (3).

TABLE 4.1. OPERATIVE CERVICAL SPINE APPROACH AND CORRESPONDING ANATOMIC LEVELS

Specific approach	Operative level	Extensile potential
Anterior		
Transoral	Clivus to upper portion of C2	Requires mandibular splitting approach
Transoral with mandibular splitting	Clivus to the subaxial cervical spine	Yes—to the cervicothoracic junction
High retropharyngeal	C1–2 lateral mass articulations to the C2–3 disc space	Yes—to the cervicothoracic junction
Anterior for odontoid stabilization	Anterior approach to C5 for anterior odontoid screw placement	Not applicable
Anterior	C3 to C7-T1 C2–3 in edentulous patients with long, lean necks C7-T1 in patients with long, lean necks	Cranially—no Caudally—yes with clavicular-manubrium resection
Anterior with clavicle-manubrium resection	C7-T4	Cranially into the subaxial cervical spine Caudally—no
Posterior		
Midline	Occiput to the thoracic spine	Yes
Paramedian incisions at the cervicothoracic level	Required for C1–2 transarticular screw insertion	Not applicable

Indications for anterior approaches include decompressive, fusion, debridement, and corrective procedures. Clinical conditions include disc herniation, spondylosis with radiculopathy or myelopathy, kyphosis, metastatic and primary neoplastic disease, trauma, discitis and osteomyelitis, rheumatoid arthritis, and neck pain. Indications for posterior approaches include decompressive, fusion, and corrective procedures. Clinical conditions include far-lateral or foraminal disc herniations or spondylosis, myelopathy, kyphosis, metastatic and primary neoplastic disease, trauma, rheumatoid arthritis, and epidural hematoma or abscess. Discitis and osteomyelitis is rarely treated via posterior approaches unless a supplemental posterior stabilization procedure is required.

The posterior approach is extensile—the occiput to the cervicothoracic junction can be exposed through the same midline incision. Anterior approaches, however, have limited extensile potential. Therefore, the surgeon must consider which vertebral levels need to be exposed and the patient's body habitus when planning the approach. The anterior approach, utilizing the interval between the sternocleidomastoid muscle and carotid sheath laterally and the midline neck structures medially, can access C3 through C7. If a patient's mandible is small or is edentulous, the C2–3 disc can be accessed through this approach. A long-necked, lean individual can have the C7-T1 interspace exposed through this approach. Conversely, a short-necked, burly individual may be difficult to expose even at the C6–7 level. Further caudal exposure below T1 may require partial resection of the medial head of the clavicle and manubrium. Extension below T3–4 is limited by the great vessels.

Anterior exposure of the upper cervical spine is achieved through either the high retropharyngeal or transoral approaches. The high retropharyngeal approach will access the C1–2 lateral mass articulations, C2 body, and C2–3 disc space. The transoral approach will allow exposure from the clivus to the upper portion of the C2 body. The transoral approach becomes extensile to C3 and lower by combining it with the mandibular splitting approach. The retropharyngeal approach is extensile to the cervicothoracic junction.

A summary of approaches and corresponding levels can be found in Table 4.1.

CONTRAINDICATIONS

There are very few contraindications for the various approaches to the cervical spine. There are basically two contraindications to a posterior approach: the inability of the patient to medically tolerate prone positioning, and active posterior infection. Relative contraindications include patients with significant deficiencies in the posterior soft tissue envelope from multiple procedures, burns, or postradiation muscle fibrosis with skin reactive changes. Recent radiation therapy (i.e., within 2 weeks of surgery) may also be a relative contraindication. These relative contraindications can be overcome if the surgeon and the patient are prepared to utilize soft tissue transfer procedures should a significant infection or soft tissue defect occur.

Contraindications to anterior procedures depend on the specific approach. Transoral procedures require that a supplemental airway (i.e., tracheostomy) be available (4–6). Nasopharyngeal infection and radiation changes can also be problematic. Should vascular structures such as the vertebral or basilar artery lie within or anterior to the lesion to be addressed, the transoral approach should not be used. Finally, intradural lesions represent a relative contraindication for the transoral approach given the risk of persistent cerebrospinal fluid leak and meningitis associated with the frequent inability to maintain a watertight dural repair in this region.

The high retropharyngeal approaches are technically challenging (7,8). These approaches are contraindicated if the surgeon or surgical team is not completely aware of the regional anatomy, including the external carotid artery and its branches, upper laryngeal vessels and nerves, the hypoglossal nerve, and submaxillary gland, when proceeding medial to the carotid sheath. When proceeding posterior to the carotid sheath, the spinal accessory nerve is at risk. In patients receiving prior head and neck radiation therapy, this approach may be relatively contraindicated if these structures cannot be identified and protected. Active infection is also a contraindication, with the exception of using the approach to drain and debride an infectious process.

The anterior approach to the cervical spine possesses very few contraindications as well. Once again, patients who have received significant amounts of radiation therapy as well as those with prior radical neck dissections may represent a relative contraindication if safe mobilization and protection of the midline neck structures and carotid sheath cannot be achieved. Penetrating trauma resulting in esophageal perforation and gross contamination of the prevertebral space is a contraindication for this approach unless an emergent clinical scenario arises. If so, the use of internal fixation should be avoided. Active head and neck infections also represent a contraindication unless the approach is being used to address the infection itself (9). The surgeon may wish to avoid the use of anterior instrumentation in favor of posterior stabilization, if necessary, when treating an anterior infection.

A challenging question arises as to which side should be used in cases of revision anterior exposures. If a left-sided approach was used at the index procedure and there is no evidence of a recurrent laryngeal nerve injury, then the side for revision would be the surgeon's preference. If a left-sided approach was used at the index procedure and there is evidence of a recurrent laryngeal nerve injury, the right-sided approach is contraindicated to prevent potential bilateral recurrent laryngeal nerve deficiencies. If the index procedure was on the right and there is no evidence of a recurrent laryngeal nerve injury, then either side can be used for the revision. The revision right-sided approach, however, may have a higher incidence of recurrent laryngeal nerve injury should the nerve not be identifiable within scar tissue. If the index procedure was on the right and there is evidence of a recurrent laryngeal nerve injury, the left-sided approach is contraindicated to prevent potential bilateral recurrent laryngeal nerve deficiencies. If there is any question as to the functional status of the recurrent laryngeal nerve and vocal cords, a preoperative ENT consultation can be helpful. Direct fiberoptic laryngoscopy can visualize the vocal cords and evaluate their function.

Finally, the presence of a tracheostomy was once felt to be a contraindication to performing an anterior cervical approach. Recent studies, however, have found that anterior approaches can be performed safely if the tracheostomy site is clean and a second lateral incision is used for the surgical approach (10,11).

The anterior approach for odontoid fixation has the same contraindications as does the anterior approach to the cervical spine. In addition, the use of this approach is contraindicated when insertion of an odontoid screw is contraindicated, such as in a case where the fracture cannot be reduced or significant comminution exists (2). This approach may be relatively contraindicated in barrel-chested patients or women with pendulous breasts that prevent the surgeon from obtaining a safe drilling angle into the C2 body. A right-angle drill and guide can overcome this problem.

The anterior exposure of the cervicothoracic junction requires entering the mediastinum. The great vessels (aortic arch and superior vena cava) limit the caudal extension. In addition, the brachiocephalic trunk and carotid sheath are in the area of exposure (12,13). Therefore, one should not attempt this approach without suitable backup from either a vascular or thoracic surgeon in the event of injury to one of these structures. Esophageal perforation and gross contamination of the mediastinum, as well as active infection in the head and neck, contraindicate this approach unless the approach is being used to address the infection itself. The surgeon may wish to avoid the use of anterior instrumentation in favor of posterior stabilization, if necessary, when treating an anterior infection.

SUMMARY

Surgical exposure of the cervical spine requires the anatomic knowledge of multiple body systems: vascular, gastrointestinal, pulmonary, nervous, and, of course, musculoskeletal. Many bodily functions can be adversely affected from approach-related complications, ranging from speech, respiration, and swallowing to devastating vascular injuries resulting in stroke and death. The remaining chapters in this section will address each of these approaches in detail, starting with preoperative planning and concluding with postoperative management. The pertinent anatomy will also be reviewed. Spine surgeons should use these sections to help optimize the chance of successful functional outcomes while minimizing the chance of complications from the surgical procedure and approach of choice.

REFERENCES

1. Robinson RA, Smith GW. Anterolateral cervical disc removal and interbody fusion for cervical disc syndrome. *Bull Johns Hopkins Hosp* 1955;96:223–224.
2. Apfelbaum R. Screw fixation of odontoid fractures. In: Wilkins RH, Rengachary SS, eds. *Neurosurgery*, 2nd ed. New York: McGraw Hill, 1999:2965–2973.
3. Magerl F, Seeman PS. Stable posterior fusion of the atlas and axis by transarticular screw fixation. In: Kehr P, Weidner A, eds. *Cervical spine.* New York: Springer-Verlag, 1987:322–327.
4. Crockard HA, Pozo JL, Ransford AO, et al. Transoral decompression and posterior fusion for rheumatoid atlanto-axial subluxation. *J Bone Joint Surg Br* 1986;68:350–356.
5. Fang HSY, Ong GB. Direct approach to the upper cervical spine. *J Bone Joint Surg Br* 1962;44: 1588–1604.
6. Menezes AH, Traynelis VC, Gantz. Surgical approaches to the craniovertebral junction. *Clin Neurosurg* 1993;41:187–203.
7. Heller JG, Whitesides TE Jr. Anterior extrapharyngeal approaches to the upper cervical spine. In: Zdeblick TA, ed. *Anterior approaches to the spine.* St. Louis: Quality Medical Publishing, 1999:15–32.
8. Whitesides TE Jr. Lateral retropharyngeal approach to the upper cervical spine. In: Sherk HH, ed. *The cervical spine: an atlas of surgical procedures.* Philadelphia: JB Lippincott Co, 1994:71–77.
9. Ghanayem AJ, Zdeblick TA. Cervical spine infections. *Orthop Clin North Am* 1996;27:53–68.
10. Northrup BE, Vaccaro AR, Rosen JE, et al. Occurrence of infection in anterior cervical fusion for spinal cord injury after tracheostomy. *Spine* 1995;20:2449–2453.
11. Sustic A, Krstulovic B, Eskinja N, et al. Surgical tracheostomy versus percutaneous dilational tracheostomy in patients with anterior cervical spine fixation: preliminary report. *Spine* 2002;27: 1942–1945.
12. Daftari TK, Herkowitz HN. Transsternal, transmanubrial and transclavicular exposures. In: Zdeblick TA, ed. *Anterior approaches to the spine.* St. Louis: Quality Medical Publishing, 1999:87–104.
13. Sundaresan N, Shah J, Foley KM, et al. An anterior surgical approach to the upper thoracic vertebrae. *J Neurosurg* 1984;61:686–690.

ANTERIOR UPPER CERVICAL SPINE APPROACHES

ASHOK BIYANI
HOWARD S. AN

A variety of pathological processes can cause anterior compression of the upper cervical spine and the clivus. These include rheumatoid arthritis, congenital conditions such as Down's syndrome and epiphyseal dysplasia, collagen disorders, trauma, extradural tumors, os odontoideum, and infection. Several surgical approaches to the anterior upper cervical spine have been described to deal with ventral compression of the upper cervical spine. de Andrade and McNab (1) first described an anterior approach to the upper cervical spine to achieve occipitocervical fusion in 1969. Since then, many other authors have described other anterior approaches to the upper cervical spine, such as transoral, retropharyngeal, and transmandibular approaches.

RELEVANT ANATOMY

Most surgeons have limited experience with anterior approaches to the upper cervical spine due to the small number of cases, complexity of the approaches, and difficult perioperative management. The purpose of the exposure and the extent of the surgical procedure determine the appropriate surgical approach. A thorough understanding of the surgical anatomy is necessary for anterior approaches to the upper cervical spine to avoid potentially catastrophic complications.

Surface Anatomy

Laryngeal prominence produced by thyroid cartilage coincides with the C4–5 level. The hyoid bone is horseshoe shaped and lies at the level of the third cervical vertebra. It is easily palpable with the neck extended. It provides attachment to the muscles of the floor of the mouth (middle pharyngeal, hyoglossus, genioglossus) and all hyoid muscles (stylohyoid, thyrohyoid, geniohyoid, omohyoid, mylohyoid, and sternohyoid). The anterior tubercle on the arch of the atlas defines the midline. It can be palpated through the pharyngeal wall and is separated from the oropharynx only by oral mucosa and pharyngeal muscles. The transverse processes of the atlas are located more lateral than those of caudal vertebrae and can be palpated on a line between the angle of the mandible and a point 1 cm anterior and inferior to the tip of the mastoid process.

Fascia

There are several layers of the investing cervical fascia. The superficial fascia containing the platysma is encountered first. Superficial and middle layers of deep cervical fascia encase the sternomastoid and the strap muscles, respectively. Visceral fascia surrounds the trachea, esophagus, and the recurrent laryngeal nerve, which is present in the tracheoesophageal groove. The deep layer of the deep fascia consists of the alar fascia and the prevertebral fascia. The alar fascia joins the two carotid sheaths and fuses with the visceral fascia in the midline. The prevertebral fascia covers the longus colli and scalene muscles.

Vessels

The external carotid artery gives out eight branches. Three ventral branches include the superior thyroid, lingual, and facial arteries emerging below, at, and above the level of the greater cornu of the hyoid bone, respectively. These anterior branches and a medial ascending pharyngeal artery that supplies the pharyngeal wall require ligation during the anterior retropharyngeal approach for mobilization and lateral retraction of the carotid sheath. The remaining two dorsal and two terminal branches of the external carotid artery are usually not encountered during the anterior retropharyngeal approach. The external carotid artery may require ligation distal to the takeoff of the superior thyroid artery during the transmandibular transcervical approach.

The internal carotid artery and jugular vein are tethered to the base of the skull at their foramina and are susceptible to injury by excessive retraction or extensive dissection.

The external jugular vein forms by the confluence of the posterior auricular vein and posterior division of the retromandibular vein at the apex of the mandible. It is contained within the superficial layer of the deep fascia and runs distally superficial to the sternomastoid to drain into the subclavian vein. The external jugular vein requires ligation and division in the superior part of the incision during anterolateral retropharyngeal exposure.

Cranial Nerves

The facial nerve exits the skull at the stylomastoid foramen and enters the substance of the parotid gland, where it divides into five branches. The most caudal branch, the marginal mandibular branch of the facial nerve, is susceptible to injury during an anterior retropharyngeal approach or a transmandibular transcervical approach. Injury to this nerve may cause drooping of the lateral angle of the mouth due to paralysis of the orbicularis oris muscle.

Glossopharyngeal, vagus, and spinal accessory nerves exit the skull at the jugular foramen, and excessive retraction can cause neuropraxia. The vagus nerve travels dorsally within the carotid sheath and gives out superior laryngeal nerve immediately below the inferior vagal ganglion. The superior laryngeal nerve traverses deep to the internal and external carotid arteries, emerging anterior to the external carotid artery at the level of the superior thyroid artery. It bifurcates into smaller external laryngeal and larger internal laryngeal branches. The external laryngeal branch supplies motor innervation to inferior pharyngeal constrictors and cricothyroid muscles. Damage to these fibers can lead to early fatigue of voice and difficulty in producing high notes. The internal branch supplies sensory innervation to the laryngeal mucosa above the glottis, laceration or stretching of which may lead to aspiration due to loss of supraglottic sensation.

The glossopharyngeal nerve passes between the internal carotid artery and internal jugular vein before passing between the stylopharyngeus and styloglossus to enter the base of the tongue. The spinal accessory nerve courses through the posterosuperior corner of the carotid triangle to reach the deep surface of the sternomastoid about 3 cm from the tip of the mastoid process. It then continues through the occipital triangle to supply the trapezius.

The hypoglossal nerve exits from the hypoglossal canal just lateral to the midportion of the occipital condyle. It enters the carotid triangle deep to the posterior belly of the digastric muscle superior to the hyoid bone. It courses between the internal jugular vein and the carotid artery and lies superficial to the internal and external carotid arteries, at a level approximately 3 cm superior to the bifurcation. It then passes medially to enter the substance of the tongue. The hypoglossal nerve also gives off the superior branch of the ansa cervicalis, which innervates the strap muscles and is at risk of division during anterior extramucosal approaches and transmandibular transcervical approaches to the upper cervical spine.

The internal carotid artery and the jugular vein are just lateral to the foramen for the hypoglossal nerve. The safe working space between the midline and these structures laterally is limited to only 2 cm. Further lateral dissection or excessive stretching is likely to injure these structures. The posterior belly of digastric is an important muscle that passes obliquely beneath the angle of the mandible and protects the hypoglossal nerve, accessory nerve, vagus, and carotid sheath that lie beneath it.

TRANSORAL APPROACH

The transoral approach is relatively simple to perform and is carried out through the hypovascular midline structures. It allows somewhat limited but direct access to the anterior cervical spine from the foramen magnum to C3. Only pharyngeal mucosa and constrictor and prevertebral muscles cover the anterior aspect of the upper cervical spine. The cranial nerves and the vertebral artery are not encountered, and neurovascular retraction is not necessary. Infection and cerebrospinal fluid (CSF) leak are a major concern with transoral approaches, although their incidence has been reduced with advances in the surgical techniques and perioperative management.

Indications

The common indications for using a transoral approach are resection of odontoid process for basilar invagination due to rheumatoid disease, chronic traumatic dislocation of the odontoid, congenital deformities of the axis, infection, and removal of extradural tumors. The indications for this approach are being extended because infection and meningitis are becoming less frequent and more easily manageable. The risk of postoperative infection is diminished by gentle tissue handling, use of operative microscope, and appropriate antibiotics. With favorable experience in management of CSF leakage with fibrin glue and CSF diversion, the transoral approach has also been used for resection of intradural lesions (2).

Anterior upper cervical fusion through the transoral approach remains a controversial issue. Bone graft appears to resolve over the years with the transoral approach (3,4). However, maxillofacial surgeons frequently use bone graft around the oral cavity without significant complications, and Ashraf and Crockard (5) have reported successful transoral fusion for high cervical fractures.

Preoperative Evaluation

All patients undergoing a transoral approach should be evaluated preoperatively for comorbidities. Their preexisting medical conditions and nutritional status should be evaluated and optimized prior to surgery. Many patients are on long-term steroids and may also experience difficulty with swallowing and respiration. Every effort should be made to eradicate dental sepsis preoperatively. Nasopharyngeal and oropharyngeal cultures are obtained 3 days prior to surgery, and perioperative antibiotics are administered based on the culture and sensitivities. A minimum interdental space of 25 mm is necessary for a transoral approach. An alternative approach, such as a transmandibular approach, may be necessary if involvement of the temporomandibular joints significantly decreases the interdental interval (6–8). Normal distance from the craniocervical junction to the dental margin is approximately 100 mm in an adult (4). If this distance is decreased due to basilar invagination, the approach to the craniocervical junction may be difficult and may not provide an optimal trajectory. Additionally, significant decrease in cervical extension secondary to subaxial kyphosis may limit the usefulness of a transoral approach.

Preparation

The patient is transported to the operating room in a supine position with the head and neck in neutral position. Prophylactic intravenous cephalosporin and metronidazole are administered. A padded Mayfield headrest or a Gardner-Wells tong with 10 pounds traction are utilized with the patient supine on the operating table. A Jackson table or Stryker frame may be preferable if posterior stabilization is planned following anterior decompression. Fiberoptic nasotracheal awake intubation is recommended for the unstable cervical spine. Once the neurologic evaluation is determined to be unchanged after positioning and awake intubation, suitable anesthetic agents are administered. The patient is placed in a slight Trendelenburg position to prevent aspiration (9).

A Davis-Crowe, modified Dingman, or Spetzler-Sonntag transoral retractor is placed in the mouth to expose the posterior oropharynx. Self-retaining flexible palatal retractors are positioned to elevate the soft palate (Fig. 5.1). Alternatively, a rubber catheter sutured to the soft palate may be brought out through the nostril for palatal retraction. Another option is to divide the soft palate in line with the midline vertical incision. A throat pack is inserted to prevent blood and debris from entering the laryngopharynx and the esophagus, and the oral cavity is prepared with Betadine solution. A lateral radiograph may be obtained to verify the position of the retractors and to ensure appropriate level and trajectory of approach to the spine. The radiograph also helps determine intraoperative alignment of the upper cervical spine. The area of the incision is infiltrated with 1:200,000 adrenaline. An operating microscope is recommended for magnification and as a concentrated light source, because it greatly enhances the illumination and visualization of the operative field. Alternatively, loupe magnification and fiberoptic light

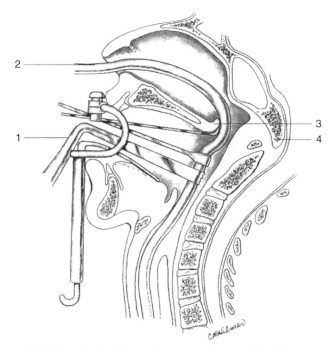

FIGURE 5.1. Sagittal view of a transoral approach with retractor blades in position. Pharyngeal retractor *(1)*, nasoendotracheal tube *(2)*, soft palate *(3)*, and anterior rim of foramen magnum *(4)* are shown. (Reprinted with permission from Howard An, MD.)

may be utilized. Stereotactic image guidance techniques have also been recommended (10,11).

Exposure

A midline 3-cm vertical incision centered over the anterior tubercle is made through the pharyngeal mucosa and musculature (Fig. 5.2). The incision is carried down to the bone, and the origin of the anterior longitudinal ligament and the longus colli muscle are divided with Bovie electrocautery. Subperiosteal dissection is carried out laterally, and pharyngeal retractors are positioned to further improve the exposure. The anterior tubercle of the arch of the atlas defines the midline (Fig. 5.3). However, the lateral mass may be mistaken for midline tubercle if C1 is rotated, which may render the vertebral artery vulnerable. Attachment of longus colli muscles on either side facilitates identification of the anterior tubercle. Care should be taken to avoid dissection more than 15 mm on either side of the midline of the atlas to avoid risk of injury to the vertebral artery, eustachian tubes, and the hypoglossal nerve superiorly (12). The safe surgical field is 14 mm at the lower border of the axis, 24 mm at the atlas, and 11 mm at the level of the foramen magnum.

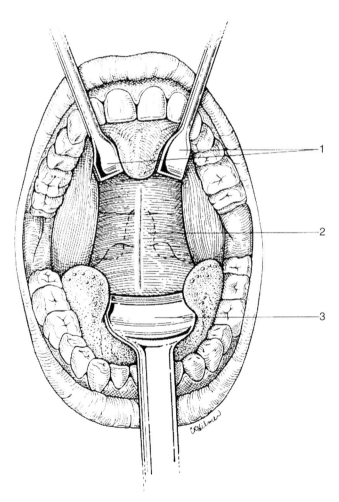

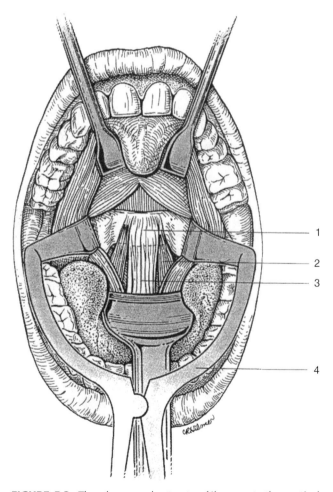

FIGURE 5.2. A 3-cm vertical midline incision is made centered on the anterior tubercle of the atlas. Soft palate retractors *(1)*, incision *(2)*, and tongue retractors *(3)* are shown. (Reprinted with permission from Howard An, MD.)

FIGURE 5.3. The pharyngeal retractor *(4)* converts the vertical incision into a hexagon and facilitates exposure of the anterior tubercle of the atlas *(1)*, longus colli muscle *(2)*, and anterior longitudinal ligament *(3)*. (Reprinted with permission from Howard An, MD.)

Removal of the central 10 to 15 mm of the anterior arch of the atlas with a high-speed air drill is necessary to perform transoral resection of the odontoid. The caudal portion of the clivus may also need to be resected (12). A large amount of pannus may be present between the anterior arch of the atlas and the odontoid in rheumatoid patients. The pannus is removed with Bovie cautery, curettes, and Leksell rongeurs. Bony compression caused by basilar invagination can be managed through a smaller opening, whereas soft tissue compression requires a larger opening. The tori tubarius limit the maximum width of exposure to 4 cm. The transverse ligament should be preserved after resection of the central portion of the anterior arch of the atlas. This ligament acts as a tie beam and prevents lateral displacement of the lateral mass and minimizes the risk of craniocervical instability.

Resection of Odontoid

Resection of the odontoid begins from cephalad to caudad using a high-speed carbide-tip burr under constant saline irrigation. Once the odontoid is reduced to a dorsal shell, the resection is completed with a diamond-tip burr, an angled curette, or Kerrison rongeur (Fig. 5.4A–C). The alar and apical ligaments are freed subperiosteally using sharp dissection. This region is often adherent to the dura mater, rendering it susceptible to development of CSF fistula (12). Resection of these ligaments is best done while the base of the odontoid is still intact and the tip of the odontoid is not floating. The odontoid should be resected to a level at least 1 cm below the slopes of the superior facets of the axis (12).

Once the odontoid resection is completed, canal compromise by residual pannus, infectious exudate, tumor, ligament, or synovial cyst is looked for. Soft tissue clearance is usually begun at the level of the lower border of C2. Soft tissues densely adherent to dura are best left alone because of the risk of dural laceration. Decompression of the tectorial membrane allows dural pulsation to return.

The transpalatal approach is an extension of the transoral approach. It provides exposure from the foramen magnum to halfway up the clivus. The soft palate incision is extended onto the hard palate in the midline for 3 cm. The mucosa is reflected laterally toward the alveolar margin, and the greater palatine vessels are preserved. A midline osteotomy of the hard palate is done with a reciprocating saw. Vomer is removed and part of the hard palate is infractured into the nasopharynx. Palatal retractors are positioned, and a midline incision is carried out through the mucosa (4).

Closure and Postoperative Care

After completion of the procedure, a Valsalva maneuver is performed to exclude a CSF leak. Meticulous hemostasis should be achieved. Wound closure begins with approximation of the longus colli muscle in the midline. The pharyngeal closure should be done in a single layer with running absorbable suture (Fig. 5.5). The throat pack is removed, and a feeding tube is placed under direct vision. A soft collar or a halo vest is applied postoperatively, and the head of the bed is elevated. The endotracheal tube is kept in place for 24 hours because of the risk of postoperative tongue swelling and airway obstruction. Postoperative massaging of the tongue and dexamethasone decrease lingual swelling and reconstitute venous and lymphatic flow. Antibiotics are continued for 3 days. Clear liquids may be allowed after 1 week, and a regular diet is permitted by 21 days. Posterior approach and C1-C2 stabilization may be performed under the same anesthetic or after 2 to 4 days, if necessary.

Complications

The transoral approach is associated with a relatively high overall complication rate. The reported complication rate is 18% to 26%, and the mortality rate is 6% (14). CSF leakage remains the most dreaded complication and can cause fistula formation, wound

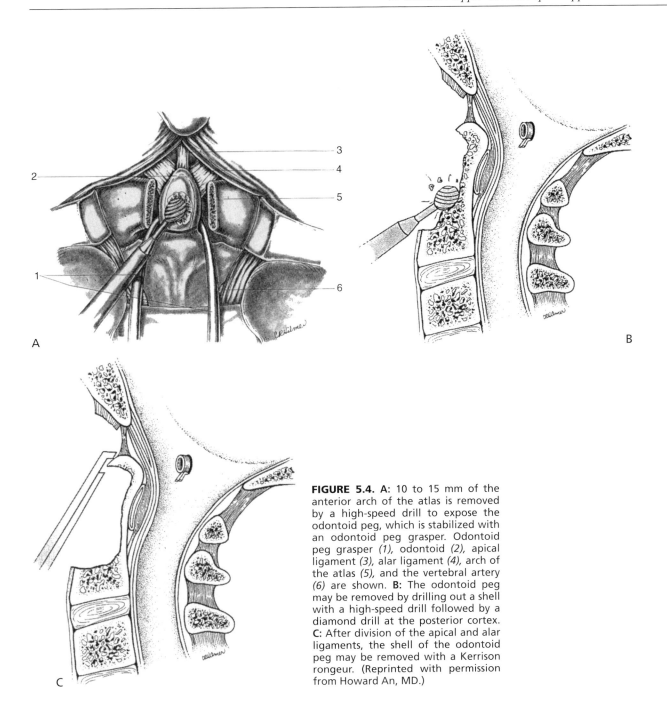

A

B

C

FIGURE 5.4. A: 10 to 15 mm of the anterior arch of the atlas is removed by a high-speed drill to expose the odontoid peg, which is stabilized with an odontoid peg grasper. Odontoid peg grasper *(1)*, odontoid *(2)*, apical ligament *(3)*, alar ligament *(4)*, arch of the atlas *(5)*, and the vertebral artery *(6)* are shown. **B:** The odontoid peg may be removed by drilling out a shell with a high-speed drill followed by a diamond drill at the posterior cortex. **C:** After division of the apical and alar ligaments, the shell of the odontoid peg may be removed with a Kerrison rongeur. (Reprinted with permission from Howard An, MD.)

breakdown, and meningitis. Repair of a dural tear is time-consuming and difficult. A dural tear is best treated by reapproximation of dura, placement of fascial graft, and fibrin glue followed by meticulous wound closure (15). A lumbar drain may also be needed postoperatively to treat a CSF fistula. Prophylactic antibiotics are given. Careful selection of the approach may avert this complication. When an intradural pathology is present, the risk for a CSF fistula is significantly reduced with a lateral transcondylar or dorsal approach (16). The incidence of meningitis associated with intradural procedures may be reduced by oral irrigation with antibiotics for 2 to 3 days preoperatively. Postoperative meningitis is treated with appropriate antimicrobial therapy.

If the midline anterior tubercle of the atlas is not palpated and the dissection is inadvertently carried out laterally, significant bleeding may be encountered from the vertebral

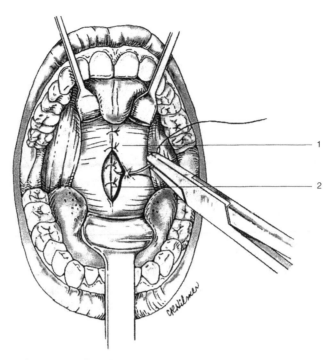

FIGURE 5.5. The pharyngeal mucosa *(1)* and muscle *(2)* are closed in two layers with interrupted 3–0 Vicryl suture. (Reprinted with permission from Howard An, MD.)

arterial branches. Meticulous hemostasis with bipolar cautery and aneurysm clips may be necessary in these circumstances.

Severe postoperative lingual swelling may be prevented by intermittent release of the tongue retractor, which decreases venous and lymphatic compression. Systemic steroids or 10% hydrocortisone cream have been recommended for controlling postoperative edema (4).

Pharyngeal wound dehiscence within the first week is usually due to inadequate wound closure. Dehiscence due to a retropharyngeal abscess usually occurs after the first week, and requires extrapharyngeal drainage. Dehiscence of soft palate repair leads to speech deficit and severe hypernasality. It also causes oronasal regurgitation on swallowing and may lead to aspiration. The palate should be repaired after the edema resolves, but excessive delay makes palatal repair difficult due to wound contraction. Lateral release incisions and fracture of the hamulus process may be needed to achieve tension-free closure (10).

Rheumatoid patients are highly susceptible to development of craniocervical instability after transoral resection of the odontoid. Unrecognized postoperative craniovertebral instability may occur in 75% of patients (17). The primary determinants of postoperative instability are the extent of the pathological bone destruction, ligamentous weakening, and operative bone removal (18). Postoperative radiographs or computed tomography (CT) scan in flexion-extension may be needed, and occipitocervical fusion may be necessary in the face of significant instability.

Neurologic deterioration may occur due to abscess, meningitis, significant loss of alignment, retained bone, inadequate decompression, postoperative hematoma, or iatrogenic injury. Neurologic injury during positioning and intubation are avoided by fiberoptic awake intubation. Preoperative and intraoperative monitoring are essential to detect neurologic compromise. If neurologic deficit is detected on extubation, an evaluation is necessary to delineate any potentially reversible causes. The neck is placed in a neutral position, and steroids are administered. Plain films are obtained to determine the relationship of C1-C2. Thin-cut CT scan helps in visualization of a hematoma or infection.

Postoperative pulmonary infection is relatively common in this patient population (14,19). Swallowing and airway protective mechanisms are compromised secondary to chronic cervicomedullary compression. Many of these patients are also on long-term steroids and are nutritionally compromised. Early patient mobilization and good pulmonary hygiene are necessary. Early posterior stabilization soon after transoral resection also facilitates pulmonary toilet by allowing discontinuation of the halo vest.

An oronasal fistula may develop due to partial dehiscence of the soft palate. This is usually treated initially with normal saline rinses, removal of nasogastric tube, and a palatal splint. Small fistulas often close with this regimen; more important, it prevents further breakdown of the wound (10). Flaps of adjacent tissue are used for closure of persistent fistulas.

Division of the soft palate and midline pharyngotomy with division of Passavant's ridge lead to some degree of velopharyngeal insufficiency in almost all patients with this approach. Most patients are able to overcome this problem within the first 3 months. Rarely, a palatal prosthesis or a push-back procedure may be needed (10).

RETROPHARYNGEAL APPROACHES

Several retropharyngeal approaches have been described that provide extramucosal anterior exposure of the upper cervical spine without risk of bacterial contamination by nasopharyngeal flora. These approaches also permit distal extension of the exposure to the lower cervical spine. Retropharyngeal approaches do not require mandibular osteotomy or division of the tongue and provide wide exposure with less morbidity than transmandibular approaches. The retropharyngeal approaches are carried out either medial or lateral to the carotid sheath.

The anterior retropharyngeal approach popularized by McAfee et al. (20) is a superior extension of the Southwick and Robinson (21) exposure to the lower cervical spine. It provides an access from the clivus to the third cervical vertebra without the need for posterior dissection of the carotid sheath and the foramina for the vagus nerve. The dissection is carried out medial to the carotid sheath, which is retracted laterally, thus permitting visualization and control of bilateral vertebral arteries. It also facilitates adequate decompression and placement of strut graft. However, this approach requires more neurovascular dissection and ligation of branches of the external carotid artery to permit lateral retraction of the carotid vessels. Higher risk of injury to the superior laryngeal nerve and glossopharyngeal nerve has also been reported with an anterior retropharyngeal approach (22).

The anterolateral retropharyngeal approach described by Whitesides and Kelly (23) is carried out lateral to the carotid sheath, thus diminishing the risk of injury to the superior laryngeal nerve, but the risk of avulsion injury to the carotid vessels and cranial nerves at the base of the skull is increased. The approach requires less neurovascular dissection than an anterior retropharyngeal approach medial to the carotid sheath. The anterolateral approach does not provide access to the contralateral vertebral artery and may be associated with a slightly higher risk of injury to the ipsilateral vertebral artery than the anterior retropharyngeal approach. Anterior decompression of the spinal cord is more difficult with the anterolateral approach because this approach provides a more lateral rather than anterior visualization. A relatively narrow interval posterolateral to the carotid vessels with this approach also makes it harder to insert long strut graft in patients with lesions extending to several vertebral levels (24).

Vender et al. (25) have described a modification of the extrapharyngeal high anterior cervical approach. They used this approach to perform fusion and instrumentation at C1 in seven patients who required a C2 corpectomy for a variety of indications. Solid fusion was obtained in six patients, and only one patient required additional posterior stabilization. An anterior approach for stabilization and instrumentation may avoid posterior fixation and preserve occipitocervical mobility. Riley (26) described an extensile retropharyngeal approach, which involved division of the stylohyoid and digastric and dislocation of the ipsilateral temporomandibular joint to mobilize the pharynx.

Indications

The primary indications for retropharyngeal approaches include decompression and stabilization of fixed atlantoaxial subluxation, resection of tumors from the anterior upper cervical spine, and debridement of infection. Both approaches may also be used for performing arthrodesis of the anterior upper cervical spine without the need for a second-stage posterior stabilization. Simultaneous anterior exposure of the upper and lower cervical spine and exposure of the vertebral arteries is also possible.

Preoperative Evaluation

In addition to a thorough neurologic examination, evaluation of nutritional status, comorbidities, swallowing, and respiratory function is mandatory. Preoperative arteriography should also be performed if there is evidence of involvement of foramen transversarium of the second cervical vertebra. Arteriography prior to tumor resection facilitates identification of feeder vessels and vascular distortion or displacement caused by the tumor.

Preparation

Preparation, positioning, and anesthesia are similar for both retropharyngeal approaches. A Gardner-Wells traction tong is placed prior to intubation. Alternatively, a halo may be applied if postoperative immobilization in a halo is planned. Ten pounds of traction is used to stabilize the upper cervical spine. A preoperative or postoperative tracheostomy may be necessary if postoperative edema or airway obstruction is a concern. Any dentures should be removed. Baseline somatosensory and motor evoked potential monitoring is obtained. With the patient awake and neural monitoring in place, maximum allowable rotation and extension of the cervical spine without untoward neurologic changes is determined. Awake fiberoptic nasotracheal intubation is performed under local anesthetic, and general anesthesia is induced if no neurologic alteration is noted on repeat examination. The mouth is kept free of all tubes, such as oral airways and esophageal stethoscopes, to avoid inferior movement of the mandible, which may render the surgical exposure more difficult. The patient is positioned in a reverse Trendelenburg position to decrease venous bleeding.

A right-sided approach is typically chosen by a right-handed surgeon. The head may be turned slightly to the left to facilitate the operative approach if such a position is deemed to not cause any neurologic deficit prior to induction. A right-sided approach that does not extend below C5 avoids iatrogenic injury to the recurrent laryngeal nerve. If the approach requires extension distal to C5, a left-sided approach may be chosen to minimize the risk of injury to the recurrent laryngeal nerve. When surgery is performed for tumor, an incision is made on the side of the tumor mass. The head is secured in the desired extension and rotation with tape. The inside and outside of the earlobe are prepped, and the earlobe is sewn anteriorly to the cheek to facilitate exposure for the anterolateral retropharyngeal approach.

ANTERIOR RETROPHARYNGEAL APPROACH (24,27–29)

Exposure

A modified transverse submandibular incision, also known as a modified Schobinger incision (24), is made from the tip of the mastoid process to the level of the hyoid bone. A longitudinal incision along the anterior border of the sternomastoid may be made if simultaneous exposure of the lower cervical vertebrae is needed (Fig. 5.6). The platysma and superficial fascia are incised and the skin flaps are mobilized deep to the platysma. The marginal mandibular branch of the facial nerve is identified with the aid of a nerve

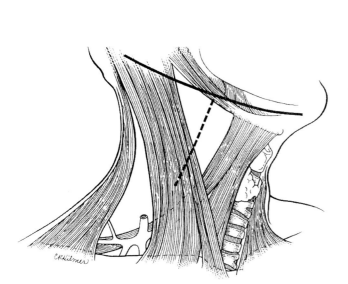

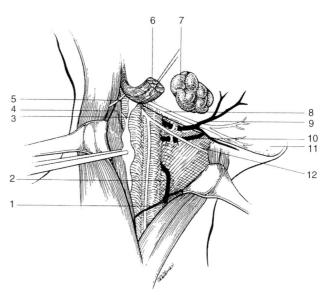

FIGURE 5.6. A submandibular incision on the right side is made for anterior retropharyngeal approach. Additional vertical incision may be made if exposure to the midcervical spine is desired. (Reprinted with permission from Howard An, MD.)

FIGURE 5.7. Initial dissection: The submandibular gland is resected and the diagastric muscle is divided. Sternomastoid branch of superior thyroid artery *(1)*, superior thyroid artery *(2)*, internal jugular vein *(3)*, sternocleidomastoid muscle *(4)*, accessory nerve *(5)*, divided stylohyoid and diagastric muscle *(6)*, resected submandibular gland *(7)*, mandibular branch of the facial nerve *(8)*, facial artery *(9)*, lingual artery *(10)*, mandible *(11)*, and hypoglossal nerve *(12)* are shown. (Reprinted with permission from Howard An, MD.)

stimulator as it courses superiorly, superficial to the retromandibular vein. Injury to this nerve can give rise to drooping of the lateral angle of the mouth due to paralysis of the orbicularis oris muscle. The retromandibular vein is usually continuous with the common facial vein, and it is ligated as it joins the internal jugular vein via the common facial vein.

Further dissection is performed deep and inferior to the ligated retromandibular vein. The anterior facial vein should be ligated and divided below the inferior border of the submandibular gland, leaving the tails of the ligature on the superior stump of the vein. This maneuver facilitates superior retraction of the superficial fascia of the submandibular gland and protects the marginal branch of the mandibular nerve, which is present within this fascia. The submandibular gland is now dissected and mobilized. The confluence of digastric and stylohyoid muscles is divided and tagged for later repair (Fig. 5.7).

Beginning inferiorly and progressing superiorly, the superior thyroid, lingual, and facial branches of the external carotid artery and their accompanying veins are ligated and divided. Identification of these vessels can be facilitated by their location below, at the level, and just above the hyoid bone, respectively. Care should be taken to avoid injury to the superior laryngeal nerve because it runs in close proximity to the superior thyroid artery (Fig. 5.8A,B).

After the superficial layer of the deep fascia is incised along the anterior border of the sternomastoid, the carotid sheath is localized by palpation of the carotid pulse. The hypoglossal and superior laryngeal nerves are identified, mobilized, and protected. The remaining branches of the carotid artery and jugular vein are ligated at this time to allow retraction of the carotid sheath posteriorly and laterally while the pharynx is mobilized medially. Excessive anterior retraction of the pharynx should be avoided because it can cause neuropraxia of the laryngeal and pharyngeal branches of the vagus nerve. The submandibular gland may be resected if mobilization and retraction of the gland does not

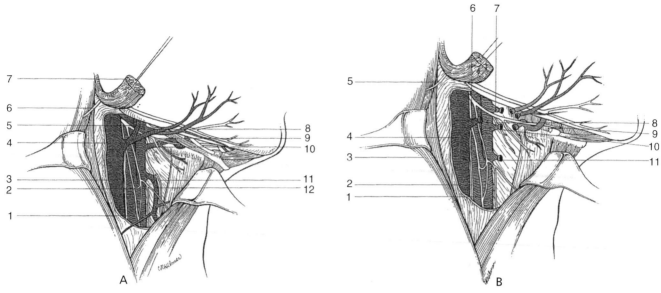

FIGURE 5.8. A: Anterolateral anatomy of the upper cervical spine, showing initial dissection and deeper neurovascular structures. Common carotid artery *(1)*, ansa cervicalis *(2)*, internal jugular vein *(3)*, common facial vein *(4)*, retromandibular vein *(5)*, spinal accessory nerve *(6)*, divided diagastric muscle *(7)*, facial artery *(8)*, hypoglossal nerve *(9)*, lingual artery *(10)*, superior laryngeal nerve *(11)*, and superior thyroid artery *(12)* are shown. **B:** Intermediate dissection: The superior thyroid artery and vein are ligated after the superficial layer of the deep cervical fascia is incised along the anterior border of the sternocleidomastoid. The hypoglossal and superior laryngeal nerves are mobilized. Additional branches of the carotid artery and internal jugular vein are ligated to allow mobilization between the carotid sheath laterally and the pharynx, larynx, and the esophagus medially. Common carotid artery *(1)*, vagus *(2)*, sternocleidomastoid muscle *(3)*, internal jugular vein *(4)*, spinal accessory nerve *(5)*, superior root of ansa cervicalis *(6)*, facial artery *(7)*, superior laryngeal nerve *(8)*, hypoglossal nerve *(9)*, lingual artery *(10)*, and superior thyroid artery *(11)* are shown. (Reprinted with permission from Howard An, MD.)

provide sufficient exposure. If the submandibular gland is resected, its salivary duct, which runs parallel to the tongue to open in the mouth, should be ligated to avoid a fistula formation. Lymph nodes in the submandibular and carotid triangles may be excised as they are encountered and may be sent for a frozen section if a neoplasm is suspected.

Division of the posterior belly of the digastric and stylohyoid muscles facilitates mobilization of the hyoid bone medially and anteriorly, which in turn allows mobilization of the pharynx. Care should be taken to avoid retraction of the posterior belly of the digastric and stylohyoid muscles near their origin to avoid neuropraxia of the facial nerve as it exits the base of the skull. The hypoglossal nerve is now completely mobilized from the base of the skull to the anterior border of the hypoglossal muscle and is retracted superiorly. Blunt finger dissection is performed to develop the plane between the carotid sheath laterally and the larynx and pharynx, and the retropharyngeal space is exposed. Small branches of the ascending pharyngeal vessels may need ligation. The superior laryngeal nerve is identified with the nerve stimulator throughout its course from its origin near the nodose ganglion of the vagus nerve to its entrance into the larynx.

The alar and prevertebral fascia are palpated and split longitudinally to expose the longus colli muscle. The midline of the spine may be determined by noting the superior attachment of the longus colli muscles on the anterior tubercle of the atlas. Any axial rotation of the head during positioning of the patient or any deformity should be remembered and can be determined by palpating the mental protuberance of the mandible. Any undesirable rotation should be corrected at this time if arthrodesis involving the clivus or C1 is being performed. The anterior longitudinal ligament is posterior to the longus colli muscles. A midline incision is made down to the bone, and the muscle and the ligament are elevated subperiosteally and laterally using sharp dissection to expose the bone. The anterior atlantooccipital membrane should not be violated.

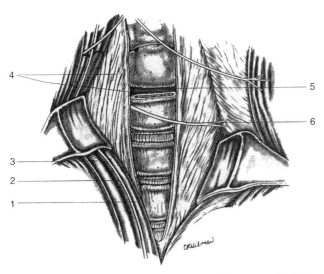

FIGURE 5.9. Initial spinal decompression: The prevertebral fascia is split longitudinally between the longus colli muscles, exposing the anterior atlas and C2 body. Discectomy at the C2–3 level is initially performed to obtain orientation to midline, lateral, and posterior extent of the vertebral body. (Reprinted with permission from Howard An, MD.)

The decompression is begun initially by performing a discectomy at C2–3 or the first normal disc at the inferior aspect of the lesion, which allows visualization of the posterior longitudinal ligament and the uncovertebral joints. The latter determine the lateral limits of decompression (Fig. 5.9). A corpectomy of C2 is done with a high-speed burr. The odontoid is removed in rheumatoid patients and in tumor cases. If there is no significant cranial settling, the tip of the odontoid may be retained to secure a clothespin-shaped strut graft, which can be wedged superiorly into the arch of the atlas and the remainder of the odontoid. Alternatively, the graft may be wedged into the clivus.

ANTEROLATERAL RETROPHARYNGEAL APPROACH LATERAL TO THE CAROTID SHEATH (22,23)

Exposure

A hockey stick–shaped incision is made along the anterior border of the sternomastoid and extended transversely and posteriorly over the mastoid process (Fig. 5.10). The platysma is divided, which exposes the wide sheathlike superficial layer of deep fascia. The external jugular vein, which is contained within this fascial layer toward the superior part of the incision, is ligated and divided. The greater auricular nerve runs parallel and posterior to the external jugular vein within the superficial layer of the deep fascia and supplies sensation over the gland and around the ear. The terminal anterior branches of this nerve may need to be divided (Fig. 5.11). The sternomastoid muscle is then detached from its origin from the mastoid process. Underlying splenius capitis muscle is partially divided to improve the exposure. The anterior border of the sternomastoid is mobilized by carrying out a combination of blunt and sharp dissection of the investing superficial layer of the deep fascia. The spinal accessory nerve runs anteroinferiorly, deep to the sternomastoid, and enters its musculature in the upper third, approximately 3 cm distal to the tip of the mastoid process. The accessory nerve should be mobilized and protected throughout the procedure (Fig. 5.12A,B). The sternomastoid branch of the occipital artery that runs close to the accessory nerve should be ligated.

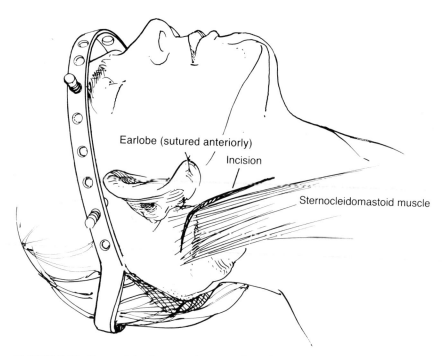

FIGURE 5.10. The earlobe is sutured anteriorly and a hockey-stick incision is made for anterolateral pharyngeal approach. (From Whitesides TE. Lateral retropharyngeal approach to the upper cervical spine. In: Sherk HH, ed., *The cervical spine: an atlas of surgical procedures.* Philadelphia: JB Lippincott Co, 1994:71–77, with permission.)

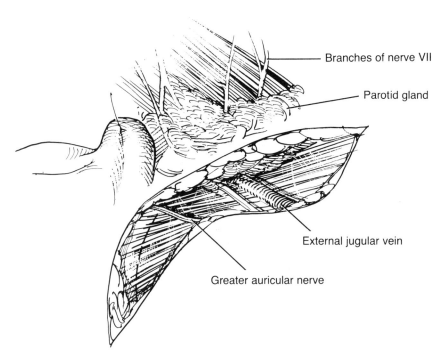

FIGURE 5.11. Greater auricular nerve is identified and subcutaneous tissue flaps are raised. (From Whitesides TE. Lateral retropharyngeal approach to the upper cervical spine. In: Sherk HH, ed., *The cervical spine: an atlas of surgical procedures.* Philadelphia: JB Lippincott Co, 1994:71–77, with permission.)

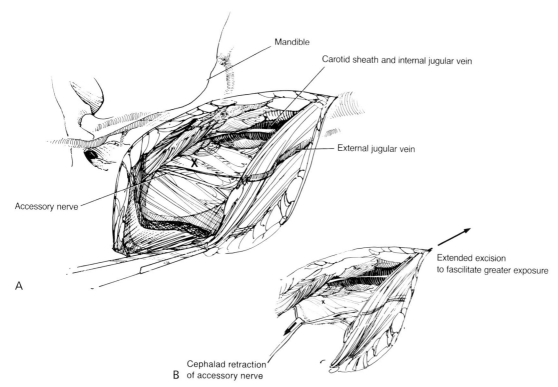

Mandible

Carotid sheath and internal jugular vein

External jugular vein

Accessory nerve

Extended excision
to fascilitate greater exposure

A

Cephalad retraction
B of accessory nerve

FIGURE 5.12. A: The sternocleidomastoid muscle is detached from the mastoid process. *X* denotes where the lateral process of C1 can be palpated. **B:** Accessory nerve is identified as it enters the sternocleidomastoid and is protected. (From Whitesides TE. Lateral retropharyngeal approach to the upper cervical spine. In: Sherk HH, ed., *The cervical spine: an atlas of surgical procedures.* Philadelphia: JB Lippincott Co, 1994:71–77, with permission.)

A plane is developed between the carotid sheath anteromedially and the sternomastoid and accessory nerve posterolaterally. The transverse processes of the cervical vertebrae can be palpated in the depth of this interval. The transverse process of C1 is most easily palpable because it extends more laterally than the caudal vertebrae. The plane between the alar and prevertebral fascia is then developed with sharp and finger dissection of the anterior aspect of the transverse processes and the longus colli and longus capitis muscles. Any large jugular or other lymph nodes may be resected if encountered during dissection. The sympathetic trunk lies within the longus capitis muscle and is not disturbed by careful blunt dissection anterior to the longus colli and capitis muscles. The ring of the atlas and its tubercle may then be palpated, which allows identification of the vertebral levels (Fig. 5.13A,B). A midline incision is made over the vertebrae, and sharp subperiosteal dissection is carried out laterally to expose the upper cervical spine. Malleable retractors are useful in retracting the esophagus and improving the exposure by levering the retractor against the contralateral transverse processes.

Alternatively, the longus colli and capitis muscles may be detached from their insertions on the transverse processes and retracted anteriorly to expose the nerve roots and the vertebral artery. However, this approach disrupts the sympathetic plexus contained within the longus capitis muscle and may cause Horner's syndrome.

Wound Closure and Postoperative Care

After completion of the planned surgery, closure is begun by reapproximating the digastric tendon. The sternomastoid is sutured back in place over a Hemovac following anterolateral exposure (Fig. 5.14). Hemovac drains are placed in the retropharyngeal space and in the subcutaneous layer. The platysma and the skin are closed in a routine manner.

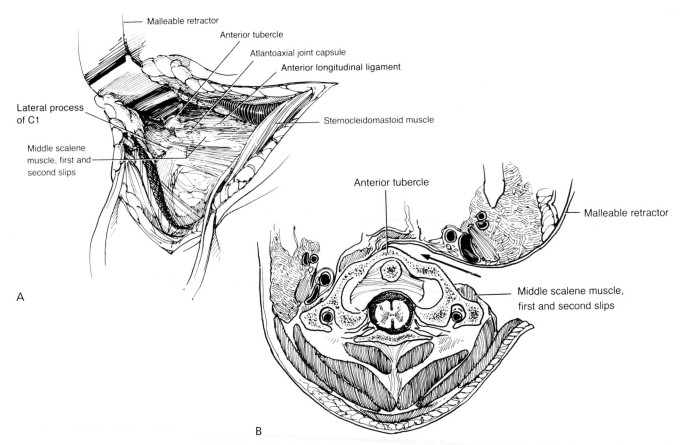

FIGURE 5.13. A: The lateral process of C1 is exposed and the retropharyngeal space is entered to expose the prevertebral fascia. **B:** Cross section showing anterolateral retropharyngeal approach to the upper cervical spine. (From Whitesides TE. Lateral retropharyngeal approach to the upper cervical spine. In: Sherk HH, ed., *The cervical spine: an atlas of surgical procedures.* Philadelphia: JB Lippincott Co, 1994:71–77, with permission.)

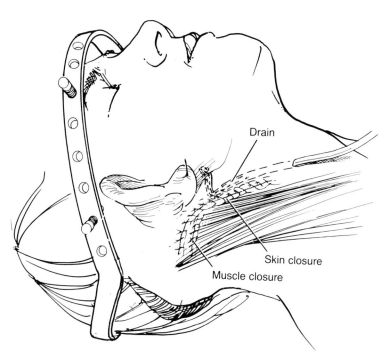

FIGURE 5.14. After completion of the procedure, the sternomastoid is reattached and the wound is closed over a Hemovac. (From Whitesides TE. Lateral retropharyngeal approach to the upper cervical spine. In: Sherk HH, ed., *The cervical spine: an atlas of surgical procedures.* Philadelphia: JB Lippincott Co, 1994:71–77, with permission.)

Halo skull traction is maintained for 2 to 4 days in 30 degrees of head elevation to reduce laryngeal edema. The patient is awakened in a supine position, and a neurologic examination is performed. The patient is transferred to the intensive care unit, and nasal intubation is maintained for 2 to 3 days. A flexible nasopharyngoscopy may be done to evaluate the laryngeal edema at the time of extubation. If intubation is considered necessary for more than 2 to 3 days, consideration should be given to tracheostomy. A halo vest is secured after 2 to 4 days of halo traction. Halo immobilization is usually needed for approximately 3 months.

Complications

If the pharynx or the esophagus has been entered inadvertently, a nasogastric tube is placed under direct vision intraoperatively to ensure that the tube bypasses the rent, which is then repaired in two layers with absorbable suture. The nasogastric tube should be left in place for 7 to 10 days to prevent leakage and to avoid fistula formation. Antibiotics are administered parenterally to cover the aerobic and anaerobic oral flora.

Neuropraxia of the hypoglossal nerve or glossopharyngeal nerve may occur, which usually resolves in 3 months. The mandibular branch of the facial nerve or superior laryngeal nerve may also be stretched or lacerated during the anterior retropharyngeal approach. The former causes paralysis of the orbicularis oris and drooping of the angle of the mouth, and the latter produces loss of supraglottic sensation and high-pitch phonation. The spinal accessory nerve may be damaged as the sternomastoid is detached from the tip of the mastoid process and mobilized during the anterolateral retropharyngeal approach.

Airway obstruction may occur due to traumatic edema or venous congestion of the larynx or upper pharynx. Postoperative intubation or tracheostomy are necessary to avert this complication. Other potential complications include hematoma formation, loosening of strut graft, and halo-related complications.

TRANSMANDIBULAR APPROACHES

Transmandibular approaches provide the widest access to the midline structures, including the nasopharynx, clivus, anterior foramen magnum, and the upper cervical spine. However, these approaches are associated with significant morbidity and should be reserved only for instances requiring extensile exposure to the craniocervical region. The transmandibular approaches are performed with or without midline division of the tongue.

Indications

Transmandibular approaches provide anterior exposure from the clivus to C6. These approaches are particularly useful when wide access to the craniocervical region is needed in patients who have temporomandibular ankylosis with reduced interdental interval, or when subaxial kyphosis limits cervical extension. Common indications include bony lesions of posterior aspect of the bodies of C2–3 or progressive kyphosis with neurologic deficit in patients with prior cervical laminectomy.

Preparation

Preoperative intravenous antibiotics, including cephalosporins and metronidazole, are administered. A tracheostomy is performed as an initial step, and general anesthesia is administered through a cuffed tracheostomy tube. The mouth is kept free of all tubes, and dentures, if any, are removed. A Mayfield headrest may be necessary for immobilization of the craniocervical region. The patient is placed in a reverse Trendelenburg position to minimize excessive venous bleeding, and spinal cord monitoring is employed to minimize the risk of neurologic deterioration.

MEDIAN LABIOMANDIBULAR GLOSSOTOMY APPROACH (6,30,31)

Exposure

A midline incision is made from the lower lip to the level of the hyoid bone. The skin at the vermilion border of the lower lip should be marked with methylene blue to facilitate precise reapproximation of the vermilion border during closure. A Z-shaped zigzag incision is made between the lower lip and the mentum to minimize scar contracture. The incision is then extended in a curvilinear manner around the lateral aspect of the chin to produce a more cosmetically appealing scar. Sharp dissection is carried through labial mucosa and gingiva down to the periosteum, which is reflected.

A stair-step anterior mandibulotomy is then performed with an oscillating power saw. The lower central incisor may need to be removed in some cases to facilitate mandibular osteotomy. Predrilling of the mandible may be done to facilitate internal fixation of the mandibular osteotomy (Fig. 5.15A.B). Care should be taken to prevent injury to the apices of the anterior central incisors while performing mandibular osteotomy or making drill holes for fixation of the mandible. The approach is continued through the midline of the floor of the mouth, following the lingual frenulum and the septum of the tongue back to the level of the epiglottis and down to the hyoid bone. Care should be taken to avoid laceration of the papillae of the submandibular gland ducts, which are present on either side of the frenulum of the tongue. Silk traction sutures are placed through both sides of the tip of the tongue, which is divided through

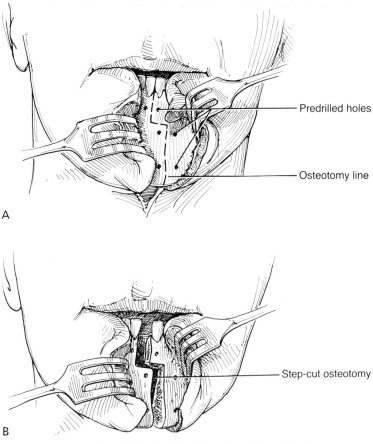

A

Predrilled holes

Osteotomy line

B

Step-cut osteotomy

FIGURE 5.15. **A:** A lip-splitting incision is made and mandibular osteotomy site is predrilled for a transmandibular approach. **B:** A step-cut osteotomy of the mandible is completed. *Continued.*

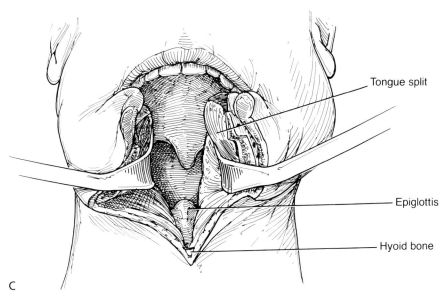

FIGURE 5.15. *(continued)* **C:** The tongue is split in the midline and access to posterior pharyngeal wall is facilitated. (From Stauffer ES. Open-mouth and transmandibular approaches to the cervical spine. In: Sherk HH, ed., *The cervical spine: an atlas of surgical procedures.* Philadelphia: JB Lippincott Co, 1994:79–91, with permission.)

the avascular midline septum using a needle-tip Bovie electrocautery. The exposure may be improved by dividing the soft palate in the midline proximally and the hyoid bone distally. The two halves of the mandible and tongue are manually retracted, and self-retaining retractors are applied to expose the epiglottis and palate (Fig. 5.15C). Packing of the lower pharynx is done to prevent the debris from entering the esophagus and trachea. The posterior pharyngeal wall may then be incised in the midline or as an inferiorly based apron flap with Bovie electrocautery. Exposure can be achieved laterally out to the uncus and posteriorly to the posterior longitudinal ligament.

TRANSMANDIBULAR TRANSCERVICAL APPROACH WITHOUT MIDLINE GLOSSOTOMY (32)

Exposure

A curvilinear incision is made extending from the mastoid tip to a point 4 cm below the mandible, just above the hyoid bone. The marginal mandibular branch of the facial nerve is identified and protected as the superficial fascia of the submandibular gland is elevated. The digastric tendon and the stylohyoid muscle are detached from their attachments to the hyoid bone and reflected superiorly with the submandibular gland. The submandibular gland is then carefully mobilized, and underlying lingual and hypoglossal nerves in the floor of the submandibular triangle are identified. The common and internal carotid arteries and internal jugular vein are preserved. The external carotid artery may either be retracted posteriorly or ligated and divided distal to the takeoff of the superior thyroid artery. The cervical incision is then extended to include a lip-splitting incision. After predrilling screw holes, a stair-step mandibular osteotomy is performed. Alternatively, a lateral osteotomy of the mandible may be done; however, this sacrifices the inferior alveolar nerve.

The tongue is retracted contralaterally, and an incision is made in the floor of the mouth in the gingivoglossal sulcus toward the anterior tonsillar pillar. Postganglionic fibers of the lingual nerve to the submandibular and sublingual glands are divided. The lip-splitting and neck incisions are then connected and the hemimandible is swung laterally to create one surgical space. The entire oropharynx and nasopharynx are retracted contralaterally, thus exposing the anterior surface of the clivus through C3.

Closure and Postoperative Care

After completion of the procedure, the posterior pharyngeal wall is closed in a single layer with a running absorbable suture, followed by repair of the tongue and floor of the mouth in layers. The mandibular osteotomy is internally fixed with a compression plate using the previously drilled holes. Alternatively, the mandible may be reapproximated with wire sutures. A Hemovac drain is brought out through the submental region. The skin is closed with interrupted nonabsorbable sutures. Halo vest immobilization is preferred because it avoids pressure on the mandible and provides access to the incision site and evaluation of healing of the pharynx. Tube feeding is necessary for the first 7 to 10 days. The tracheostomy tube may be removed after approximately 1 week when laryngeal edema resolves and the pharyngeal incision has healed.

Complications

Complications of transmandibular approaches include formation of orocervical fistula, mandibular malunion, parapharyngeal abscess, and cranial nerve injury. Significant epidural venous bleeding may be encountered as the posterior longitudinal ligament is removed to decompress the neural elements. Serous otitis media may necessitate insertion of a ventilation tube. Dysphagia, neuromuscular incoordination in swallowing, and recurrent aspiration are rare complications and may require temporary percutaneous gastrostomy (33).

REFERENCES

1. de Andrade JR, MacNab I. Anterior occipito-cervical fusion using an extra-pharyngeal exposure. *J Bone Joint Surg Am* 1969;51:1621–1626.
2. Crockard HA, Sen CN. The transoral approach for the management of intradural lesions at the craniovertebral junction: review of 7 cases. *Neurosurgery* 1991;28:88–97.
3. Bonney G, Williams JPR. Trans-oral approach to the upper cervical spine. A report of 16 cases. *J Bone Joint Surg Br* 1985;67:691–698.
4. Crockard HA. Midline ventral approaches to the craniocervical junction and upper cervical spine. In: Sherk HH, ed. *The cervical spine: an atlas of cervical procedures.* Philadelphia: JB Lippincott Co, 1994:93–112.
5. Ashraf J, Crockard HA. Transoral fusion for high cervical fractures. *J Bone Joint Surg Br* 1990; 72:76–79.
6. Hall JE, Denis F, Murray J. Exposure of the upper cervical spine for spine decompression by a mandible and tongue-splitting approach. Case report. *J Bone Joint Surg Am* 1977;59:121–123.
7. Honma G, Murota K, Shiba R, et al. Mandible and tongue-splitting approach for giant cell tumor of axis. *Spine* 1989;14:1204–1210.
8. Shaha AR, Johnson R, Miller J, et al. Transoral-transpharyngeal approach to the upper cervical vertebrae. *Am J Surg* 1993;166:336–340.
9. Mendoza N, Crockard HA. Anterior transoral procedures. In: An HS, Riley LH III, eds. *An atlas of surgery of the spine.* London: Martin Dunitz, 1998:55–69.
10. Welch WC, Ragoowansi A, Carrau RL. Transoral resection of the odontoid. *Operative Tech Orthopaedics* 1998;8:8–12.
11. Pollock IF, Welch W, Jacobs GB, et al. Frameless stereotactic guidance, an intraoperative adjunct in the transoral approach for ventral cervicomedullary decompression. *Spine* 1995;20:216–220.
12. Clark CR, Menezes AH. Rheumatoid arthritis: surgical considerations. In: Herkowitz HN, Garfin SR, Balderstone RA, et al., eds. *The spine,* 4th ed. Philadelphia, WB Saunders, 1999:1281–1301.
13. Menezes AH. Complications of surgery at the craniovertebral junction: avoidance and management. *Pediatr Neurosurg* 1991;17:254–266.
14. Crockard HA, Calder I, Ransford AO. One-stage transoral decompression and posterior fixation in rheumatoid atlanto-axial subluxation. *J Bone Joint Surg Br* 1990;72:682–685.
15. Menezes AH. Transoral approaches to the clivus and upper cervical spine. In: Menezes AH, Sonntag VKH, Benzel EC, et al., eds. *Principles of spinal surgery.* New York: McGraw-Hill, 1996:1241–1251.

16. Zileli M, Naderi S, Benzel EC, et al. Preoperative and surgical planning for avoiding complications. In: Benzel EC, ed. *Spine surgery. Techniques, complication avoidance and management.* Philadelphia: Churchill Livingston, 1999:135–142.

17. Menezes AH. Indications and techniques for transoral and foramen magnum decompression. In: Bridwell KH, DeWald RL, eds. *The textbook of spine surgery,* 2nd ed. Philadelphia: Lippincott–Raven Publishers, 1997:1011–1026.

18. Dickman CA, Locantro J, Fessler RG. The influence of transoral odontoid resection on stability of the craniovertebral junction. *J Neurosurg* 1992;77:525–530.

19. Merwin GE, Post JC, Sypert GW. Transoral approach to the upper cervical spine. *Laryngoscope* 1991;101:780–784.

20. McAfee PC, Bohlman HH, Riley LH, et al. The anterior retropharyngeal approach to the upper part of the cervical spine. *J Bone Joint Surg Am* 1987;69:1371–1383.

21. Southwick WO, Robinson RA. Surgical approaches to the vertebral bodies in the cervical and lumbar regions. *J Bone Joint Surg Am* 1957;39:631–644.

22. Whitesides TE. Lateral retropharyngeal approach to the upper cervical spine. In: Sherk HH, ed. *The cervical spine: an atlas of cervical procedures.* Philadelphia: JB Lippincott Co, 1994:71–77.

23. Whitesides TE, Kelly RP. Lateral approach to the upper cervical spine for anterior fusion. *South Med J* 1966;59:879–883.

24. Cappuccino A, McAfee PC, Gastein CD. Anterior retropharyngeal approach to the upper cervical spine. In: Bridwell KH, DeWald RL, eds. *The textbook of spine surgery,* 2nd ed. Philadelphia: Lippincott–Raven Publishers, 1997:227–236.

25. Vender JR, Harrison SJ, McDonnell DE. Fusion and instrumentation at C1–3 via the high anterior cervical approach. *J Neurosurg (Spine 1)* 2000;92:24–29.

26. Riley LH. Surgical approaches to the anterior structures of the cervical spine. *Clin Orthop Related Res* 1973;91:16–20.

27. Bailey RW, Badgley CE. Stabilization of the cervical spine by anterior fusion. *J Bone Joint Surg Am* 1960;42:565–594.

28. Komisar A, Tabaddor K. Extrapharyngeal (anterolateral) approach to the cervical spine. *Head Neck Surg* 1983;6:600–604.

29. McNulty PS, McAfee PC. Anterior retropharyngeal exposure of the upper cervical spine. In: An HS, Riley LH III, eds. *An atlas of surgery of the spine.* London: Martin Dunitz, 1998:71–82.

30. Moore LJ, Schwartz HC. Median labiomandibular glossotomy for access to the cervical spine. *J Oral Maxillofac Surg* 1985;43:909–912.

31. Stauffer ES. Open-mouth and transmandibular approaches to the cervical spine. In: Sherk HH, ed. *The cervical spine: an atlas of cervical procedures.* Philadelphia: JB Lippincott Co, 1994:79–91.

32. Biller HF, Shugar JM, Krespi YP. A new technique for wide-field exposure of the base of the skull. *Arch Otolaryngol* 1981;107:698–702.

33. Jyung RW, Specter JG. Anterior approaches to the cervical spine. In: Bridwell KH, DeWald RL, eds. *The textbook of spine surgery,* 2nd ed. Philadelphia: Lippincott–Raven Publishers, 1997:217–225.

6

ANTERIOR AND ANTEROLATERAL, MID AND LOWER CERVICAL SPINE APPROACHES: TRANSVERSE AND LONGITUDINAL (C3 TO C7)

JEFF S. SILBER
TODD J. ALBERT

The anterior and anterolateral approaches to the cervical spine expose the anterior aspects of the cervical vertebral bodies and intervening intervertebral discs from C3 to T1. These approaches are most useful for anterior cervical decompression of the spinal cord and nerve roots, although they can be used to access the anterior aspect of the cervical spine for any reason. They exploit the internervous plane between the sternocleidomastoid muscle (accessory nerve) and the strap muscles (segmental innervation from C1, C2, and C3) and then deeper between the left and right longus colli muscles (segmental innervation from C2 through C7) (Fig. 6.1). These approaches are potentially expansile

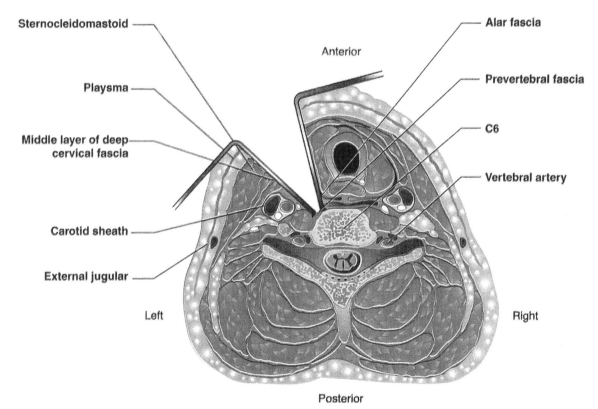

FIGURE 6.1. Cross-sectional anatomy of the neck showing the surgical approach to the anterior aspect of the C6 vertebral body as well as the relevant anatomical structures.

and allow the following: (a) excision of herniated discs, (b) vertebral corpectomies, (c) interbody fusions, and (d) excision of tumors, infections, and other pathological processes. These atraumatic and generally safe approaches, when extended, can expose the anterior cervical spine from C3 to T1, allowing the removal of multiple discs and vertebral bodies with the placement of strut grafting and anterior cervical instrumentation.

RECOMMENDED POSITIONING

The patient is placed supine on the operating table. Before the operation is initiated, the awake patient is asked to actively extend his or her head. If there are any myelopathic complaints reported, an awake intubation should be considered in the patient with spinal cord compression. Electrophysiologic monitoring in the form of motor evoked potentials, somatosensory evoked potentials, and dermatomal evoked potentials is invaluable for any anterior cervical procedure. Leads are best placed in the preoperative holding area in order to lessen operative time. After the patient demonstrates appropriate cervical extension without neurologic changes, asleep intubation is undertaken.

A rolled towel or 1-liter intravenous bag placed in a pillow case is positioned either longitudinally between or transversely across the shoulder blades. This will allow the head and cervical spine to maximally extend (always with monitoring in the asleep patient), allowing an easier exposure. The head is also slightly rotated away from the planned incision to provide better access to the operative side of the neck. A second bump can be placed under the desired donor hip in larger patients, if iliac crest bone graft is to be taken. If a multiple-level procedure is planned (a three-level corpectomy or more), Garner-Wells tongs may be used for intraoperative traction for decompression and graft placement. For less than a three-level corpectomy, we prefer use of the Caspar distractor. The arms are padded with gel wraps and then tucked to the patient's sides using prior placed sheets from under the patient. The shoulders are pulled caudally and held with 3-inch tape, allowing for both appropriate radiographic imaging of the lower cervical spine and patient stabilization, thus enhancing the exposure. The entire anterior aspect of the neck is prepped from lateral to both sternocleidomastoid muscles and from below the clavicles up to the chin. An appropriate area for the procurement of the iliac crest or for a fibula graft is prepped accordingly.

In revision cases, the patient should be endoscopically evaluated for vocal cord function. If the vocal cords on the side of the prior incision are functioning properly, either a right- or a left-sided approach can be used. If the vocal cords on the side of a prior incision are not functioning properly, it is best to use that incision so as to avoid potential injury to the only remaining intact opposite vocal cord. Our preference is to use the contralateral exposure, if possible, allowing for a safer, less traumatic dissection.

SKIN INCISIONS

It is recommended that a transverse incision be utilized for up to three disc levels without instrumentation. For procedures exposing three or more disc levels and more than two vertebral bodies (corpectomies) with instrumentation, an oblique longitudinal incision along the anterior border of the sternocleidomastoid muscle is used. The appropriate level for placement of a transverse incision is determined by palpating superficial landmarks. With the head hyperextended, the superficial landmarks may be displaced in the cephalad direction. To account for this, either deeper landmarks are used or the incision is placed in a slightly cephalad position, or both. Often in the asleep patient, the carotid (Chassaignac's) tubercle, a reliable deep landmark, can be palpated on the transverse process of the C6 cervical vertebrae.

The transverse incision for a one- or two-level discectomy or a one-level corpectomy is approximately 2 to 3 inches long (Fig. 6.2A). It runs from midline or just past the midline of the neck medially to just up to or slightly past the anterior border of the sternocleidomastoid muscle laterally and is placed in or parallel to a skin crease. Extending the incision too far laterally may result in skin puckering at the border of the sternocleidomastoid muscle and an unsightly scar. Palpable superficial landmarks for both a transverse or longitudinal incision include the following: (a) the clavicle (inferior), chin (superior), anterior border of the sternocleidomastoid muscle (lateral), and trachea (medial) for the operative site prepping borders, (b) sternal notch (inferior) and thyroid notch (superior) to assess for midline, and (c) hyoid cartilage (just above the C3–4 vertebral bodies), thyroid cartilage (overlying the C5–6 vertebral bodies), and cricoid cartilage (overlying the C5–6 interspace) (Fig. 6.3A). Palpable deep landmarks include the following: (a) the carotid tubercle located at the C6 transverse process and (b) vertebral body osteophytes that may be palpated in the asleep thinner patient (Figs. 6.2A and 6.3A). We

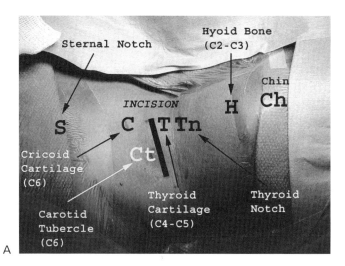

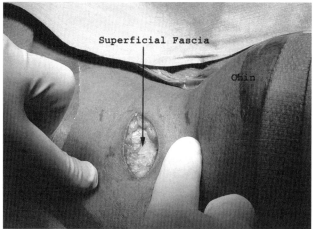

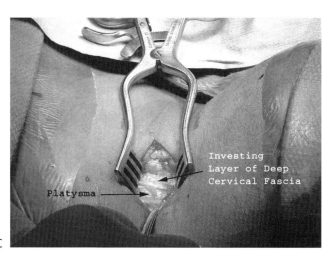

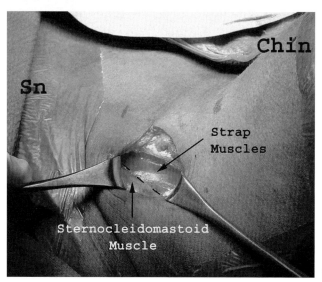

FIGURE 6.2. A: Palpable landmarks for an anterior (transverse) approach to the cervical spine are shown. **B:** After the skin incision is made and the subcutaneous fat wiped off the platysma muscle, the superficial fascia is identified. **C:** After sectioning the superficial fascia, the platysma muscle is divided, revealing the investing (first) layer of the deep cervical fascia. **D:** Once the investing layer is sectioned along the sternocleidomastoid muscle, the internervous interval between the strap muscles and sternocleidomastoid muscle is identified. SN, sternal notch. *(continued)*

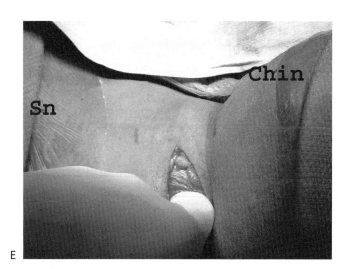

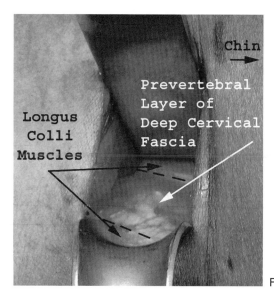

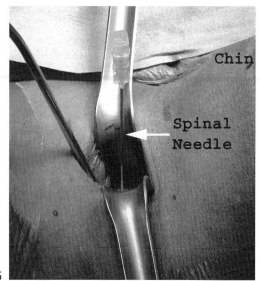

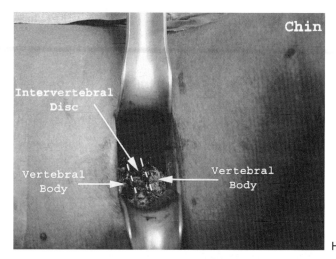

FIGURE 6.2. *(continued)* **E:** Next, finger palpation of the carotid artery followed by medially directed superior and inferior blunt dissection of the middle layer of the deep cervical fascia is performed. **F:** Handheld retractors are placed medially and laterally, exposing the longus colli muscles, the deepest layer of the deep cervical fascia, and the anterior longitudinal ligament. **G:** A spinal needle is placed in the disc space for radiographic determination of the desired cervical level(s). **H:** Once the proper level or levels are identified, the longus colli muscles and anterior longitudinal ligament are released, exposing the vertebral bodies and disc spaces.

prefer a left-sided approach because of the more reliable anatomy of the recurrent laryngeal nerve on this side as compared with the right side.

SURGICAL EXPOSURE

After proper prepping and draping, the chosen incision is drawn with a sterile marking pen. The dermal skin layer is then infiltrated with a local aesthetic and epinephrine. The first incision is made down to subcutaneous fat with either a no. 10 or no. 15 scalpel blade, and all skin bleeders are controlled with electrocautery. Gauze is used to wipe the fat off the superficial fascia containing the platysma muscle and external jugular vein (Fig. 6.2B). The superficial fascia and platysma muscle are divided transversely or longi-

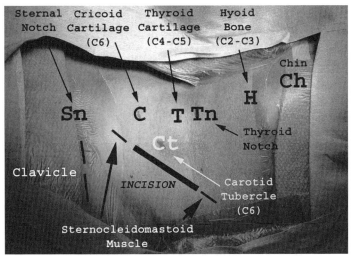

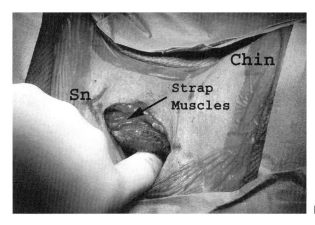

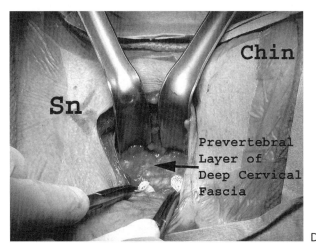

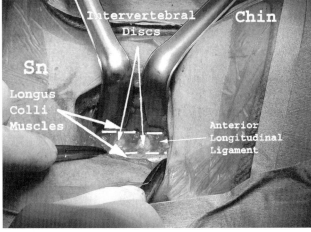

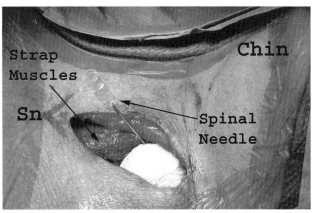

FIGURE 6.3. A: Palpable landmarks for an anterolateral (longitudinal) approach to the cervical spine are shown. **B:** After dissection is carried out as with the transverse incision, blunt dissection of the middle layer of the deep cervical fascia is performed. SN, sternal notch. **C:** Occasionally the omohyoid muscle is released to aid exposure. **D:** Following blunt dissection of the middle layer of the deep cervical fascia, handheld medial and lateral retractors are placed, exposing the deepest (pretracheal and prevertebral) layer of the deep cervical fascia overlying the anterior longitudinal ligament and vertebral bodies. **E:** The deepest layer of deep cervical fascia is released with peanut dissectors, exposing the anterior longitudinal ligament, vertebral bodies, and longus colli muscles. **F:** A spinal needle is placed in the disc space for radiographic determination of the desired cervical level(s). Thrombin-soaked gauze can be placed in the wound to aid in coagulation while awaiting development of the intraoperative radiograph. *(continued)*

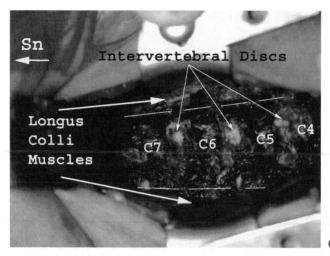

G

FIGURE 6.3. *(continued)* **G:** Once the proper level or levels are identified, the longus colli muscles and anterior longitudinal ligament are released, exposing the desired vertebral bodies and disc spaces.

tudinally with either electrocautery or sharply with a scalpel. This layer too is wiped and rolled with gauze for later closure.

This will expose the next layer, consisting of the superficial (investing) layer of the deep cervical fascia (the first of the four deep layers of cervical fascia), covering both the strap and sternocleidomastoid muscles (Fig. 6.2C). With fine-toothed forceps and blunt dissecting scissors, the superficial fascia is divided transversely over the entire extent of the incision. This layer must be completely released in order to mobilize the soft tissue for adequate exposure. One may encounter the anterior jugular or external jugular vein or both during this step, and they may need to be coagulated or ligated to improve exposure. Next, the fascia is dissected longitudinally along the sternocleidomastoid muscle to expose the next-deeper middle layer of the deep cervical fascia. To expose the middle layer, fascia along the sternocleidomastoid muscle must also be completely released both inferiorly to the clavicular head and superiorly as needed for adequate exposure (Fig. 6.2D). Blunt finger dissection can often be used; one should avoid past pointing with the dissecting scissors since this may result in inadvertent bleeding. This step develops a potential space directly deep to the sternocleidomastoid muscle referred to as Burn's space. Cushing vein retractors are useful when used superiorly and inferiorly to apply longitudinal retraction during release of this layer. When exposing the C3 vertebral level, the superior thyroid artery may be identified. Care must be taken because the superior laryngeal nerve often accompanies this artery and vigorous retraction and dissection may injure this nerve.

Once this layer is released, the carotid artery situated in the carotid sheath is finger palpated deep and medial to the sternocleidomastoid muscle. Once palpated, the same finger is directed in a medial direction to the anterior aspect of the cervical spine (Figs. 6.2E and 6.3B). A Richardson appendiceal retractor is placed medially to the finger for retraction of the trachea and esophagus in a medial direction. The layer now viewed is the middle layer of deep cervical fascia. If exposure includes the C5–6 and C6–7 levels, the omohyoid muscle can be identified (Fig. 6.3C). Rarely, this muscle must be released to aid in exposure. This is usually done with a right-angle retractor placed around the muscle, which is divided by electrocautery. The middle layer of fascia is violated with a Leiter dissector; the easiest place to accomplish this is along the border of the omohyoid muscle, which it invests.

After violation of the middle layer is carried out and extended, the alar fascia comes into view. This is really a confluence of the pretracheal and prevertebral fascia (the two deepest layers) overlying the anterior longitudinal ligament and vertebral bodies. This thick fascia is bluntly dissected from the anterior aspect of the vertebral bodies in an inferior and superior direction with peanut dissectors (Figs. 6.2F and 6.3D). If tenacious, a rent in this layer can be started with blunt scissors followed by peanut dissection. Whether a transverse or longitudinal approach is utilized, this results in an exposure with the trachea and esophagus medially and the carotid sheath and sternocleidomastoid muscle laterally. Now identified is the anterior longitudinal ligament. This usually results in full longitudinal exposure of the anterior vertebral bodies and intervening discs (Fig. 6.3E). Palpation of the carotid tubercle may assist placement of an 18-gauge spinal needle with two 90-degree bends into the desired disc level (Figs. 6.2G and 6.3F). The bends should not be too long to avoid deep penetration into the spinal canal. A lateral intraoperative cervical radiograph is then obtained to confirm the level. We prefer to expose and procure bone graft while waiting for the marker film to be developed.

After the desired level is confirmed radiographically, the longus colli muscles running longitudinally along the anterolateral border of the cervical spine are released. This is best accomplished with a small-bore Frazier sucker tip acting as a retractor, and electrocautery while the assistant uses handheld retractors medially and laterally. Care must be taken not to wander too far laterally, especially at the disc level, to avoid inadvertent injury to the vertebral artery. Elevating the longus colli subperiosteally will allow protection of the esophagus and carotid artery from retractor injury (Figs. 6.2H and 6.3G). This step is invaluable, and it cannot be overemphasized that it must be done properly to place the retractors well under the longus colli muscles. The dissection is always best started at the midvertebral body level for vertebral artery protection and full definition of any osteophytes anteriorly.

After longus colli elevation, blunt-toothed Cloward self-retaining retractors are placed in the medial/lateral position underneath them. Each retractor is placed individually under direct visualization and attached to the self-retaining articulation. The medial side of the retractor handle is affixed to the drapes to help prevent the blade from riding up and penetrating into the esophagus. One or 2 pounds of weight can also be tied to the medial/lateral retractors with sterile umbilical tape to keep them from migrating. Smooth toothless retractors are placed in the superior/inferior positions with the handle situated opposite the surgeon. In procedures involving multiple levels, the retractors may have to be repositioned either superiorly or inferiorly during the case for adequate exposure at the level to be worked upon. At times, the use of rolled gauze placed behind either the superior or inferior retractor blade may help situate the retractor in a more desirable superior or inferior position. At this point, after complete exposure, the surgeon may begin the desired procedure, usually at the lowest level first if more than one level is to be approached. This prevents rundown bleeding from interfering with the next level of the procedure.

CLOSURE

Closure is best performed in three layers over a drain (surgeon preference). We prefer a no. 7 round Jackson-Pratt drain coming out directly through the skin incision. The platysma muscle is approximated with interrupted 2.0 Vicryl sutures. Next the subcutaneous tissue is closed with interrupted 3.0 Vicryl sutures followed by a running 4.0 Vicryl or 5.0 Prolene pullout stitch in a subcuticular fashion. Adhesive strips are applied, followed by a sterile dressing and, if used, a proper prefitted cervical orthosis is placed. If Gardner-Wells tongs are used, the pin sites are checked and dressings applied with pressure if bleeding occurs.

Postoperatively, the head of the bed is elevated 45 degrees to aid in hematoma drainage. We prefer pneumatic compression boots and immediate ambulation when possible (for deep vein thrombosis prevention) as opposed to chemical anticoagulation in order to help avoid or limit postoperative hematoma formation. Patients are kept intubated overnight after prolonged multilevel procedures and if a difficult intubation led to repeated attempts at endotracheal tube placement, with the potential for excessive soft tissue swelling.

COMPLICATIONS

Complications with anterior cervical approaches are rare but have the potential to be devastating. Injury to the vital neurovascular structures may occur and often must be repaired. Esophageal injury usually results from improper placement of the self-retainer retractor blades above the longus colli muscle or from overzealous retraction as well as from high-speed or sharp instruments such as burrs. When recognized intraoperatively, an esophageal injury should be primarily repaired with nasogastric suction applied until closure. Unrecognized esophageal injuries may result in a retropharyngeal abscess or mediastinitis, or both, with a dismal prognosis. Routine surveillance can prevent this catastrophic complication. We prefer an orogastric tube; at the end of the case, the tube is pulled back until it is digitally palpated in the neck and flooded with 60 mL of diluted indigo carmine. The wound is checked for any dark blue color representing dye leakage; its absence represents an intact esophagus at the surgical site.

Recurrent laryngeal nerve injury may lead to postoperative voice changes or swallowing difficulties. We recommend a left-sided approach where the nerve course is more constant in an attempt to decrease the chance of injury. Recent studies have suggested that letting down the endotracheal tube cuff and reinflating it after positioning of the medial/lateral retractors may also help to prevent a recurrent laryngeal nerve palsy. Nonetheless, injury can occur; it usually results from a traction injury and not from direct trauma. Injury to the sympathetic nerves and stellate ganglion may occur, leading to a postoperative Horner's syndrome. This can be avoided with subperiosteal dissection of the longus colli muscles without exposing too far laterally onto the transverse processes.

The carotid sheath (carotid artery, internal jugular vein, and vagus nerve) is protected by the anterior border of the anterior sternocleidomastoid muscle. Avoiding the placement of retractors in this area will avoid inadvertent injury. The use of rounded handheld retractors in addition to the self-retaining retractors may aid in additional visualization and protection during certain aspects of the procedure. The vertebral artery runs longitudinally along the lateral aspect of the vertebrae within the foramen transversarium located in the transverse processes of C2 through C6. The C7 vertebrae has a foramen, although the vertebral artery does not course through it in the majority of patients. Not straying too far laterally will avoid injury to this structure.

RECOMMENDED READING

Afelbaum RI, Kriskovich MD, Heller JR. On the incidence, cause and prevention of recurrent laryngeal nerve palsies during anterior cervical spine surgery. *Spine* 2000;22:2906–2912.

Albert TJ. Anterior middle and lower cervical exposures. In: Albert TJ, Balderston RA, Northrup BE, eds. *Surgical approaches to the spine.* Philadelphia, WB Saunders, 1997:9–24.

Heller JG, Pedlow FX Jr. Anatomy of the cervical spine. In: Clark CR, ed. *The cervical spine,* 3rd ed. Philadelphia: Lippincott–Raven Publishers, 1998:3–36.

Hoppenfeld S, deBoer P. Cervical spine anterior approach. In: Hoppenfeld S, deBoer P, eds. *Surgical exposures in orthopaedics: the anatomic approach,* 2nd ed. Philadelphia, Lippincott–Raven Publishers, 1994:263–275.

Robinson RA, Southwick WO. Surgical approaches to the cervical spine. *Instr Course Lect* 1960; 17:299–330.

ANTERIOR APPROACHES TO THE CERVICOTHORACIC JUNCTION

CHETAN K. PATEL
HARRY N. HERKOWITZ

Of the many approaches spine surgeons perform, the anterior approach to the cervicothoracic junction is the least familiar. Pathology in this region tends to consist of trauma, tumors, and infections that are relatively rare. The great vessels, clavicle, and the sternum obstruct a direct view of the spine through extension of the usual anterior approach to the cervical spine. Kyphosis of the thoracic spine makes visualization difficult while attempting to extend the exposure distally in the upper thoracic spine.

Four approaches to this region are described, each offering a different perspective of the spine along with different extents of exposure.

OVERVIEW OF PERTINENT ANATOMY

A thorough knowledge of anatomy in this region will help provide ease and confidence with any of the approaches described here.

Osseous Anatomy

Approach to this region is through the thoracic outlet, which is defined by the sternoclavicular joints anteriorly, first rib laterally, and the C7 to T2 vertebrae posteriorly. As the cervical spine transitions into the thoracic spine, articulations are noted for rib attachments (Fig. 7.1). The superior portion of the sternum is known as the

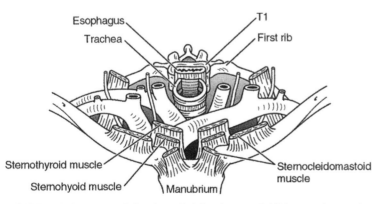

FIGURE 7.1. Anatomy of the thoracic inlet. (From Zdeblick TA, ed. *Anterior approaches to the spine*. St. Louis: Quality Medical Publishers, 1999, p. 76, with permission.)

manubrium, which articulates with the clavicles superiorly and with the costal cartilage of the first rib inferiorly. The clavicle is held to the sternum by strong anterior and posterior sternoclavicular ligaments along with the capsule. Muscular attachments also help stabilize this articulation. The sternal head of the sternocleidomastoid attaches anterior to the sternoclavicular joint, while the sternohyoid and sternothyroid attach posteriorly. The clavicles are held together medially by the interclavicular ligaments that reside in the suprasternal notch. The costoclavicular ligament is another strong stabilizer between the medial end of the clavicle and the first costal cartilage. The first costal cartilage laterally transitions into the first rib, which posteriorly articulates with the first thoracic vertebrae along its superior-most aspect. The costovertebral ligaments anchor the rib head to the superior endplate of the vertebrae above, the annulus of the disc above, and the superior endplate of the corresponding vertebrae.

Muscular Anatomy

The sternocleidomastoid is the large, most discernible muscle that guides much of the dissection in the anterior approaches of the upper spine. As the name suggests, the two heads arise from the sternum (upper manubrium) and the medial third of the clavicle, traversing obliquely and posteriorly to attach to the mastoid process (Fig. 7.2). Superficial to this is the platysma, which is located immediately deep to the subcutaneous tissue. Deeper muscles of the anterior neck are the infrahyoid muscles, which attach to the hyoid, sternum, clavicle, and scapula. The sternohyoid muscle originates from the posterior aspect of the manubrium and medical clavicle and attaches to the hyoid bone (Fig. 7.2). The omohyoid passes superiorly and obliquely from the scapula to attach to the hyoid. Finally, deep to the sternohyoid is the sternothyroid muscle, which originates from the manubrium to attach to the thyroid cartilage (Fig. 7.2). The subclavius muscle originates from the first costal cartilage and attaches to the inferior lateral half of the clavicle. The anterior and middle scalene muscles originate from the transverse processes of the cervical vertebrae and attach to the first rib, compartmentalizing the neurovascular bundle that exits from the thorax into the upper extremity. The anterior scalene travels between the subclavian vein and artery, while the medial scalene is posterior to the artery.

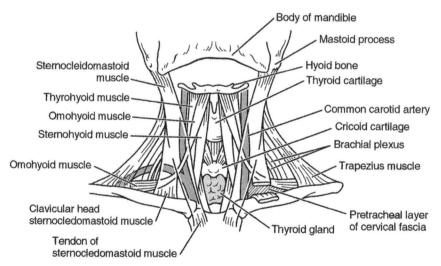

FIGURE 7.2. Superficial and deep muscles of the neck. (From Zdeblick TA, ed. *Anterior approaches to the spine.* St. Louis: Quality Medical Publishers,1999, p. 89, with permission.)

If a thoracotomy approach is chosen, then a knowledge of the muscular attachments to the scapula becomes necessary. Superficially, the trapezius and the latissimus dorsi are encountered. Superiorly, the trapezius originates from the spinous processes and attaches to the crest of the scapula. Inferiorly, the latissimus dorsi similarly originates from the spinous processes and traverses superior obliquely to attach onto the proximal humerus. Deep to this layer are the rhomboid major and minor originating from the spinous processes of C7-T5 and attaching to the medial border of the scapula.

The longus colli form the deepest layer of muscles, being encountered anterolaterally on both sides immediately superficial to the spine. The vertical portion originates from the first three thoracic vertebrae, which can be a useful landmark.

Vascular Anatomy

The great vessels are present in the mediastinum at the inferior aspect of the dissection (Figs. 7.1 and 7.3). The aorta ascends from the heart, then curves and descends at approximately the T3-T4 level. This limits the inferior extent of the dissection in these approaches. The aorta sequentially branches into the innominate artery, the left common carotid artery, and the left subclavian arteries to supply the head, neck, and the upper extremities. The innominate artery branches into the right carotid and the right subclavian artery to mirror the blood supply of the left side of the body. The subclavian vessels along with the brachial plexus emerge between the clavicle and the first rib to supply the upper extremities. They are compartmentalized by the scalene muscles as described previously. The carotid artery travels in the carotid sheath along with the internal jugular vein and the vagus nerve deep to the sternocleidomastoid and can be easily identified. The veins in the thoracic inlet are generally superficial to the arteries. The internal jugular veins combine with the subclavian veins to form the brachiocephalic trunks, which combine to form the superior vena cava.

Nervous Anatomy

The vagus nerve descends in the carotid sheath and branches into the laryngeal nerves that are at risk during the anterior approaches. The recurrent laryngeal nerve branches

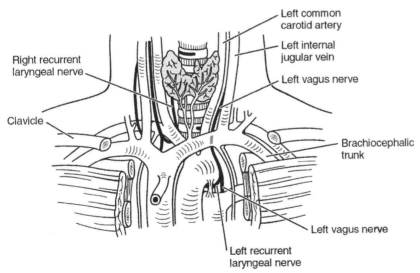

FIGURE 7.3. Nerves, arteries, and veins at the cervicothoracic junction. (From Zdeblick TA, ed. *Anterior approaches to the spine.* St. Louis: Quality Medical Publishers, 1999, p. 77, with permission.)

high in the neck but continues to descend in the carotid sheath until it loops around the subclavian artery on the right and the aortic arch on the left to ascend proximal and medial behind the esophagus (Fig. 7.3). This means that the recurrent laryngeal nerve on the right recurs more proximally at approximately the T3 level and is more likely to be encountered and damaged during a right-sided approach. The nerve travels more obliquely on the right before entering the plane between the trachea and the esophagus, which may also place it at more of a risk. Another possible disadvantage of a right-sided approach is that in 1% to 3% of the population, the right recurrent laryngeal nerve is not recurrent and crosses directly medial, making it more likely to be encountered during the surgical approach.

Lymphatic Anatomy

The thoracic duct ascends in the chest on the left side of the esophagus, passing behind the left subclavian artery. It ascends as high as C7/T1 behind the carotid sheath prior to turning forward to empty into the internal jugular vein. It is found in the triangle formed inferiorly by the first rib, medially by the longus colli and esophagus, and laterally by the anterior scalene muscle. There is no counterpart of the thoracic duct on the right side of the body.

LOW ANTERIOR SMITH-ROBINSON APPROACH

A standard left-sided Smith-Robinson anterior approach to the cervical spine can be used to expose distally to the T1 level with an oblique incision paralleling the medial border of the sternocleidomastoid (1) (Fig. 7.4). The inferior thyroid vessels may be seen in the surgical field and may have to be ligated. The vessels should be ligated laterally to avoid inadvertent injury to the recurrent laryngeal nerve. The remainder of this approach is the standard Smith-Robinson anterior cervical approach (Fig. 7.5). The wound is closed in the usual manner by reapproximating the platysma and the skin.

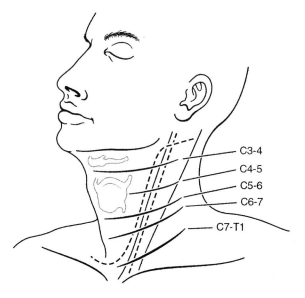

FIGURE 7.4. Skin incisions for the traditional anterior Smith-Robinson approach. (From Benzel EC, ed. *Spine surgery: techniques, complications, avoidance, and management.* Philadelphia: Churchill Livingstone, 1999, p. 1168, with permission.)

C3-4
C4-5
C5-6
C6-7
C7-T1

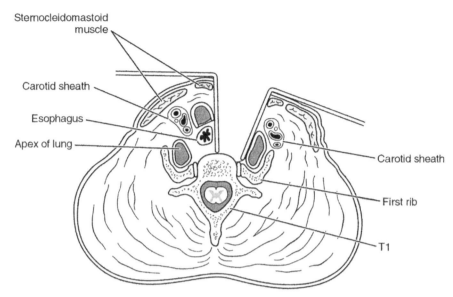

FIGURE 7.5. A cross section demonstrating the low anterior Smith-Robinson approach. (From Zdeblick TA, ed. *Anterior approaches to the spine.* St. Louis: Quality Medical Publishers, 1999, p. 79, with permission.)

MODIFIED ANTERIOR APPROACH

Limits of Exposure

In order to improve the visualization provided by the Smith-Robinson approach, transsternoclavicular approaches were devised (2). The variations have included osteotomy of the medial clavicle and manubrium, bilateral clavicular osteotomy, and a transverse manubrial osteotomy (3,4). Kurz et al. (5) described removing the medial one-third of the clavicle unilaterally without resecting any part of the sternum. This approach is described in this section and allows visualization distally to the T4 level.

Positioning

The patient is placed supine on the operating table with a roll towel between the scapulae. The neck should be slightly hyperextended and rotated to the right.

Skin Incision

An angled skin incision is made at the base of the left neck anteriorly (Fig. 7.6). The vertical limb of the incision starts distally at the base of the manubrium and extends 1 inch proximal to the clavicle prior to angling and becoming parallel to the clavicle. This transverse limb of the incision ends at the lateral border of the sternocleidomastoid.

Deep Dissection and Retractor Placement

The subcutaneous tissue is divided, platysmal flaps are raised, and the superficial veins are ligated. The medial supraclavicular nerve and the external jugular vein can usually be safely retracted without impeding the exposure. The two heads of the sternocleidomastoid are visible at this point and are released from their insertion on the

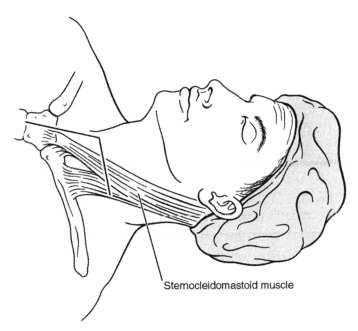

Sternocleidomastoid muscle

FIGURE 7.6. Skin incision for modified anterior approach to the cervicothoracic junction. (From Albert TJ, Balderston RA, Northrup BE. *Surgical approaches to the spine.* Philadelphia: Saunders, 1997, p. 62, with permission.)

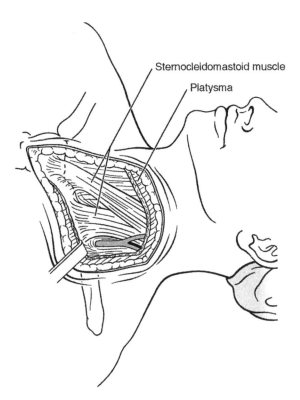

Sternocleidomastoid muscle

Platysma

FIGURE 7.7. Exposed sternocleidomastoid and strap muscles that need to be released. (From Albert TJ, Balderston RA, Northrup BE. *Surgical approaches to the spine.* Philadelphia: Saunders, 1997, p. 63, with permission.)

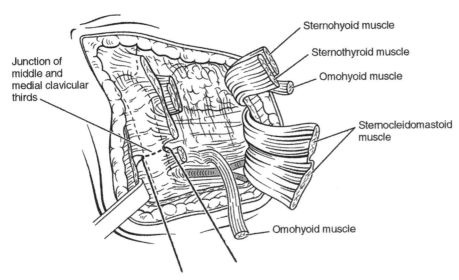

FIGURE 7.8. The subperiosteally dissected clavicle is resected with a Gigli saw. (From Albert TJ, Balderston RA, Northrup BE. *Surgical approaches to the spine.* Philadelphia: Saunders, 1997, p. 66, with permission.)

manubrium and clavicle (Fig. 7.7). They are retracted superiorly and laterally. The sternohyoid and sternothyroid muscles are next cut at the level of the clavicle. The clavicle and the sternoclavicular joint are next subperiosteally dissected, and the clavicle is resected with a Gigli saw at the junction of the medial and the middle third (Fig. 7.8). The subclavian vein lies under the clavicle, and thus extreme care must be used to keep the dissection in the subperiosteal plane around the clavicle. The subclavius muscle is located between the clavicle and the subclavian plane, which should be preserved to create a safe plane. The clavicle is removed by sharp disarticulation from the manubrium. The removed portion of the clavicle can serve as a good source of autogenous bone graft.

In the proximal portion of the wound, a plane can be developed lateral to the trachea and the esophagus while remaining medial to the carotid sheath in the usual fashion. The inferior thyroid vessels may be encountered ascending in the field and may need to be ligated. The spine is exposed by retracting the trachea, esophagus, and strap muscles medially while retracting the carotid sheath and the sternocleidomastoid laterally. The recurrent laryngeal nerve is retracted with the medial structures. The subclavian vein and the brachiocephalic vessels are next retracted inferomedially to visualize the vertebral body and the longus colli muscles, which are present anterolaterally on both sides distally to the T3 level (Fig. 7.9).

Closure

The sternocleidomastoid is reattached to the clavicular periosteal flap, followed by closure of the platysma and the skin.

Dangers of Approach

Resection of the clavicle carries the theoretical risk of weakness in the shoulder girdle; however, this has not been reported as a clinically significant problem. Injury to the great vessels, the subclavian vein, the recurrent laryngeal nerve, and the thoracic duct are all possibilities.

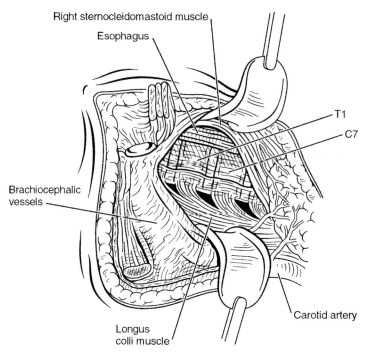

Right sternocleidomastoid muscle

Esophagus

T1

C7

Brachiocephalic
vessels

Carotid artery

Longus
colli muscle

FIGURE 7.9. The exposure obtained after deep retractor placement. (From Albert TJ, Balderston RA, Northrup BE. *Surgical approaches to the spine.* Philadelphia: Saunders, 1997, p. 69, with permission.)

HIGH THORACOTOMY

Limits of Exposure

This approach differs from the standard thoracotomy in that the scapula must be freed from its muscular attachments to be retracted. Entrance through the third or fourth rib allows exposure of the spine distally to the T4 level (6). Proximally, the C7 level can be reached, although with some difficulty. Portions of the proximal ribs may be removed to enhance the proximal exposure. A right-sided approach is typically used to avoid the proximity of the heart on the left.

Positioning

The patient is placed in the left lateral decubitus position, and the table is rolled 30 degrees toward the supine position.

Skin Incision

A curved skin incision is made starting proximally at the lateral border of the paraspinal muscles, curving distally and anteriorly over the inferior angle of the scapula, and ending at the anterior axillary line over the third or fourth rib (Fig. 7.10).

Deep Dissection and Retractor Placement

The subcutaneous tissue is next divided in line with the skin, allowing visualization of the trapezius and the latissimus dorsi (Fig. 7.11). The trapezius and the latissimus dorsi are divided in line with the skin incision, exposing the scapula along with the rhomboid

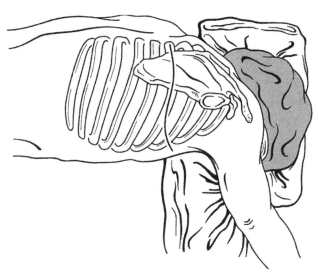

FIGURE 7.10. Skin incision for a high thoracotomy. (From Albert TJ, Balderston RA, Northrup BE. *Surgical approaches to the spine.* Philadelphia: Saunders, 1997, p. 70, with permission.)

major and minor attaching to its medial border, which can be divided to enhance the exposure if needed (Fig. 7.12). The scapula is retracted forward and anterior to allow access to the subscapular space and the chest wall.

Next the first rib is located, allowing identification of the third and the fourth rib. If some slips of serratus anterior cover the ribs, they have to be released. The rib is then subperiosteally dissected and removed (Fig. 7.13). The rib should be sectioned as far anterior and posterior as possible to optimize the exposure. The pleura is incised and a rib spreader is used to enlarge the opening. The lung is retracted anteriorly to allow visualization of the upper thoracic vertebrae, which are exposed by cutting the overlying parietal pleura (Figs. 7.14 and 7.15). The segmental vessels lie over the vertebral bodies and may

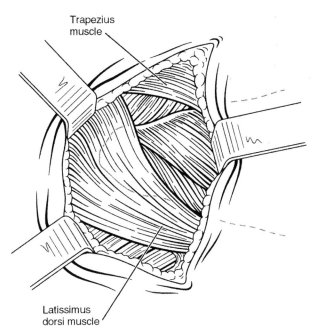

Trapezius
muscle

Latissimus
dorsi muscle

FIGURE 7.11. Exposed trapezius and latissimus dorsi that need to be transected. (From Albert TJ, Balderston RA, Northrup BE. *Surgical approaches to the spine.* Philadelphia: Saunders, 1997, p. 71, with permission.)

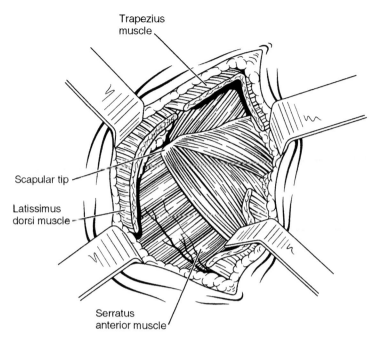

FIGURE 7.12. Release of trapezius and latissimus dorsi allows retraction of the scapula, exposing the chest wall. (From Albert TJ, Balderston RA, Northrup BE. *Surgical approaches to the spine.* Philadelphia: Saunders, 1997, p. 72, with permission.)

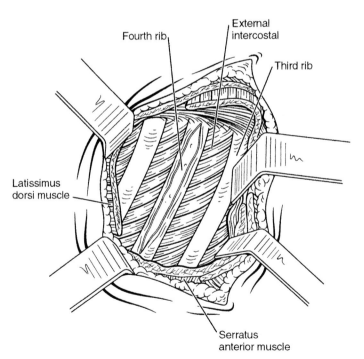

FIGURE 7.13. The rib is subperiosteally dissected. (From Albert TJ, Balderston RA, Northrup BE. *Surgical approaches to the spine.* Philadelphia: Saunders, 1997, p. 73, with permission.)

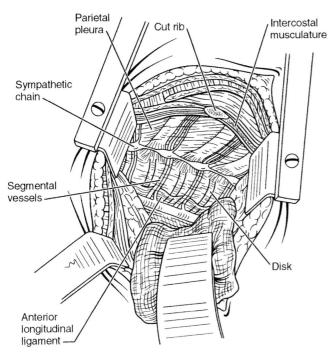

FIGURE 7.14. Resection of the rib exposes and retraction of the lung allows visualization of the spine through the parietal pleura. (From Albert TJ, Balderston RA, Northrup BE. *Surgical approaches to the spine.* Philadelphia: Saunders, 1997, p. 74, with permission.)

have to be ligated depending on the needs of the procedure (Fig. 7.16). The course of the azygous vein and the right superior intercostal vein is variable, and thus any vertical venous structures encountered must be handled with care to avoid significant blood loss.

Closure

The chest wall may be closed in a standard manner over a chest tube.

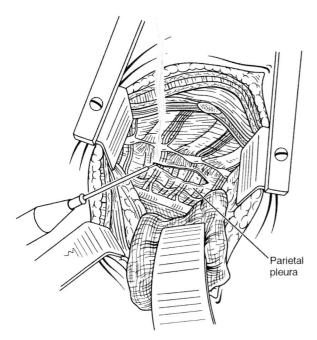

FIGURE 7.15. The parietal pleura is cut, exposing the spine. (From Albert TJ, Balderston RA, Northrup BE. *Surgical approaches to the spine.* Philadelphia: Saunders, 1997, p. 75, with permission.)

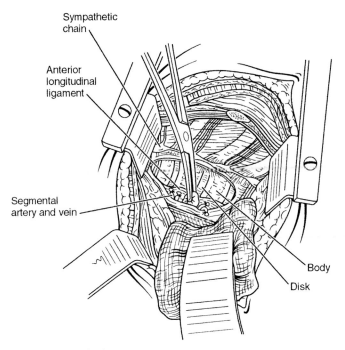

FIGURE 7.16. Final exposure demonstrating the dissection of the vertebral body by ligating the segmental vessels. (From Albert TJ, Balderston RA, Northrup BE. *Surgical approaches to the spine.* Philadelphia: Saunders, 1997, p. 75, with permission.)

Dangers of Approach

The risks are those of any standard thoracotomy approach.

STERNAL SPLITTING APPROACH

Limits of Exposure

The midline sternal splitting approach is typically used with the modified anterior approach described earlier to provide an extensile exposure from C4 to T4 (2,3,5,7).

Positioning

The patient is positioned supine in a fashion similar to the modified anterior approach.

Skin Incision

A skin incision is made in the midline directly over the sternum, starting proximally in the sternal notch (Fig. 7.17). An angled skin incision is made paralleling the clavicle and meeting the proximal sternal incision to perform the modified anterior approach.

Deep Dissection and Retractor Placement

After dividing the subcutaneous tissue, the sternum is subperiosteally exposed and split longitudinally in the midline with a saw. The sternum is retracted, allowing exposure of the thoracic inlet. The dissection described previously for the modified anterior approach is performed. Blunt dissection along the inferior aspect of the wound allows the identification of the left brachiocephalic vein, which is retracted to allow inferior exposure to T4. The trachea and the esophagus are retracted medially, and the carotid sheath and the left subclavian artery are retracted laterally (Fig. 7.18).

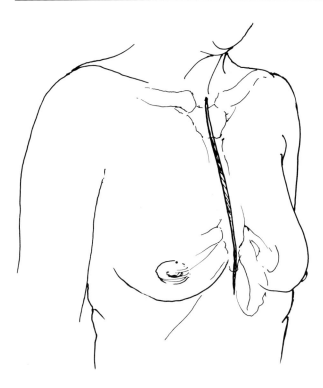

FIGURE 7.17. Skin incision for a sternal splitting approach.

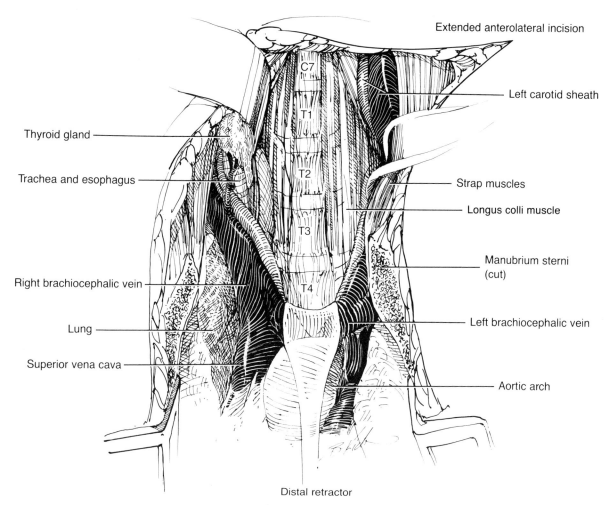

Extended anterolateral incision

C7

T1

Left carotid sheath

Thyroid gland

T2

Trachea and esophagus

Strap muscles

Longus colli muscle

T3

Right brachiocephalic vein

Manubrium sterni (cut)

T4

Lung

Left brachiocephalic vein

Superior vena cava

Aortic arch

Distal retractor

FIGURE 7.18. Exposed spine after deep retractor placement.

Closure

The sternum is reapproximated with wires, and a standard closure for the modified anterior approach is performed.

Dangers of Approach

In addition to the risks described for the modified anterior approach, malunion and nonunion of the sternum are a concern. The pleural cavity may also be inadvertently entered, requiring the placement of a chest tube.

CONCLUSION

Many different approaches are available to expose the cervicothoracic junction, each providing differing visualization of the anatomy. The surgeon must consider the extent of exposure required preoperatively in addition to the risks of each approach to select the most appropriate approach for the patient.

REFERENCES

1. Southwick WO, Robinson RA. Surgical approaches to the vertebral bodies in the cervical and lumbar regions. *J Bone Joint Surg Am* 1957;39:631–644.
2. Sundaresan N, Shah J, Foley KM, et al. An anterior surgical approach to the upper thoracic vertebrae. *J Neurosurg* 1984;61:686–690.
3. Sundaresan N, Shah J, Feghali JG. A transsternal approach to the upper thoracic vertebrae. *Am J Surg* 1984;148:473–477.
4. Lesoin F, Thomas CE III, Autricque A, et al. A transsternal biclavicular approach to the upper anterior thoracic spine. *Surg Neurol* 1986;26:253–256.
5. Kurz LT, Pursel S, Herkowitz HN. Modified anterior approach to the cervicothoracic junction. *Spine* 1991;16(suppl):S542–S547.
6. Hodgson AR, Stock FE, Fang HSY, et al. Anterior spinal fusion: the operative approach and pathologic findings in 412 patients with Pott's disease of the spine. *Br J Surg* 1960;48:172–178.
7. Fang HSY, Ong GB, Hodgson AR. Anterior spinal fusion, the operative approaches. *Clin Orthop* 1964;35:16–33.

8

POSTERIOR APPROACH: OCCIPUT TO T1

CHRISTOPHER M. BONO
CHRISTOPHER P. KAUFFMAN
STEVEN R. GARFIN

The posterior approach to the occiput and cervical spine is useful for decompression, instrumentation, and fusion procedures. The midline exposure exploits a relatively avascular plane at the decussation of the paraspinal neck musculature and ligamentum nuchae. Careful positioning and operative setup is crucial. A thorough familiarity with regional anatomy, particularly in the upper cervical region, is requisite to minimize the risk of vascular and neurologic injury. Positioning and planning for intraoperative imaging should also be done before draping to help with effective and safe surgery.

ANATOMY

Occipitocervical Region

The occipital bone is the diploic posteroinferior aspect of the cranium that cradles the cerebellum and brainstem. At its anterior and inferior aspect it forms the posterior part of the foramen magnum, which houses the junction between the spinal cord in the spinal canal and the brain. The occiput has several bony structures that are useful surgical landmarks. At its topographical center, the external occipital protuberance (EOP) is a dense uprising that marks the thickest portion of the bone (Fig. 8.1). The superior nuchal line is a ridge that extends medial and lateral from the EOP. The inferior nuchal line is a similar condensation running parallel and below its superior counterpart. Though not a useful surgical landmark, the lambdoidal suture denotes the borders of the occipital bone at its fused junctions with the temporal and maxillary bones. The occiput curves sharply anterior from the superior nuchal line to the foramen magnum. This feature makes accurate contouring of implants, to match the skeletal geometry, challenging. The occiput interacts with the cervical spine through bilateral articular condyles on either side of the foramen magnum. Together with the posterior and anterior ligaments, the occipitoatlantal joints stabilize the head on the neck. Motion at this junction is minimal, allowing 13 degrees of flexion/extension, 8 degrees of lateral bending, and no rotation (1).

The occipitocervical region is stabilized by numerous ligaments. A durable capsule stabilizes the articulation of the occipital condyles to the atlas. A broad sheet of fibrous tissue extends from the posterior border of the foramen magnum to the superior surface of the C1 ring. This is the posterior atlantooccipital (tectorial) membrane. This is analogous to the ligamentum flavum at other levels. Entering this membrane approximately 1.5 cm from the midline is the vertebral artery (Fig. 8.2). The artery arises lateral and posterior from the transverse foramen of the atlas. This vessel can be injured with extensive exposure of the posterior ring. The ligamentum nuchae is a thick condensation of

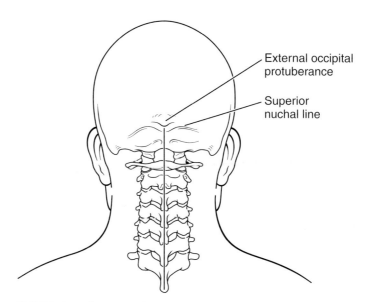

FIGURE 8.1. The external occipital protuberance (EOP) can be palpated in the midline of the skull. This represents the thickest aspect of the posterior cranium and provides an excellent point of fixation with either screws or wires. The superior nuchal line is the thickened ridge that extends laterally from the EOP.

supraspinous fibrous bands. This structure overlays the spinous processes of the cervical vertebrae and extends from the EOP to C7.

There are few muscles that directly span between the occiput and the atlas. The superior obliquus capitis muscle spans from the lateral aspect of the superior nuchal line to the transverse process of C1. Medially, the rectus capitis posterior minor attaches to the superior nuchal line and the C1 spinous process. The rectus capitis posterior major muscle extends from the superior nuchal line to the spinous process of C2. Spanning from the mastoid process of the skull, the longissimus capitis blends with the deep muscles of the upper thoracic paraspinal region.

Atlantoaxial Region

The upper cervical vertebrae are unique compared with the subaxial spine. The atlas has large broad-based articular processes to interface with the occipital condyles superiorly and the axis inferiorly. An articular surface on the posterior aspect of the anterior arch faces the odontoid process of the axis. The posterior ring of C1 is quite thin, with no discrete spinous process. The axis articulates with C1 at three points: broad bilateral supe-

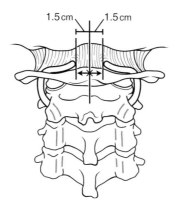

FIGURE 8.2. The vertebral artery takes a medial turn at the level of the C1 ring. It lies over the posterior ring approximately 1.5 centimeters lateral to the midline. It can be endangered with lateral dissection.

rior articular surfaces and the odontoid process. By its morphology, it allows approximately 47 degrees of rotation (50% of axial rotation of the entire cervical spine), while limiting flexion/extension to 10 degrees (1). Virtually no lateral bending is permitted at the atlantoaxial articulation. The axis marks the transition between the upper and lower cervical spine. In so doing, the inferior articular processes of C2 are offset posteriorly. Because of this offset, the pars interarticularis sustains high shear forces with axial loading, predisposing it to the classic hangman's fracture pattern. A foramen in the transverse processes transmits the ascending vertebral artery. The second cervical nerve roots exit through foramina formed by adjacent superior and inferior pedicle walls. The ligamentum flavum proper is first encountered at this level, extending from the inferior ring of C1 to the superior ring of C2. The flavum attaches more anterior (deep) on the C1 ring and more posterior on the C2 ring. This is an important consideration when elevating this membrane to expose the bony lamina for decompression.

Several muscles connect the atlas and axis (2). As in other spinal regions, small bilateral interspinalis muscles span between spinous processes. The inferior obliquus capitis extends from the transverse process of C1 laterally to the spinous process of C2 medially. It is at the inferior border of this muscle that the greater occipital nerve exits posteriorly, traveling cranial and medial to lie superficial to the rectus capitis posterior minor and obliquus capitis superior muscles. Finally, it exits the trapezius near the midline over the EOP and can be injured with lateral dissection at this level. Nerve injury can lead to dysesthesia of the posterior scalp, which can be troublesome to some patients.

Subaxial Region

Subaxial anatomy is more uniform than at the upper two cervical levels. The posterior vertebral ring is formed from two posteromedially projecting laminae that form a bifid midline spinous process. The laminae attach to the lateral mass, the complex of articular processes, pedicles, and transverse processes. A transverse foramen transmits the vertebral artery from C1 to C6. At C6, the vessel enters the cervical spine as a branch from the first part of the subclavian artery. Pedicles connect the facet to the vertebral body. Between the upper and lower facets of the same vertebra lies a dense pars interarticularis. It is in this region that lateral mass screws are inserted. Facet joints are formed between adjacent articular processes. The superior articular surface from cephalad vertebrae is angled approximately 45 degrees posterior. This is matched by an underlying inferior articular surface from the adjacent caudal segment. Together, they form a stable joint that allows motion mostly in the sagittal plane. Each level contributes approximately 10 degrees of rotation to supplement the majority of torsional movement at the atlantoaxial articulation. Intervertebral ligaments include the ligamentum flavum, articular capsules, and ligamentum nuchae.

In the deep layer of muscle, small intervertebral ligaments extend from the spinous processes of cephalad vertebrae to the transverse processes of caudal vertebrae. These are the rotatores cervicis muscles longus and brevis. The thin spinalis cervicis connects the spinous processes of C2 to C7. In the superficial layer, the semispinalis capitis is a confluence of the semispinalis thoracis. The muscle extends cranially to broadly insert onto the superior nuchal line. The splenius capitis is the more superficial and lateral, spanning from the upper thoracic spinous processes to the superior nuchal line. The trapezius is the most superficial. It inserts on the midline ligamentum nuchae in the cervical region and onto the spinous processes in the thoracic region. The skin over the midline cervical region is innervated by the medial cutaneous branches of the dorsal rami of cervical nerves 3, 4, 5, and 6.

Cervicothoracic Region

The seventh cervical vertebra marks the transition between the cervical and thoracic regions. In some cases there is a cervical rib that articulates with it. At this level the spinous process is no longer bifid and is morphologically similar to the thoracic vertebrae. It is usually the only subcutaneously easily palpable prominent cervical vertebra and represents a helpful surface landmark during posterior surgery. Because it connects a stiff thoracic region to a relatively flexible cervical region, it is a frequent site of injury with acceleration/deceleration mechanisms.

PREOPERATIVE CONSIDERATIONS

A detailed preoperative neurologic examination should be performed just before surgery. In the unstable upper cervical spine, an awake fiberoptic intubation is recommended. Excessive extension of the neck, often required for standard intubation maneuvers, could lead to subluxation and neurologic injury.

OPERATIVE SETUP AND POSITIONING

In the supine position, baseline somatosensory and motor evoked potentials can be obtained. In some cases awake positioning is done so the patient's neurologic status can be assessed after positioning. Before induction of general anesthesia, the patient is then logrolled prone onto a radiolucent spine table with well-padded bolsters. This should be performed under the coordination of the surgeon, with the anesthesiologist caring for endotracheal tube position and ventilation. Bilateral bolsters should extend from the anterior aspect of the clavicles to the anterior superior iliac spine. The face, nipples, abdomen, and genitals must be free of any undue pressure. Positioning the table and the patient so that the head and posterior aspect of the neck are higher than the heart helps decrease epidural bleeding. Taping down the shoulder also helps with the approach and radiographic imaging of the lower cervical spine.

If cervical tongs were not in place preoperatively, they may be applied in the operating room (Fig. 8.3). This is best performed in the supine position, after intubation and light sedation given for patient comfort. In some cases, a halo ring can be used so that it may be incorporated into a halo vest postoperatively. Alternatives such as Mayfield tong head holders, horseshoe headrests, or sponge-type head holders on the table can all be used, depending on cervical stability, radiographic requirements, and surgeon preference. The patient is then turned prone (Fig. 8.4). The position of the neck should be noted. Neutral flexion/extension is optimal, especially if occipitocervical fusion is planned, since this will most likely be the final fused position. Gross neurologic assessment or evoked potentials or both can be repeated if awake positioning was performed. With confirmation of the neurologic status, general anesthesia can then be initiated.

A C-arm or regular radiographs can be used to confirm that adequate imaging is possible prior to skin preparation. Often, a free electrocardiogram lead or an inadvertent piece of table hardware can obscure imaging views. If a reduction is being performed, se-

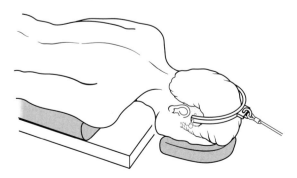

FIGURE 8.3. Cervical tongs can be applied preoperatively or in the operating suite. This can be used in conjunction with a padded horseshoe rest to support the head during posterior cervical surgery.

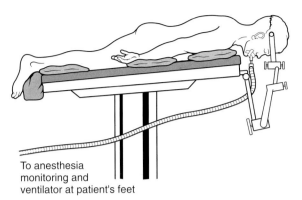

To anesthesia
monitoring and
ventilator at patient's feet

FIGURE 8.4. The patient is carefully log-rolled onto the operating table. The anesthesia monitor and ventilator are placed at the foot of the table, allowing the surgeons and C-arm easier access to the operative region. Special consideration for increased dead space with longer ventilator tubing must be taken. The bed is angled into slight reverse Trendelenburg to position the heart lower than the head, helping decrease epidural venous congestion. Pillows are placed under the legs to slightly flex at the knee, relieving undue tension on the sciatic nerve.

quential lateral views must be possible. Intraoperatively, a cross-table lateral plain radiograph is obtained to confirm the level of surgery. Adequate visualization of all radiographic landmarks is important. This may be difficult at the C7/T1 junction. Setup adjustments should be made prior to sterile preparation.

RECOMMENDED INSTRUMENTS

In addition to standard surgical instruments, an electrocautery and bipolar cautery must be available. Cobb elevators facilitate tissue retraction during periosteal elevation. Sharp-tipped, deep-bladed (e.g., Adson-Beckman, cerebellar, or angled Wiltse) retractors are placed to maintain exposure. Large rongeurs are used to remove the posterior spinous processes to the level of the laminae. Small and medium-sized Kerrison rongeurs are useful for laminectomy. A no. 3 or 4 Penfield retractor or Freer elevator can be used to free the dura from the bony surface.

SURGICAL APPROACH

The posterior scalp and neck are shaved in the region of surgery. Useful surface landmarks include the EOP and the spinous process protuberans at C7. If occipitocervical dissection is necessary, the surgical field should be extended 4 cm above the EOP/superior nuchal line. For surgery at the cervicothoracic junction, the field should include the T4 spinous process caudally. After standard surgical scrub and prep, the field is draped with sterile sheets. An iodine-impregnated adhesive film can be placed to seal the edges of the surgical working area.

Using a no. 10 scalpel blade, a midline incision is created over the desired region (Fig. 8.1). Sharp dissection is carried through the subcutaneous tissue down to the midline trapezius fascia. Since palpation of the spinous processes is still difficult because of the thick layers of overlying muscles, visualization of the decussation of tendon fibers confirms the midline. The fascia is incised with electrocautery, maintaining a relatively avascular plane through the ligamentum nuchae. With tension applied anterolaterally to the muscles using a flat periosteal elevator, this white midline band usually stands out.

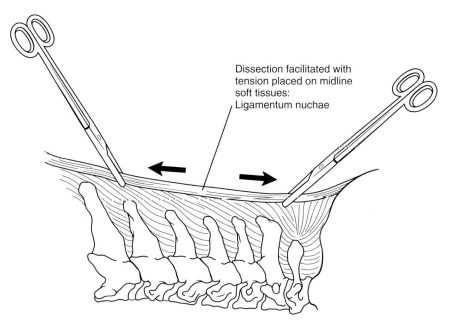

FIGURE 8.5. Once the white condensation of midline ligaments (ligamentum nuchae) has been identified, Kocher clamps can be placed proximally and distally to provide tension. This facilitates lateral dissection of the paraspinal muscles while maintaining the integrity of the midline structures.

Alternatively, Kocher clamps can be used to provide longitudinal tension on the midline structures (Fig. 8.5). Once the tips of the spinous processes are visualized, dissection is continued laterally, maintaining the interspinous ligaments (Fig. 8.6). At this time, the proposed level of surgery is marked with either a spinal needle or a clamp. A cross-table lateral radiograph is made to confirm the correct surgical level.

Periosteal dissection is carried anteriorly along the spinous processes and then laterally, elevating the paraspinal muscles off the laminae (Fig. 8.7). The subaxial vertebrae should be visualized to the facet joint. Care is taken to leave the facet capsule intact until, or if, exposure and decortication for fusion has been decided at that level. Deep cerebellar retractors can be placed to maintain exposure (Fig. 8.8). Dissection lateral to the facet joint risks destabilization of the joint and bleeding from small vessels laterally. *Caution:*

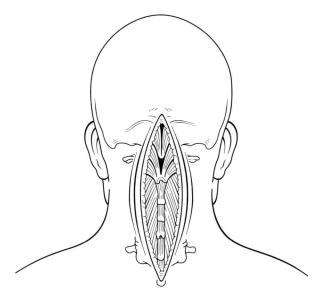

FIGURE 8.6. Once the tips of the spinous processes are visualized, dissection is continued laterally, maintaining the interspinous ligaments. The length of dissection is determined by the number of vertebral levels necessitating exposure. A localizing intraoperative radiograph can be taken to verify the correct level and exposure.

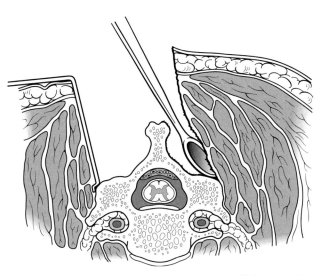

FIGURE 8.7. Parapsinal muscles are elevated off the posterior bone using a Cobb elevator or (the authors' preference) electrocautery. Care is taken to not sacrifice the facet capsules during exposure. In addition, the interlaminar spaces are not violated because this can endanger the neural elements and cause undue epidural bleeding.

The ring of C1 should not be exposed more than 1.5 cm from the midline because of risk of injury to the vertebral artery (Fig. 8.2). In the occipital region, the surgical dissection is carried down to the bone in the midline. The EOP is visualized and the periosteal exposure is continued along the superior nuchal line as needed. *Caution:* Lateral dissection or retraction at the level of the EOP can injure the greater occipital nerve. Care must be taken to maintain instruments at the subperiosteal level. They should be intermittently released every 1 to 2 hours to allow reperfusion of the underlying tissue. Bone wax can be used to control focal points of bone bleeding, but should be removed before fusion.

Decompression can be performed at this stage. The spinous processes can be removed to the level of the laminae. Using sharp, curved curettes, the ligamentum flavum

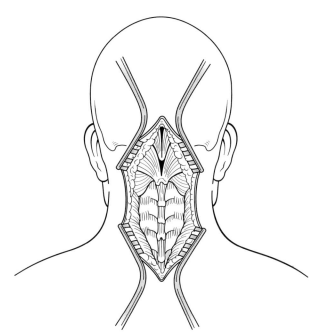

FIGURE 8.8. Deep retractors are placed to maintain exposure while bony work is performed. Cerebellar retractors are usually sufficient, although Adson-Beckman devices may be necessary in larger patients.

is carefully elevated from the inferior borders of the cervical lamina. A regular rongeur, followed by a Kerrison rongeur, is used to remove the lamina. At each level the ligamentum should be teased off the underlying dura, as it may be adherent. In the occipitocervical region, the borders of the tectorial membrane are elevated in a similar manner. If necessary, partial resection of the posterior foramen magnum can also be performed for decompression.

After laminectomy, a clear view of the dural covering of the spinal cord is afforded. Decompression of the nerve roots necessitates foraminotomy. The roots exit the spinal cord at the level of the foramen. The foramen is bounded superiorly and inferiorly by adjacent pedicles. Visualization of the nerve root foramen necessitates at least partial removal of the articular processes. A no. 4 Penfield can be used to develop a plane between the dura and the cortical walls of the foramen. Hemostasis in the area of the cord and root is achieved with bipolar electrocautery and with hemostatic agents as necessary.

Retraction and exposure of the dura can cause small tears that are difficult to detect. Before wound closure, a Valsalva maneuver should be performed to check for cerebrospinal fluid leaks. Tears should be repaired with 4–0 or 6–0 monofilament suture.

The wound is irrigated with copious amounts of warmed normal saline solution. If desired, a medium-sized drain can be placed deep to the fascia layer. Closure of all layers (muscle, fascia, subcutaneous tissue, and skin) is routine.

LIMITATIONS OF EXPOSURE

The posterior approach is extensile. It can be carried as far caudad as needed. It relies on the same avascular plane at the decussation of cervical, thoracic, and lumbar paraspinal muscles. In the thoracolumbar region, overlying layers of the latissimus, periscapular, and costal muscles must be considered. Structures anterior to the cord cannot be visualized through the approach.

POSTOPERATIVE CARE

The type of external orthotic, if any, depends on the procedure and postoperative cervical stability. With rigid internal fixation, external adjuncts may not be necessary. Often a soft cervical collar is applied for patient comfort during the immediate perioperative period. Prophylactic antibiotic coverage with a first-generation cephalosporin is maintained for 24 to 48 hours after surgery. If concomitant injuries permit, the patient can be mobilized on postoperative day 1. Drains are removed the next day.

REFERENCES

1. White A, Panjabi M. The clinical biomechanics of the occipitoatlantoaxial complex. *Orthop Clin North Am* 1978;9:867–878.
2. Hoppenfeld S, deBoer P. *Surgical Exposures in Orthopaedics.* Philadelphia: JB Lippincott Co., 1994.

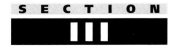

DECOMPRESSION

CONCEPTS OF CERVICAL DECOMPRESSION

ANTHONY J. MATAN
PATRICK J. CONNOLLY

CLINICAL PRESENTATION OF RADICULOPATHY AND MYELOPATHY

Patients with cervical degenerative disease can present with symptoms of nerve root compression, spinal cord compression, axial neck pain, or any combination of the three. Radiculopathy typically is described as arm pain in a dermatomal distribution. The pain is frequently burning in nature and accompanied by an uncomfortable dysesthesia. The dermatomal distributions of the specific cervical nerve roots have been well described (Fig. 9.1). Compression of each nerve root affects a specific portion of the upper extremity: The C5 nerve root will affect the lateral arm, the C6 nerve root will affect the lateral forearm and hand, the C7 nerve root will affect the middle of the hand and the middle finger, the C8 nerve root will affect the medial hand and forearm, and the T1 root will affect the medial arm. The classic presentation of cervical radiculopathy has been described as neck pain with paresthesia distally; however, there is much variation between patients. In addition, there is a great deal of overlap between the dermatomes, and patients often present with pain in two or more dermatomes, even with compression of a single nerve root.

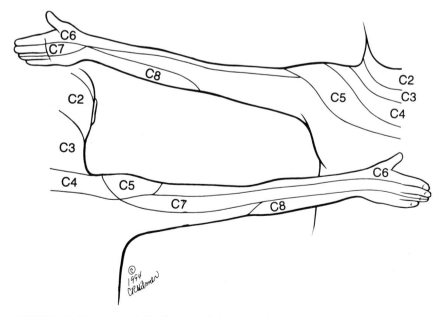

FIGURE 9.1. Dermatomal distribution of the cervical nerve roots.

Sensory symptoms and radicular pain can often be elicited by extremes of range of motion. Patients complain of pain in a dermatomal distribution with rotation of the head or lateral bending of the neck. Spurling's test is a provocative maneuver that is based on the irritation of a nerve root by cervical rotation. The test, as described by Spurling, involves axial compression with lateral bending of the neck. A positive result is reproduction of the patient's radicular symptoms (1). Spurling's test is only moderately sensitive but is quite specific (2).

Nerve root compression due to cervical spondylosis can result in muscular weakness, which, if present, is more specific than sensory dysfunction for identification of a neurologic level. A specific motor dysfunction is usually caused by compression of a specific nerve root: deltoid and biceps weakness from C5 compression, wrist extensors from C6, triceps from C7, finger flexors from C8, and interossei muscles from compression of T1. The clinically useful reflexes of the lower extremities are the C5 biceps reflex, the C6 brachioradialis reflex, and the C7 triceps reflex. Neurologic examination of a patient with severe nerve root compression will reveal lower motor neuronal dysfunction with decreased tone, atrophy of skeletal muscle, and hyporeflexia.

Cervical spondylosis can also cause spinal cord compromise, or myelopathy. Myelopathy is characterized by motor weakness, which is frequently greater in the upper extremities than in the lower extremities. Ataxia can occur and the patient will typically walk with a broad-based, shuffling gate. Intrinsic weakness and atrophy are typical findings in the hand. Intrinsic weakness causes the small finger to abduct. This is known as the *finger escape sign*. Physical examination will reveal findings of lower motor neuron dysfunction at the level of the lesion and upper motor neuron dysfunction below the level of the lesion. Upper extremity reflexes may be hypoactive due to nerve root compression, whereas lower extremity reflexes may be hyperactive due to spinal cord compression. Babinski's sign is positive if stroking the plantar aspect of the foot causes extension of the great toe. A positive Babinski's sign or a positive Hoffmann's sign is indicative of upper motor neuron dysfunction. Clonus is another finding indicative of spasticity. Lhermitte's sign is present if flexion of the neck produces radiating dysesthesia into the lower extremities.

PATHOPHYSIOLOGY AND PATHOANATOMY OF RADICULOPATHY AND MYELOPATHY

Cervical radiculopathy and myelopathy can result from any process that compromises the cervical nerve root or the spinal cord. Figure 9.2 illustrates the relationship between the neural structures and the bony elements in the cervical spine. Pathological compression of the cord or nerve roots can occur from acute herniation of nuclear material or from degenerative changes in the vertebral disc, endplates, uncovertebral joint, or facet joint. Less common causes include acute or chronic traumatic changes and neoplastic compression of neural structures.

Acute disc herniation causes direct mass effect upon the nerve and also causes the onset of an inflammatory cascade. The disc leaks neuromodulating substances such as phospholipase A_2, cytokines, and substance P, which cause direct irritation of the nerve root, generating a chemical radiculitis (3–5). Hasue (3) has described a proposed pathomechanism for radicular pain. Compression of the nerve root causes circulatory changes as well as inflammation, as described earlier. Compression also disturbs cerebrospinal fluid (CSF) flow to the nerve root and exacerbates circulatory and inflammatory changes and leads to malnutrition of the root. Persistence of the compression over a prolonged period then leads to demyelination, electrophysiologic changes, and hypersensitivity of the nerve root, all leading to radicular pain.

Several authors have described the pathoanatomy of acute cervical disc herniation. Three types of soft disc herniation have been described. Intraforaminal herniation causes radiculopathy due to compression of the nerve root and the dorsal root ganglion.

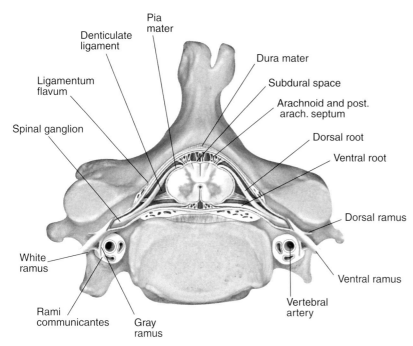

FIGURE 9.2. Cross section of the cervical spine showing the spinal cord, nerve roots, and bony elements.

Posterolateral herniation compresses the anterior horn of the spinal column and causes lower motor neuron findings of flaccid weakness and atrophy. Midline disc herniations compress the cord and cause myelopathy.

Cervical degenerative spondylosis results from a combination of events that begins with the degeneration of the intervertebral disc. The initial degeneration is insidious and may or may not be symptomatic. Early degeneration of the disc is marked by dehydration of the normally well-hydrated nucleus. This is caused by a relative loss of hydrophilic molecules that are abundant in the normal nucleus. In addition, as the disc loses height, the annular fibers become redundant and the posterior annulus bulges outward. This annular bulging is the first of several anatomic encroachments into the neural space caused by the developing spondylosis. The dehydrated nucleus loses volume as it loses its water content and begins to shrink. The dehydrated disc can no longer perform its biomechanical function of dispersing compressive loads, and the loads begin to concentrate along the vertebral endplates. The abnormal proximity of the two vertebral endplates leads to a reactive osteophytosis. The osteophyte formation commonly occurs at the posterior vertebral endplates and expands the diameter of the endplate at that site. This posterior bony bar can compromise the anterior aspect of the neural canal as well as the neural foramina. The collapse of the intervertebral disc also initiates the degeneration of the uncovertebral joint. As the two vertebral bodies become abnormally close, the uncinate process impinges upon the opposing surface known as the echancrure. This causes abnormal concentration of forces across the articulation, and uncovertebral degeneration ensues with reactive osteophyte formation as well as protrusion of hypertrophied soft tissue into the medial aspect of the neuroforamen.

There are a number of vascular changes that contribute to cervical spondylotic myelopathy (6). The anterior spinal artery supplies 60% to 75% of the cord tissue and is situated in the midsagittal plane directly anterior to the cord. Its branches consist of the sulcocommissural or direct sagittal branches as well as branches to the vascular plexus within the leptomeninges that surround the cord. Neuroischemic myelopathy can occur by several mechanisms. The anterior spinal artery can be directly compressed by midline pathologic structures such as osteophytes or disc herniations. Degenerative pathology can also encroach upon the medullary branches off of the anterior spinal artery. These medullary branches are significant sources of blood supply to the spinal cord. A study of 235 postmortem specimens showed that the cervical spinal cord may have up to seven branches from the anterior spinal artery but usually only has two or three. The segmental levels that most frequently contained a branch artery to the cord were C3 and C6 (7).

The greatest risk to the vascular supply to the cord is in the region from C4 to C7. Above C4 there are anastomoses with intracranial arteries branching off of the vertebral arteries that support the medullary branches off of the anterior spinal artery and provide collateral flow in the case of compromise to the anterior spinal artery. Below C4 the spinal cord tissue supported by the anterior spinal artery would be more directly at risk of ischemic insult should degenerative pathology cause impingement upon the anterior spinal artery because this region lacks the anastomoses with the intracranial vasculature (8). The lower cervical vasculature is supported to some degree by anastomoses with upper thoracic arteries, but these arteries have been shown to be particularly susceptible to atherosclerotic occlusive disease (9).

It is possible to develop a purely ischemic myelopathy of the cervical spinal cord in the absence of significant spinal cord compression. This occurs by way of isolated compression of an essential branch of the anterior spinal artery that is acting as the sole feeder to a significant portion of the cervical cord (6). The symptoms are identical to those seen with thrombosis of the anterior spinal artery. The upper extremities show a flaccid paralysis, while the lower extremities demonstrate spastic diplegia.

ANTERIOR APPROACH FOR RADICULOPATHY AND MYELOPATHY

The anterior approach to the cervical spine allows direct access to the compressive structures, which lie anterior to the cord and nerve roots (Fig. 9.3). The anterior cervical discectomy and fusion was described by Robinson and Smith (10) in 1955. They recognized that the anterior approach allowed indirect decompression of the nerve root and spinal cord by distraction of the disc space. The anterior approach was an improvement over the earlier posterior approaches because it did not require manipulation of the spinal cord. In 1958, Cloward (11) published his technique of anterior discectomy with

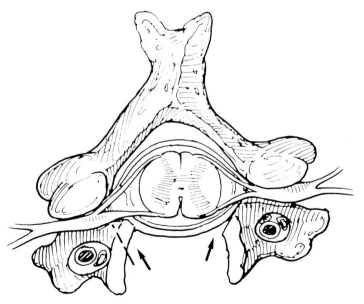

FIGURE 9.3. The anterior approach to the cervical spine allows decompression of both the spinal cord and the nerve roots.

direct decompression of compressed neurologic structures. The technique of Robinson and Smith did not require direct decompression of the neural elements (12). The intervertebral disc was removed only to the extent necessary to prepare the endplates and apply the intervertebral graft. Stabilization of the motion segment then allowed regression and resorption of the posterior and posterolateral osteophytes. In contrast, Cloward described direct decompression of the spinal cord and nerve roots by visualization and removal of offending posterior and posterolateral osteophytes (13).

Numerous authors have described the indications for anterior cervical discectomy and fusion in patients with cervical radiculopathy (12–14). These include radiculopathy that is disabling and persists despite at least 6 weeks of conservative treatment; radiculopathy with severe episodic recurrences; an acute or progressive motor deficit; or spinal instability in conjunction with radiculopathy. In all cases, there must be symptoms and findings referable to specific nerve roots and there should be anatomic imaging demonstrating compression of the nerve roots in question. Surgical success is most likely when the operative level is the only level showing significant spondylosis. Surgical success is least likely when the levels adjacent to the operative level show significant spondylosis (14).

Anterior cervical discectomy and fusion has a high success rate that is well documented for the treatment of cervical radiculopathy. Numerous authors have reported their results with various surgical techniques in the literature. This has engendered certain controversies regarding the technical aspects of the surgery. One of the earliest controversies surrounding anterior cervical discectomy, a controversy that survives today, concerns the need for complete decompression of the neurologic structures. The difference of opinion on this matter dates back to the original techniques of Cloward (11) as well as Robinson and Smith (10). Cloward described anterior discectomy followed by removal of the posterior longitudinal ligament, direct visualization of compressed neurologic structures, and excision of endplate and uncovertebral osteophytes that are causing compression. The technique of Robinson and Smith requires excision of disc to create an adequate bed for bony fusion. There is no attempt to directly decompress the nervous structures. It is assumed that a solid arthrodesis across the disc space will result in resorption of the posterior osteophytes that are causing compression.

Numerous series have reported success with either technique. Mosdal (15) reported in 1984 on 755 cases performed by the Cloward technique over an 18-year period. The initial success rate with regard to radicular pain was 83%, although there was some deterioration of benefits at long-term follow-up. The overall complication rate was 4%. Mosdal found that short duration of symptoms, the finding of free intraspinal disc fragments, and single-level surgery all correlated with favorable outcome. Likewise, numerous authors report success with the Robinson and Smith technique. For example, Bohlman et al. (16) reported in 1993 on use of the Robinson method on 122 patients with cervical radiculopathy. At long-term follow-up averaging 6 years, 93% of patients had either no pain or mild pain and were categorized with a good or excellent result. Pseudarthrosis occurred in 13% of patients (the same rate reported by Robinson et al. [17] in 1962), and the authors found that pseudoarthrosis was the greatest risk factor for a negative outcome. They found that risk of pseudoarthrosis was greater with multilevel fusion surgery. The literature demonstrates ample support for either complete decompression of neurologic compression or for discectomy and fusion without direct decompression in the treatment of cervical radiculopathy. It is left up to the preferences and training of the operating surgeon to decide which technique is applicable to a given case.

Anterior decompression and fusion is also documented to work very well for cervical spondylotic myelopathy (Fig. 9.4). In 1998, Emery et al. (18) reported on 108 patients with cervical myelopathy treated with anterior decompression and fusion. The surgical technique consisted of simple Smith-Robinson discectomy and fusion if the compressive lesion was predominately soft disc herniation. If posterior osteophytes from the vertebral endplates were causing compression, they were removed via a partial corpectomy; if multiple levels were involved, then a standard corpectomy was performed. The patients were followed for 2 to 17 years, with an average of 4.5 years. Postoperative follow-up showed

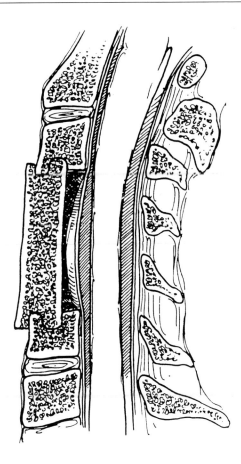

FIGURE 9.4. The anterior approach allows excellent decompression of anterior pathology for treatment of cervical spondylotic myelopathy.

that 38 of the 82 patients who had a gait abnormality preoperatively had a normal gait postoperatively, and 33 had a significant improvement of their gait. Of the 87 patients who had a preoperative motor deficit, only 7 failed to improve or got worse, whereas 54 had complete recovery and 26 had partial recovery. Only 5 patients had recurrent myelopathy, with 3 of them having neurologic compression at the site of a surgical nonunion. New stenotic lesions at different levels occurred in 2 patients with recurrent myelopathy. The best predictive factor with respect to recovery from the myelopathy was the preoperative status of the patient. Those patients with the most severe myelopathy were the least likely to recover postoperatively, and those with the best preoperative function were the most likely to achieve maximum recovery. Pain relief was very consistent in the postoperative patients: 87% had no or mild postoperative pain at latest follow-up. Other authors have documented similar successful outcomes for anterior decompression and fusion for cervical myelopathy (19–21).

Many controversies remain surrounding the anterior approach. One controversy that is relatively long-standing concerns the need for fusion after an anterior discectomy and decompression. In 1960, Hirsch (22) reported on his series of 35 patients who underwent anterior cervical discectomy without fusion (ACD). All patients developed a fibrous union at the operative site, and 29 of the 35 patients had a good to excellent result. Numerous other authors have reported clinical results without fusion that rival the clinical results of anterior surgery with fusion (22–34). Most of these studies demonstrate success rates of approximately 90%.

Watters and Levinthal (32) retrospectively compared outcomes of surgery with and without fusion in 126 patients treated with anterior discectomy for radiculopathy. The fusion group included 64 patients who underwent complete discectomy under magnification, and fusion (ACF) without plating using tricortical iliac autograft. The nonfusion group (ACD) of 62 patients had an identical discectomy without the fusion. Most patients in both groups had single-level surgery. The authors found that the ACD group had a hospital stay of 2.5 days, compared with a stay of 3.7 days in the ACF group. On the other hand, the ACF patients had a significantly faster resolution of neck pain following surgery: 27 days compared with 70 days ($p < .001$). The ACF group had a much higher perioperative complication rate, but this was associated mainly with graft site complications. One patient in the ACD group required reoperation for kyphosis and neck pain 5 weeks after ACD. The authors felt that the primary benefit of ACD was the elimination of graft site morbidity. The primary benefit of ACF was significantly faster resolution of symptoms. The authors were unable to draw definitive long-term conclusions because half of the patients in both groups were lost after the short-term follow-up. They felt that neither procedure was clearly superior in treating cervical radiculopathy.

Critics of ACD cite concerns over neck pain and kyphotic deformity. These concerns are supported by the long-term results reported by Yamamoto et al. (34). The authors reported on 55 consecutive patients who underwent ACD with 100% long-term follow-up of 2 to 13 years with a mean of just over 5 years. The indications for surgery included radiculopathy, myelopathy, or myeloradiculopathy. Forty-eight patients had single-level surgery, and the rest had two-level surgeries. At long-term follow-up, 18% of patients had no improvement and 35% of patients had deteriorated. Deterioration was related to spinal instability, aggravation of myelopathy due to kyphosis, recurrence of radiculopathy, and severe neck or intrascapular pain. The most troublesome complication was pain persisting for greater than 1 year: This complication was found in 11 of the 55 patients (20%). Likewise, approximately 20% of the patients demonstrated a significant kyphotic deformity at long-term follow-up. The authors stated that they prefer ACF for cervical spondylotic disease.

Another area of controversy in the arena of anterior cervical discectomy and fusion is the use of allograft versus autograft bone as a fusion material. Bone graft ideally acts as both a source of bone-producing cells and as a mechanical support at the site of fusion. Autograft fulfills both of these roles yet is complicated by the graft harvest. Complications of anterior iliac crest harvest for cervical surgery are reported to range from 6.3% to 36%. These complications include infection, hematoma, graft site discomfort, meralgia paresthetica, graft site fracture, and dehiscence of the wound (32,35,36). Fibular autograft has even more significant donor site morbidity, including tibial stress fractures and long-term pain or neurologic deficits (37,38).

Allograft bone requires no harvest, yet has a number of inherent disadvantages as a graft material when compared with autograft. Allograft is incorporated more slowly and less completely, probably as a result of host immune response to antigens within the allograft (39,40). The processes of sterilization also negatively affect allograft. Both freeze-drying and irradiation significantly decrease the strength of allograft bone compared with autograft. Torsional and bending strength are weakened most, but compressive strength is also affected (41,42). Allograft carries a risk of transmitting infection from donor to host. Fresh-frozen bone caused two cases of human immunodeficiency virus (HIV) transmission in the earliest stages of the AIDS epidemic. In the past decade, screening of donors has been rigorous, including testing for hepatitis B and hepatitis C and polymerase chain reaction testing for HIV. With current screening, the risk of transmission of HIV from fresh-frozen allograft bone is probably less than 1 in a million (43,44).

The major practical advantage of autograft bone is that it has been clearly shown to yield very high fusion rates. The fusion rate of iliac crest bone autograft is well documented. Over the past four decades, numerous studies have shown the rate of fusion for a single noninstrumented level with iliac crest autograft to be just below 90% (16,35,45). Several authors have modified the Smith-Robinson technique and have increased fusion rates for a single level to around 95% (46,47). It is not clear that the increased fusion rate translated into improved clinical success. The modified technique described by Brodke and Zdeblick (46) also had good success with multilevel fusions. In this group of patients, 30 of 32 double-level and 5 of 6 triple-level fusions were successful. Autograft iliac crest deserves to be called the gold standard grafting material for anterior column support in the cervical spine (48).

Allograft bone has been used in cervical fusion for a number of years, and significant clinical experience with this technique has been developed. In 1999, Martin et al. (49) reviewed a single surgeon's experience with 317 consecutive patients who received freeze-dried fibula for one- to three-level surgery. All surgeries were done for degenerative spondylosis and all were without instrumentation. Of the 319 patients, 289 (91%) had 2 years follow-up and were included in the study group. Lucency at any level classified a case as a nonunion. The overall fusion rate was 88%, with 90% of single-level cases, 72% of two-level cases (13 of 18), and 0% (0 of 2) of three-level cases achieving fusion. This study suggests that two-level cases have a higher nonunion rate, but the number of two-level cases was too small for the difference to reach statistical significance.

In an earlier study with smaller numbers, Zdeblick and Ducker (50) compared patients with iliac crest allograft to those undergoing an identical Smith-Robinson procedure using iliac crest autograft. These authors also found a high single-level allograft fusion rate of 95% that compares favorably with the better-published rate for autograft (and was identical to the fusion rate for their autograft group). Similar to Martin et al., they found that the fusion rate drops off significantly with two-level procedures: Autograft two-level fusion rate was 95%, whereas allograft two-level fusion rate was 83%. It appears that allograft fibula or iliac crest is equivalent to autograft bone for single-level surgery. For noninstrumented fusions involving multiple levels, autograft iliac crest is the graft choice with the best track record in the literature.

A further controversy with respect to the anterior approach centers on the use of instrumentation in the setting of anterior fusions. As discussed earlier, the fusion rate for multilevel cervical surgery has been high. This has led surgeons to postulate that the addition of instrumentation might increase these rates. In 1991, Fernyhough et al. (51) reported on 126 cases of multilevel discectomy and vertebrectomy, comparing allograft fibula with autograft fibula used without plating. They found that the nonunion rate was high in both groups: 27% for autograft and 41% for allograft. The nonunion rate was significantly higher for allograft than for autograft, but the authors felt that lack of rigid stabilization contributed to the high nonunion rate in both groups.

Subsequent studies suggest that the addition of plating increases the success rate of multilevel cervical fusions. Shapiro et al. (52) reported on 246 consecutive patients who underwent ACF with allograft fibula and plating and compared them with 111 consecutive patients with autologous iliac crest grafts without plating. They found that 99.6% of the patients with allograft and locking plate had documented fusion at an average follow-up of 5 years. Connolly et al. (53) reported in 1996 on a series of 43 patients treated surgically for cervical spondylosis with Smith-Robinson discectomy and fusion using iliac crest autograft. Group I consisted of 25 consecutive surgical cases using the Morscher titanium hollow screw plate system. Group II consisted of 18 cases performed without plate fixation. The fusion rate of the single-level fusions was 100% with plating and 88% without plating. However, the clinical success of the two groups was similar, with the plated group having a slightly lower success rate. Despite the fact that the overall clinical results were not significantly different between the two groups, some trends did emerge. The authors found that the fusion rate for multilevel fusions was better in the group of patients receiving plate fixation. They also found that the overall complication rate of multilevel fusion surgery, which they defined as pseudoarthrosis plus delayed union plus graft collapse, was lower in the group of patients receiving anterior plate fixation. Their report suggested that anterior plate fixation might decrease the complication rate in multilevel fusions.

Wang et al. (54–56) have published a series of reports detailing the effect of cervical plating on one-, two- and three-level anterior cervical discectomy and fusions. Their group first reported on the effect of cervical plating on one-level surgeries (54). They compared outcomes in 80 patients treated with single-level anterior cervical discectomy and fusion. Forty-four had cervical plates, while 36 did not. The authors reported a fusion rate of 42 of 44 with plating and 33 of 36 without plating. The group with plating had a slightly higher clinical success rate and a slightly lower incidence of graft subsidence and kyphosis; however, none of these differences was either statistically or clinically significant. The addition of plating did not increase the complication rate of the procedure.

Wang et al. (55) next reported on the effect of plating on two-level anterior cervical discectomy and fusion. This report detailed 60 patients undergoing anterior discectomy and fusion at two levels. Thirty-two were plated, and 28 were not. At a mean 2.7 years follow-up, the pseudoarthrosis rates were significantly different in the two groups. There was no pseudoarthrosis in the 32 plated patients, and there were 7 cases in the 28 patients who were not plated. In contrast to the findings in single-level surgeries, there was significantly decreased collapse and significantly decreased kyphosis in the plated group versus the nonplated group. The authors found no complications related specifically to the plating. Most recently (56), this group reported on 59 patients who underwent three-level anterior cervical discectomy and fusion for spondylosis at a mean 3.2 year follow-up. The nonunion rate in the plated group was 7 of 40 (18%), and the nonunion rate in the nonplated group was 7 of 19 (37%). Thus, fusion rate was improved with the use of a plate, although the number of patients was not large enough to allow significance. As in their other groups, there were no complications specific to the plate itself. These studies add to the body of literature that suggests that anterior cervical plate fixation is a safe way of decreasing complication rates in multilevel anterior cervical fusions. In contrast, the plating of single-level surgeries has not been shown to improve outcomes, although it has been associated with a slight trend toward lower nonunion rates.

POSTERIOR APPROACH FOR RADICULOPATHY

Posterior surgery for treatment of cervical radiculopathy is well reported in the literature (Fig. 9.5) (57–72). Numerous authors have documented the efficacy of the posterior approach in the treatment of lateral disc herniations and osteophytes causing nerve root compression within the neural foramen. There appears to be agreement in the literature that radiculopathy caused by central or paracentral disc herniations or osteophytes is best treated by anterior decompression. The treatment of lateral herniations or osteophytes is more controversial, and there are proponents of both the anterior and the posterior approaches.

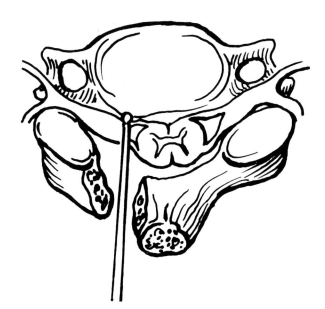

FIGURE 9.5. The posterior foraminotomy allows decompression of the nerve root and removal of an accessible disc herniation.

The posterior approach used for decompression of the nerve root is the lamino-foraminotomy. If a lesion lies within the axilla of the nerve root or lateral to the axilla, it can be reached via this approach. If the lesion lies medial to the axilla, most authors agree that a posterior approach is not indicated (57,58,60,65). The reason for this is simply that medial retraction of the dura is necessary in order to access a central disc or osteophytic lesion. This retraction causes compression of the cord and undue risk of iatrogenic neurologic injury. Thus, the anterior approach is preferred for removal of central disc herniations.

For a disc herniation lying within the axilla of the nerve root or lateral to the axilla, many authors do recommend a posterior approach (57–59,62,63,66–68,72). A lamino-foraminotomy with gentle retraction of the nerve root will allow access to the anterior pathology for removal of soft disc herniation or uncovertebral osteophyte.

The advantage of the posterior approach is that it does not require fusion of the motion segment and therefore preserves motion at the operative level. Numerous authors have described their operative technique, and most emphasize preservation of the facet joint as the key to maintaining stability at the operative level. Most state that with proper technique a laminotomy can be combined with a medial facetectomy that involves more undercutting of the anterior aspect of the facet joint than actual removal of facet joint (57–59,62,63,66–68,72). This allows preservation of the mechanical integrity of the joint. Zdeblick et al. (71) demonstrated *in vitro* that mechanical stability is lost if more than 50% of the facet joint is removed in the performance of this operation. However, they demonstrated in the same study that at least 25% of the joint can be removed without sacrificing stability at that level. This validates the recommendation of the authors, who suggest a laminoforaminotomy that only removes the medial edge of the facet joint and then proceeds with undercutting the remainder of the facet without actually violating the capsule or articulation any further.

Zeidman and Ducker (72) give an excellent summary of the technical requirements of successful posterior cervical laminoforaminotomy. They describe their methods of handling the rich venous plexus surrounding the axilla of the nerve root, which is commonly encountered during this approach. This venous plexus raises the possibility of significant bleeding, in addition to a risk for embolization of air. Zeidman and Ducker, as well as other authors, recommend that this surgery be performed with the patient in the sitting position to maximize venous drainage and cut down problems with epidural bleeding (58,63,67,72). This does lead to an increased relative risk of air embolism, and numerous techniques are advocated for intraoperative diagnosis and treatment of air embolism. Zeidman and Ducker (72) recommend precordial Doppler monitoring to listen for air. More aggressive monitoring has been suggested—such as transthoracic echocardiogram to allow visualization and intraatrial catheterization to allow diagnosis and removal of air in the heart—but most authors agree that routine use of such measures is unnecessary as long as the surgical team aggressively monitors the clinical status of the patient (57,58,63,67,72). Not surprisingly, the reported rate of air embolism seems to be highest in those groups that monitor aggressively for it; however, it is rarely reported to be clinically significant.

Posterior surgery for radiculopathy has been carried out for many decades in North America. As a result, there are a number of series with large numbers of patients and sufficient postoperative follow-up. These studies show that this approach can be extremely effective in treating radiculopathy. For example, Henderson et al. (63) published, in 1983, their experience with 846 consecutive cases performed from 1963 to 1980 with a mean follow-up of about 2.5 years. They found that 91% of patients self-reported good to excellent postoperative relief of symptoms. They found no difference in outcome between patients with hard disc and those with soft disc herniations. Williams (67) reported his results in 235 patients with 585 symptomatic levels. He found 100% had complete pain relief, with only a 1% recurrence rate. Zeidman and Ducker (72) reported on 172 patients operated on over a 7-year period. They reported 97% pain relief at final follow-up. Numerous other smaller series have been published, and most have found similarly high rates of pain relief (57,61,62,66,68,70).

The posterior approach involves a more direct confrontation with the neurologic structures than does a Smith-Peterson anterior surgery and therefore raises concerns of increased risk of neurologic injury. The major risk of neurologic injury is due to retraction of the cord and development of cord injury. Central cord syndrome has been reported, and any surgeon undertaking this approach must apprise patients of this risk (72). Many authors have presented sizable series of posterior approaches that suggest that the incidence of severe iatrogenic neurologic changes, although small, is slightly higher with this approach than with the standard anterior approaches, even in the most experienced hands (63,67,72).

There are clearly advantages and disadvantages of both the anterior and the posterior approaches for the treatment of radiculopathy, and there are ample retrospective studies that describe good results with both approaches in large series of patients. A few studies attempt to directly compare the two prospectively in a well-matched group of patients. Herkowitz et al. (65) reported a prospective study in which 28 patients with cervical soft disc herniations underwent anterior discectomy and fusion, while 16 underwent posterior laminotomy-foraminotomy. The authors operated on all central disc herniations via an anterior approach. Seventeen patients with single-level lateral soft disc herniations underwent surgery via an anterior approach, while 16 patients with the same diagnosis underwent surgery via the posterior approach. The authors found a higher rate of excellent to good results in the anterior group: 16 of 17 (94%), compared with 12 of 16 (75%). The authors argue that the posterior approach should be reserved for revision cases or for patients with disc herniations at levels that are difficult to access from the front.

In summary, the posterior approach for spondylotic radiculopathy appears to have an excellent success rate for relief of radicular arm pain. It removes the need for fusion and also eliminates the potential complications of the anterior approach. Posterior surgery, however, has a slightly higher risk of serious intraoperative neurologic complications, specifically central cord syndrome, compared with the anterior surgery. The spinal surgeon treating this disease process should be competent in both approaches and should choose the appropriate approach for each individual patient.

LAMINECTOMY VERSUS LAMINOPLASTY FOR CERVICAL SPONDYLOTIC MYELOPATHY

The role of the isolated posterior cervical laminectomy in the treatment of cervical spondylotic myelopathy is controversial because the occurrence of postoperative kyphosis and its concomitant morbidity is quite high with isolated laminectomy (Fig. 9.6). Kaptain et al. (73) reported that 21% of their patients with laminectomy had kyphotic deformity postoperatively. Patients with normal preoperative alignment have the lowest risk, while those with preoperative kyphosis have the highest risk of progressive kyphotic deformity. Skeletal immaturity at the time of laminectomy is a large risk factor for the development of kyphosis (74). The rate of reported kyphosis after multiple laminectomies in children varies between studies, but most report at least one-third of patients, and many higher. Bell et al. (75), for example, reported an incidence of 37%. Another risk factor for the development of kyphosis is aggressive resection of the facet joints at the level of the laminectomy. Nowinski et al. (76) examined the biomechanical effect of resecting portions of the facet in a cadaveric laminectomy model. They found that resection of 25% or more of the facet adversely affects stability in the sagittal plane. These data are confirmed by clinical studies of the role of facetectomy in postoperative kyphotic deformity. Herkowitz (64) found a 25% incidence of postoperative kyphotic deformity in patients with bilateral facetectomy. Clinically, postoperative kyphosis presents as delayed onset of postoperative sagittal plane decompensation, neck pain, fatigue, and, frequently, neurologic progression (77). The surgical correction of postlaminectomy kyphosis—generally by anterior or combined anterior and posterior revision—is well described, with all authors suggesting that prevention of deformity should be the primary goal of treatment (77–79).

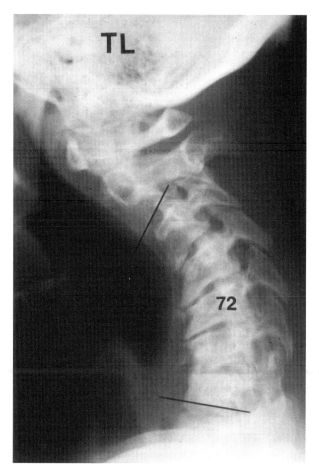

FIGURE 9.6. Radiograph demonstrating postlaminectomy kyphosis of the cervical spine.

Combining posterior fusion with cervical laminectomy appears to prevent the development of postoperative kyphosis. Kumar et al. (80) reviewed 25 patients treated for cervical spondylotic myelopathy with laminectomy and fusion with lateral mass instrumentation using lateral mass plates. There were no cases of late kyphosis and no cases of neurologic deterioration. This is a study of a small group of patients, with no control group. However, the patients were followed closely for almost 4 years and they demonstrated reasonably good outcomes on standard outcome scales. The results in this group were similar to those published for anterior decompression and fusion for the same diagnosis (81). Successful results have been reported with laminectomy and fusion using various other techniques, such as cervical pedicle screws, cervical Luque wires, and Luque rectangle, as well as noninstrumented fusion with anchoring of the laminae to the lateral masses (82–84). All of these techniques afford resistance to the distraction of the posterior column, which can otherwise result in kyphosis in the postlaminectomy patient without fusion.

Anterior cervical decompression and fusion and posterior laminectomies with fusion are both considered reasonable treatment options for a patient with cervical spondylotic myelopathy. A third treatment option for these patients is the use of cervical laminoplasty. Laminoplasty was developed in Japan in response to the poor results with isolated laminectomy. The concept of laminoplasty is to expand the epidural canal while leaving the facet joints intact and functional. Thus, laminoplasty is designed to both prevent late kyphotic deformity as well as retain motion throughout the operative levels. The North American literature has a good number of reports from Japan of the clinical efficacy of laminoplasty (85–89). There have been fewer reports of the North American results, but some centers have built up considerable experience and have results rivaling those in the Japanese literature (90–92). Lee et al. (91) reviewed the results of 105 patients with a modified cervical laminoplasty. They were evaluated with at least 6 months' follow-up and a mean follow-up of 18 months. The authors found no cases of segmental instability and no evidence of recurrent stenosis. Edwards et al. (90) reported their results with 18 patients who underwent laminoplasty with a threaded T-saw. They found that none of their patients had worsening of neurologic symptoms. Bladder and bowel symptoms resolved in 5 of 6 patients, while approximately two-thirds had improvement of motor deficits. Two of the 18 patients developed small kyphotic deformities; one patient had a C5 deficit that developed in the first 24 hours after the procedure. The patient with the C5 deficit had complete loss of deltoid function and motion in the biceps, but not against gravity.

Baisden et al. (93) studied a laminoplasty model in the goat by performing laminectomies on five and laminoplasty on five. It was noted that in the laminectomy group there was a progressive kyphosis, with a 70% decrease in the normal curvature. The laminoplasty group showed no change in its lordotic curvature. Sagittal plane laxity was increased in the animals with laminectomy, whereas it remained normal in the animals with laminoplasty. This study provides a reasonable rationale for the claims made that laminoplasty preserves motion without creating segmental instability.

There has been some attempt in the North American literature to compare the efficacy of laminoplasty with other forms of surgical treatment for cervical myelopathy (94–96). Heller et al. (95) reviewed the results of 13 patients who underwent laminoplasty and paired them in matched sets with patients who underwent laminectomy and fusion. These patients were examined 2 years after surgery. There were no complications in the laminoplasty group, whereas the laminectomy and fusion group had numerous complications, such as progression of myelopathy, nonunion, instrumentation failure, development of kyphosis, and transition syndrome.

In summary, laminoplasty can compare favorably to posterior decompression and fusion for cervical spondylotic myelopathy. Published reports of postoperative kyphosis or radicular injury reinforce that the surgeon must be familiar with the technical requirements of the procedure. The spinal surgeon treating cervical spondylotic myelopathy should be competent in more than one approach to this difficult problem; this will allow the surgeon to perform the procedure that best fits the needs of each individual patient.

REFERENCES

1. Spurling R. Lateral rupture of the cervical intervertebral discs. *Surg Gynecol Obstet* 1944;78: 350–358.
2. Viikari-Juntura E, Porras M, Laasonen EM. Validity of clinical tests in the diagnosis of root compression in cervical disc disease. *Spine* 1989;14:253–257.
3. Hasue M. Pain and the nerve root: an interdisciplinary approach. *Spine* 1993;18:2053–2058.
4. Marshall LL, Trethewie ER, Curtain CC. Chemical radiculitis: a clinical, physiological, and immunological study. *Clin Orthop* 1977;129:61–67.
5. Saal JS, Franson RC, Dobrow R, et al. High levels of inflammatory phospholipase activity in lumbar disc herniations. *Spine* 1990;15:674–678.
6. Parke W. Correlative anatomy of cervical spinal myelopathy. *Spine* 1988;13:831–837.
7. Mannen T. Vascular lesions in the spinal cord of the aged. *Geriatrics* 1966;21:151–160.
8. Taylor A. Vascular factors in the myelopathy associated with cervical spondylosis. *Neurology* 1964; 14:62–68.
9. Jellinger K. Spinal cord arterioscleroses and progressive vascular myelopathy. *J Neurol Neurosurg Psychiatry* 1967;30:195–206.
10. Robinson R, Smith G. Anterolateral cervical disc removal and interbody fusion for cervical disc syndrome. *Bull Johns Hopkins Hosp* 1955;96:223–224.
11. Cloward R. The anterior approach for removal of ruptured cervical disks. *J Neurosurg* 1958;15: 602–617.
12. Albert TJ, Murrell S. Surgical management of cervical radiculopathy. *JAAOS* 1999;7:368–376.
13. Whitecloud T, Werner J. Cervical spondylosis and disc herniation: the anterior approach. In: Frymoyer J, ed. *The adult spine: principles and practice,* 2nd ed. Philadelphia: Lippincott–Raven Publishers, 1997:1357–1379.
14. Clements D, O'Leary P. Anterior cervical discectomy and fusion. *Spine* 1990;15:1023–1025.

15. Mosdal C. Cervical osteochondrosis and disc herniation. Eighteen years' use of interbody fusion by Cloward's technique in 755 cases. *Acta Neurochir* 1984;70:207–225.
16. Bohlman HH, Emery SE, Goodfellow DB, et al. Robinson anterior cervical discectomy and arthrodesis for cervical radiculopathy. *J Bone Joint Surgery Am* 1993;75:1298–1307.
17. Robinson R, Walker A, Ferlic D, et al. The results of anterior interbody fusion of the cervical spine. *J Bone Joint Surgery Am* 1962;44:1569–1587.
18. Emery SE, Bohlman HH, Bolesta MJ, et al. Anterior cervical decompression and arthrodesis for the treatment of cervical spondylotic myelopathy. Two to seventeen-year follow-up. *J Bone Joint Surgery* 1998;80:941–951.
19. Bernard TN Jr, Whitecloud TS III. Cervical spondylotic myelopathy and myeloradiculopathy. Anterior decompression and stabilization with autogenous fibula strut graft. *Clin Orthop Related Res* 1987:149–160.
20. Ebersold MJ, Pare MC, Quast LM. Surgical treatment for cervical spondylitic myelopathy. *J Neurosurg* 1995;82:745–751.
21. Yonenobu K, Hosono N, Iwasake M, et al. Neurologic complications of surgery for cervical compression myelopathy. *Spine* 1991;16:1277–1282.
22. Hirsch C. Cervical disc rupture: diagnosis and therapy. *Acta Orthop Scand* 1960;30:172–186.
23. Bertalanffy H, Eggert H. Clinical long-term results of anterior discectomy without fusion for treatment of cervical radiculopathy and myelopathy. A follow-up of 164 cases. *Acta Neurochir* 1988;90:127–135.
24. Bertalanffy H, Eggert H. Complications of anterior cervical discectomy without fusion in 450 consecutive patients. *Acta Neurochir* 1989;99:41–50.
25. Cuatico W. Anterior cervical discectomy without interbody fusion: an analysis of 81 cases. *Acta Neurochir* 1981;57:269–274.
26. Dunsker S. Anterior cervical discectomy with and without fusion. *Clin Neurosurg* 1977;24:516–521.
27. Kelft EVd, Vyve Mv, Selosse P. Postsurgical follow-up by MRI of anterior cervical discectomy without fusion. *Eur J Radiol* 1992;15:196–199.
28. Martins A. Anterior cervical discectomy with and without interbody bone graft. *J Neurosurg* 1976;44:290–295.
29. Maurice-Williams R, Dorward N. Extended anterior cervical discectomy without fusion: a simple and sufficient operation for most cases of cervical degenerative disease. *Br J Neurosurg* 1996;10:261–266.
30. Rosenorn J, Hansen E, Rosenorn M. Anterior cervical surgery with and without fusion. A prospective study. *J Neurosurg* 1983;59:252–255.
31. Savitz M. Anterior cervical discectomy without fusion or instrumentation: 25 years' experience. *Mt Sinai J Med* 2000;67:314–317.
32. Watters W, Levinthal R. Anterior cervical discectomy with and without fusion. Results, complications, and long-term follow-up. *Spine* 1994;19:2343–2347.
33. Wilson D, Campbell D. Anterior cervical discectomy without bone graft. Report of 71 cases. *J Neurosurg* 1977;47:551–555.
34. Yamamoto I, Ikeda A, Shibuya N, et al. Clinical long term results of anterior discectomy without interbody fusion for cervical disc disease. *Spine* 1991;16:272–279.
35. Depalma A, Rothman R, Lewinnek G, et al. Anterior interbody fusion for severe cervical disk degeneration. *Surg Gynecol Obstet* 1972;134:755–758.
36. Schnee C, Freese A, Weil R, et al. Analysis of harvest morbidity and radiographic outcome using autograft for anterior cervical fusion. *Spine* 1997;22:2222–2227.
37. Emery S, Heller J, Petersilge C, et al. Tibial stress fracture after a graft has been obtained from the fibula: a report of five cases. *J Bone Joint Surg Am* 1996;78:1248–1251.
38. Vail T, Urbaniak J. Donor site morbidity with use of vascularized autogenous fibular grafts. *J Bone Joint Surg Am* 1996;78:204–211.
39. Bos GD, Goldberg VM, Powell AE, et al. The effect of histocompatibility matching on canine frozen bone allografts. *J Bone Joint Surg* 1983;65:89–96.
40. Goldberg VM, Stevenson S. Natural history of autografts and allografts. *Clin Orthop Related Res* 1987:7–16.
41. Pelker RR, Friedlaender GE. Biomechanical aspects of bone autografts and allografts. *Orthop Clin North Am* 1987;18:235–239.
42. Pelker RR, Friedlaender GE, Markham TC. Biomechanical properties of bone allografts. *Clin Orthop Related Res* 1983:54–57.
43. Musculoskeletal Transplant Foundation. Donor services: screening and testing [online]. 2002. Available at: http://www.mtf.org/tissueservices/process.html. Accessed March 9, 2002.
44. Asselmeier M, Caspari R, Bottenfield S. A review of allograft processing and sterilization techniques and their role in transmission of the human immunodeficiency virus. *Am J Sports Med* 1993;21:170–175.
45. Riley L, Robinson R, Johnson K, et al. The results of anterior interbody fusion of the cervical spine. *J Neurosurg* 1969;30:127–33.

46. Brodke DS, Zdeblick TA. Modified Smith-Robinson procedure for anterior cervical discectomy and fusion. *Spine* 1992;17:S427–S430.
47. Emery SE, Bolesta MJ, Banks MA, et al. Robinson anterior cervical fusion comparison of the standard and modified techniques. *Spine* 1994;19:660–663.
48. Malloy K, Hilibrand A. Autograft versus allograft in degenerative cervical disease. *Clin Orthop Related Res* 2002;1:27–38.
49. Martin GJ Jr, Haid RW Jr, MacMillan M, et al. Anterior cervical discectomy with freeze-dried fibula allograft. Overview of 317 cases and literature review. *Spine* 1999;24:852–858; discussion 858–859.
50. Zdeblick TA, Ducker TB. The use of freeze-dried allograft bone for anterior cervical fusions. *Spine* 1991;16:726–729.
51. Fernyhough J, White J, LaRocca H. Fusion rates in multilevel cervical spondylosis comparing allograft fibula with autograft fibula in 126 patients. *Spine* 1991;16(suppl):S561–S564.
52. Shapiro S, Connolly P, Donnaldson J, et al. Cadaveric fibula, locking plate, and allogeneic bone matrix for anterior cervical fusions after cervical discectomy for radiculopathy or myelopathy. *J Neurosurg* 2000;95:43–50.
53. Connolly PJ, Esses SI, Kostuik JP. Anterior cervical fusion: outcome analysis of patients fused with and without anterior cervical plates. *J Spinal Disord* 1996;9:202–206.
54. Wang JC, McDonough PW, Endow K, et al. The effect of cervical plating on single-level anterior cervical discectomy and fusion. *J Spinal Disord* 1999;12:467–471.
55. Wang JC, McDonough PW, Endow KK, et al. Increased fusion rates with cervical plating for two-level anterior cervical discectomy and fusion. *Spine* 2000;25:41–45.
56. Wang JC, McDonough PW, Kanim LE, et al. Increased fusion rates with cervical plating for three-level anterior cervical discectomy and fusion. *Spine* 2001;26:643–646; discussion 646–647.
57. Adamson T. Microendoscopic posterior cervical laminoforaminotomy for unilateral radiculopathy: results of a new technique in 100 cases. *J Neurosurg* 2001;95:51–57.
58. Burke T, Caputy A. Microendoscopic posterior cervical foraminotomy: a cadaveric model and clinical application for cervical radiculopathy. *J Neurosurg* 2000;93:126–129.
59. Chen B, Natarajan R, An H, et al. Comparison of biomechanical response to surgical procedures used for cervical radiculopathy: posterior keyhole foraminotomy versus anterior foraminotomy and discectomy versus anterior discectomy with fusion. *J Spinal Disord* 2001;14:17–20.
60. Chestnut R, Abitbol J, Garfin SR. Surgical management of radiculopathy: indications, techniques and results. *Orthop Clin North Am* 1992;23:461–474.
61. Davis R. A long-term outcome study of 170 surgically treated patients with compressive cervical radiculopathy. *Surg Neurol* 1996;46:523–530.
62. Grieve J, Kitchen N, Moore A, et al. Results of posterior cervical foraminotomy for treatment of cervical spondylitic radiculopathy. *Br J Neurosurg* 2000;14:40–43.
63. Henderson C, Hennessy R, Shuey H, et al. Posterior-lateral foraminotomy as an exclusive operative technique for cervical radiculopathy: a review of 846 consecutively operated cases. *Neurosurgery* 1983;13:504–512.
64. Herkowitz H. A comparison of anterior cervical fusion, cervical laminectomy, and cervical laminoplasty for the surgical management of multiple level spondylotic radiculopathy. *Spine* 1988;13:774–780.
65. Herkowitz H, Kurz L, Overholt D. Surgical management of cervical soft disc herniation: a comparison between the anterior and posterior approach. *Spine* 1990;15:1026–1030.
66. Rodrigues M, Hanel R, Prevedello D, et al. Posterior approach for soft cervical disc: a neglected technique? *Surg Neurol* 2001;55:17–22.
67. Williams R. Microcervical foraminotomy: a surgical alternative for intractable radicular pain. *Spine* 1983;8:708–716.
68. Witzmann A, Hejazi N, Krasznai L. Posterior cervical foraminotomy. A followup study of 67 surgically treated patients with compressive radiculopathy. *Neurosurg Rev* 2000;23:213–217.
69. Woertgen C, Holzschuh M, Rothoerl R, et al. Prognostic factors of posterior cervical disc surgery: a prospective consecutive study of 54 patients. *Neurosurgery* 1997;40:724–728.
70. Woertgen C, Rothoerl R, Henkel J, et al. Long term outcome after cervical foraminotomy. *J Clin Neurosci* 2000;7:312–315.
71. Zdeblick TA, Zou D, Warden K, et al. Cervical stability after foraminotomy. *J Bone Joint Surg Am* 1992;74:22–27.
72. Zeidman S, Ducker TB. Posterior cervical laminoforaminotomy for radiculopathy: review of 172 cases. *Neurosurgery* 1993;33:356–362.
73. Kaptain G, Simmons N, Replogle R, et al. Incidence and outcome of kyphotic deformity following laminectomy for cervical spondylotic myelopathy. *J Neurosurg* 2001;93:199–204.
74. Cattell H, Clark G. Cervical kyphosis and instability following multiple laminectomies in children. *J Bone Joint Surg Am* 1977;59:991–1002.
75. Bell D, Walker J, O'Connor G, et al. Spinal deformity after multiple-level cervical laminectomy in children. *Spine* 1994;4:406–411.
76. Nowinski G, Heiko V, Dipl-Ing, et al. A biomechanical comparison of cervical laminoplasty and cervical laminectomy with progressive facetectomy. *Spine* 1993;18:1995–2004.

77. Albert TJ, Vacarro A. Postlaminectomy kyphosis. *Spine* 1998;23:2738–2745.
78. Heller J, Whitecloud TS III. Post-laminectomy instability of the cervical spine. In: Frymoyer J, ed. *The adult spine: principles and practice.* New York: Raven Press, 1991:1219–1239.
79. Herman J, Sonntag V. Cervical corpectomy and plate fixation for postlaminectomy kyphosis. *J Neurosurg* 1994;80:963–970.
80. Kumar V, Rea G, Mervis L, et al. Cervical spondylotic myelopathy: functional and radiographic long-term outcome after laminectomy and posterior fusion. *Neurosurgery* 1999;44:771–777.
81. Fessler R. Comments on: Cervical spondylotic myelopathy: functional and radiographic long-term outcome after laminectomy and posterior fusion. *Neurosurgery* 1999;44:778.
82. Abumi K, Kaneda K, Shono Y, et al. One-stage posterior decompression and reconstruction of the cervical spine by using pedicle screw fixation systems. *J Neurosurg* 1999;90:19–26.
83. Maurer P, Ellenbogen R, Ecklund J, et al. Cervical spondylotic myelopathy: treatment with posterior decompression and Luque rectangle bone fusion. *Neurosurgery* 1991;28:680–683.
84. Miyazaki K, Tada K, Matsuda Y, et al. Posterior extensive simultaneous multisegment decompression with posterolateral fusion for cervical myelopathy with cervical instability and kyphotic and/or S-shaped deformities. *Spine* 1989;14.
85. Hirabayashi K, Satomi K. Operative procedure and results of expansive open-door laminoplasty. *Spine* 1988;13:870–876.
86. Hirabayashi K, Toyama Y, Chiba K. Expansive laminoplasty for myelopathy in ossification of the longitudinal ligament. *Clin Orthop* 1999;359:35–48.
87. Kawano H, Handa Y, Ishii H, et al. Surgical treatment for ossification of the posterior longitudinal ligament of the cervical spine. *J Spinal Disord* 1995;8:145–150.
88. Kohno K, Kumon Y, Oka Y, et al. Evaluation of prognostic factors following expansive laminoplasty for cervical spinal stenotic myelopathy. *Surg Neurol* 1997;48:237–245.
89. Koshu K, Tominaga T, Yoshimoto T. Spinous process-splitting laminoplasty with an extended foraminotomy for cervical myelopathy. *Neurosurgery* 1995;37:430–435.
90. Edwards C, Heller J, Silcox. T-saw laminoplasty for the management of cervical spondylotic myelopathy. *Spine* 2000;25:1788–1794.
91. Lee T, Green B, Gromelski E. Safety and stability of open-door cervical expansive laminoplasty. *J Spinal Disord* 1998;11:12–15.
92. Lee T, Manzano G, Green B. Modified open-door cervical expansive laminoplasty for spondylotic myelopathy: operative technique, outcome and predictors for gait improvement. *J Neurosurg* 1997;86:64–68.
93. Baisden J, Voo L, Cusick J, et al. Evaluation of cervical laminectomy and laminoplasty. *Spine* 1999;24:1283–1293.
94. Edwards C, Heller J. Posterior approaches for the surgical treatment for multilevel cervical spondylotic myelopathy: laminoplasty versus laminectomy. *Curr Opin Orthop* 2001;12:224–230.
95. Heller J, Edwards C, Murakami H, et al. Laminoplasty versus laminectomy and fusion for multilevel cervical myelopathy. *Spine* 2001;20:1732–1734.
96. Hirabayashi K, Bohlman HH. Multilevel cervical spondylosis: laminoplasty versus anterior decompression. *Spine* 1995;20:1732–1734.

10

SURGICAL EXPOSURE AND DECOMPRESSION OF THE VERTEBRAL ARTERY

ALOK D. SHARAN
ALEXANDER R. VACCARO

The vertebral arteries provide the blood supply to the posterior circulation of the brain, the brainstem, and the spinal cord. The vertebral artery originates as a branch from the first portion of the subclavian artery and then ascends superiorly through the sixth cervical vertebrae within the transverse foramina (C6 through C1) into the foramen magnum, where it joins with its counterpart to form the basilar artery (1). The size of the vertebral artery ranges in diameter from 0.5 to 5.5 mm and in length from 5.0 to 35.0 cm (2). In 51% of cases the left vertebral artery is larger, and in 41% of cases the right vertebral artery is larger (2,3).

Berguer (4) classified the regional anatomy of the vertebral artery into four segments (Fig. 10.1). V1 is the proximal segment that extends from the subclavian origin to the level at which the artery enters the transverse foramen within the transverse process of C6. V2 is the interosseous segment where the artery courses through the transverse foramina within the transverse processes of C6 through C2. V3 is the segment that begins distal to C2 and terminates at the base of the skull. V4 is the final portion that begins at the atlantooccipital membrane and terminates at the basilar artery.

During anterior or anterolateral approaches to the cervical spinal cord and nerve roots, the vertebral artery is at risk, although rare, of inadvertent injury. The V2 segment of the vertebral artery is the most prone to accidental injury during these procedures. The management of an inadvertent vertebral artery injury during cervical spine surgery has been well documented in the literature (5,6). A thorough knowledge of the anatomy of the cervical spine in relation to the extracranial circulation as well as appropriate preoperative imaging studies illustrating the course of the vertebral vessels can help the spine surgeon avoid a vascular complication.

OVERVIEW OF ANATOMY

The vertebral artery enters the transverse foramen of the sixth cervical vertebra in 90% of cases, of the fifth cervical vertebra in 7%, and of the seventh cervical vertebra in 3% (7,10). It then runs superiorly through the cervical transverse foramina until it exits the first cervical vertebra prior to entering the foramen magnum. The artery is adjacent to the apophyseal joints of C6 to C3, and just lateral to the uncovertebral joints. This makes the artery prone to injury by compression, subluxation, or spondylosis at these joints (7). Running with the vertebral artery is the sympathetic nervous plexus and multiple venous plexuses.

A computed tomographic (CT) imaging study by Vaccaro et al. (8) found that the transverse foramina of the more cephalad vertebrae run more medially and posteriorly than the caudad vertebrae. This may potentially lead to a greater likelihood of injury

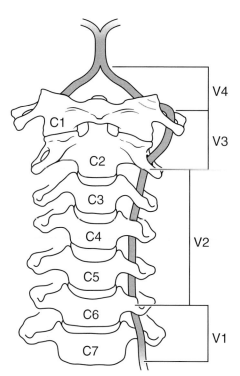

FIGURE 10.1. Anatomy of the vertebral artery and its four segments.

during decompression of the upper cervical vertebrae, especially when performing a foraminotomy or undercutting the lateral gutters during an anterior decompression.

INDICATIONS FOR VERTEBRAL ARTERY EXPOSURE AND DECOMPRESSION

The indications to expose or decompress the vertebral arteries have changed dramatically over time. Matas is credited with being the first surgeon to review his and previous surgeons' experience with vertebral artery surgery (9). Originally, vertebral artery surgery was performed for patients with traumatic bleeding from the artery or for repair of aneurysms (6,10). Today the primary indication for elective operations on the vertebral artery is to increase blood flow to the basilar territory of the brain in those patients with symptomatic vertebrobasilar ischemia (11). This limiting of blood supply is typically caused by either intrinsic or extrinsic factors, or both, affecting the vertebral artery at the V1 or V2 segment. Intrinsic factors include thrombotic embolization or atherosclerotic plaque formation. Extrinsic factors include compression by osteophytic spurs in the transverse foramen or compression by the longus colli tendon (12,13). Tendinous compression typically occurs when the vertebral artery aberrantly enters the bony canal at C4 or C5 instead of the normal C6 foramen. Accurate diagnosis of vertebral artery compression can only be made after an arteriogram is performed.

The V3 segment is most commonly affected by arterial dissections, arteriovenous fistulae, or arteriovenous aneurysms. This can lead to stenosis, thrombosis, or dilatation at this level requiring operative intervention. Once again, this can only be evaluated properly with an arteriogram.

LIMITATIONS

Exposure of the vertebral artery is typically performed at the V1 and V3 segments. Exposure of the artery within the V2 segment is difficult due to the bony covering of the transverse foramen. Fortunately, most pathology of the artery occurs at its proximal and distal segments. Injury to the vertebral artery during spinal surgery most commonly occurs when the operative surgeon decompresses too far laterally or is unaware of an aberrant coursing of the vertebral artery during cervical decompression.

PREOPERATIVE CONSIDERATIONS

Before surgery on the vertebral artery is performed electively, it is imperative that a complete angiogram be performed to accurately visualize the vertebral artery. Although rare, congenital anomalies of the vertebral arteries exist. Approximately 15% of patients have one hypoplastic vertebral artery; in 1.8% (right vertebral artery) and 3.1% (left vertebral artery), the vertebral artery does not communicate with the basilar artery (14,15). Therefore, ligation of these vessels would compromise the posterior circulation to the brain.

OPERATING ROOM SETUP AND NEEDED INSTRUMENTS

Operations on the vertebral artery are best performed with the patient under general anesthesia. The patient is positioned supine on the operating room table with the neck extended and rotated away from the planned incision.

Because of the risks for neurologic complications, intraoperative electroencephalographic monitoring is recommended, using compressed spectral analysis. Heparin is used intravenously before cross-clamping either the subclavian or vertebral artery. The instruments used are standard for vascular or cervical spine procedures. Gelfoam, Oxycel cotton, or bone wax should be available if the vertebral artery needs to be tamponaded.

TECHNIQUE GUIDE

Exposure of the V1 Segment of the Vertebral Artery

Exposure of the vertebral artery at its origin off of the subclavian artery is typically performed by surgeons to get proximal control of hemorrhage or for use as a bypass segment for arterial insufficiency. Traditionally, the exposure is accomplished using a supraclavicular or a vertical anterior cervical approach. The supraclavicular approach is used only when a limited exposure is needed of the proximal segment of the vertebral artery. The anterior cervical approach is a more practical approach to use when both proximal and distal access is needed of the vertebral artery (Fig. 10.2). This approach allows the surgeon to extend the incision for better exposure of a distal segment of the vertebral artery.

For the anterior cervical approach, the patient is placed on the operating table. The patient's neck is extended and rotated away from the planned incision site. An incision is made from the retromandibular area to the head of the clavicle, extending along the anterior border of the sternocleidomastoid muscle. This incision is then deepened through the platysma and fascia to expose the sternocleidomastoid muscle. The muscle needs to be dissected off the carotid sheath and retracted laterally. If the surgeon needs more exposure of the inferior aspect of the wound, the omohyoid muscle can be divided at this point. The carotid sheath is then dissected out by incising the fascia along the lateral border of the internal jugular vein. The sheath should be retracted medially, paying careful attention to the vagus nerve and sympathetic chain (Fig. 10.3). At this point the vertebral artery lies directly underneath the scalene fat pad and the anterior scalene muscle. The fat pad should be mobilized laterally by dissecting along its medial border. Careful attention should be given to the phrenic nerve as it crosses ventrally across the anterior scalene muscle. In addition, the inferior thyroid artery should be ligated and divided to give better exposure of the anterior scalene muscle. Retracting the muscle laterally at this point offers proper exposure of the proximal segment of the vertebral artery.

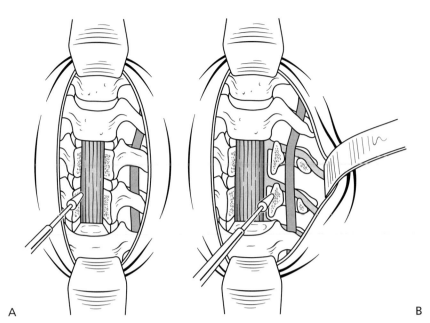

FIGURE 10.2. Anterior view of the cervical spine during a decompressive procedure. Note how easy it is to burr too far laterally during the decompression.

Exposure of the V2 Segment of the Vertebral Artery

The interosseous segment of the vertebral artery may be inadvertently exposed during cervical decompressive procedures. This may occur when the surgeon dissects too far lateral into the transverse foramen during burring of the vertebral body or removal of the

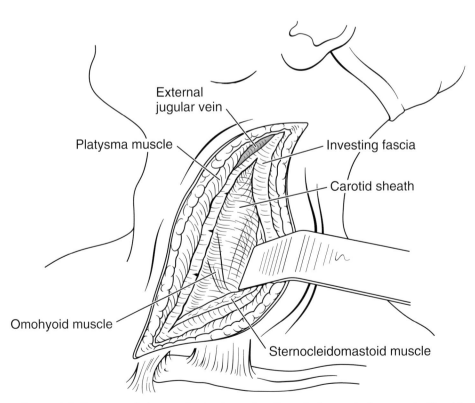

FIGURE 10.3. Exposure of the vertebral artery using the anterior cervical approach. The skin incision can be extended as distal as needed to get exposure of the entire vertebral artery.

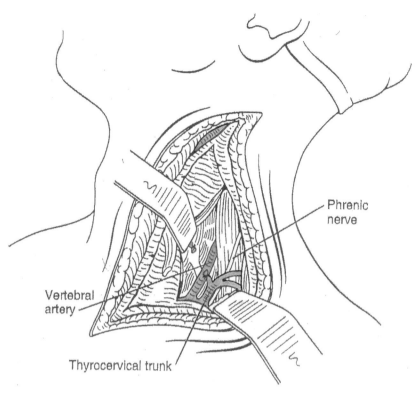

FIGURE 10.4. The carotid sheath has been retracted medially to give exposure of the vertebral artery.

intervertebral disc. If incidental penetration of the vertebral artery occurs, the vessel should be tamponaded with a combination of Gelfoam, Oxycel cotton, or bone wax, depending on the location of injury. Exposure of the artery can then be performed through the same surgical exposure (Smith-Robinson approach) by burring away the external bony boundaries of the transverse foramen above and below the level of injury (Figs. 10.4 and 10.5).

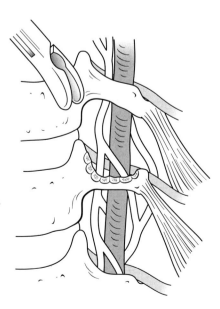

FIGURE 10.5. Removal of the bone at the transverse foramen allows for a direct exposure of the vertebral artery in the bony canal.

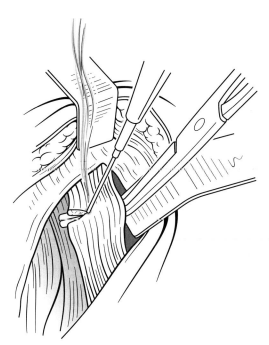

FIGURE 10.6. Division of the levator scapulae will reveal the vertebral artery underneath.

If an anterior exposure of the vertebral artery is required de novo, the standard Smith-Robinson approach to the cervical spine can be used from C2 to C6 (V2 segment). This approach involves placing the patient in a supine position on the operating table with the head turned slightly away from the side of the planned incision. The skin incision is made transversely within a neck crease at the level of the vertebral pathology. An incision in line with the skin incision is made through the fascial sheath overlying the platysma. Using blunt dissection, the platysma is split longitudinally. The sternocleidomastoid muscle is identified, and the deep cervical fascia overlying its medial border is incised longitudinally. The sternocleidomastoid muscle is retracted laterally while the sternohyoid and sternothyroid muscles are retracted laterally.

The carotid artery can now be palpated laterally within the incision. The pretracheal fascia is now incised medial to the carotid sheath, allowing the carotid artery along with the contents of the carotid sheath to be retracted laterally, with the trachea and esophagus retracted medially. This allows exposure of the cervical vertebral bodies and longus colli muscles. The longus colli muscles are then retracted laterally using a periosteal elevator. The vertebral artery itself can now be visualized between the transverse foramen. Complete exposure can then be obtained by removing the anterior wall of the transverse foramen using a small curette, rongeur, and Kerrison bone punch (Fig. 10.6).

Exposure of the V3 Segment of the Vertebral Artery

Exposure of the vertebral artery between C1 and C2 is typically performed by vascular surgeons to construct bypasses to this segment. The transverse processes of C1 and C2 are the widest in the cervical vertebrae, allowing the easiest access to the vertebral artery. The spine surgeon may have to access the vertebral artery in this region to get proximal control of bleeding that is distal to the first cervical vertebra. Ligation of the vertebral artery can be safely performed if adequate collateral circulation exists on the opposite side. This can be inferred by evaluating preoperative vascular angiography or magnetic resonance angiography to determine vessel size and collateral blood flow.

To expose the V3 segment of the vertebral artery, the patient is positioned supine on the operating table with the head turned away from the planned side of the incision. An incision is made from the level of the cricoid to the mastoid process, coursing anterior to the sternocleidomastoid muscle. The incision then proceeds through the platysma and deep cervical fascia as described previously, allowing the sternocleidomastoid muscle to be retracted laterally. The carotid sheath is identified and its contents are retracted medially. At this point the surgeon has the option of detaching the sternocleidomastoid muscle from the mastoid process, allowing for better exposure (5).

The next step involves the identification and retraction of the spinal accessory nerve anteriorly. This helps to identify the levator scapulae and the splenius cervicis muscles. These muscles cover the interspace between C1 and C2, where the vertebral artery is most accessible. The tip of the transverse process of C1 can be palpated deep to the digastric muscle. An incision is made through the prevertebral fascia posteriorly, from the transverse process of C1 running parallel to the spinal accessory nerve (16). Extending from the anterior border of the levator scapulae will be the anterior ramus of the C2 nerve root. A small retractor is placed between the nerve root and the levator scapulae and splenius cervicis muscles (17). These muscles can now be divided as close to the transverse process of C1 as possible, allowing exposure of the vertebral artery. Careful attention must be given to the C2 nerve root as it emerges posterior to the vertebral artery.

INTRAOPERATIVE AND POSTOPERATIVE COMPLICATIONS

Vertebral artery surgery has risks associated with it that are common to most vascular procedures. Because the artery is the main supply of blood to the posterior circulation of the brain, damage to it can be manifested as a cerebral ischemic event. Diaz and Ausman (18) reported on their results with 107 patients who underwent surgery on the vertebral artery. In their series, transient Horner's syndrome was the most common complication seen. Other complications due to vascular insult included quadriplegia and perioperative basilar infarction. Complications that occurred due to exposure included transient vocal cord paralysis from recurrent laryngeal nerve injury, phrenic nerve paresis, transient brachial plexus paralysis, pneumothorax, and injury to the thoracic duct. This last injury was manifested by the development of a lymphocele. If this occurs, a compression dressing can be applied over the leakage, and the patient should remain on intravenous fluids and be given a low-fat diet.

AVOIDING THE VERTEBRAL ARTERY DURING CERVICAL SPINE SURGERY

The vertebral artery is most prone to injury between the third and sixth cervical vertebrae. Surgeons are more likely to accidentally injure the vertebral artery in the more cephalad vertebrae due to its more medial and posterior location in this region. It is important that the surgeon maintain proper midline orientation while decompressing the cervical canal. We recommend using the borders of the longus colli muscles and uncovertebral joints to orient oneself to the limits of decompression, along with careful inspection of preoperative imaging studies to identify any aberrant coursing of the vertebral vessels. A marking pen can be used to mark the estimated midline of the vertebral body so that midline orientation is not lost when the longus colli muscles are retracted.

Smith et al. (19) suggested that the surgeon should decompress laterally in the subaxial spine to within approximately 3 mm of the medial border of the longus colli muscle. This would allow a 5-mm margin of safety between the foramen and the extent of lateral decompression. Unfortunately, this measurement cannot be used consistently for all cervical vertebrae because the transverse foramen moves more medially and posteriorly as it travels superiorly. The best method of safely avoiding the vertebral artery during anterior cervical spine surgery is through careful assessment of all preoperative imaging studies to carefully map out the coursing of this vessel.

REFERENCES

1. Daseler EH, Anson BJ. Surgical anatomy of the subclavian artery and its branches. *Surg Gynecol Obstet* 1959;108:149.
2. Hutchinson EC, Yates PO. The cervical portion of the vertebral artery. A clinico-pathological study. *Brain* 1956;79:319.
3. Carney AL. Vertebral artery surgery: historical development, basic concept of brain hemodynamics, and clinical experience of 102 cases. *Adv Neurol* 1981;30:249.
4. Berguer R. Vertebral artery reconstruction for vertebrobasilar insufficiency. In: Ernst CB, Stanley JC, eds. *Current therapy in vascular surgery.* Toronto: BC Decker; 1987:62
5. Golfinos JG, Dickman CA, Zabramski JM, et al. Repair of vertebral artery injury during anterior cervical decompression. *Spine* 1994;19(22):2552.
6. Pfeifer BA, Freidberg SR, Jewell ER. Repair of injured vertebral artery in anterior cervical procedures. *Spine* 1994;19(13):1471.
7. Brain L. Some unsolved problems of cervical spondylosis. *Br Med J* 1963;1:771.
8. Vaccaro AR, Ring D, Scuderi G, et al. Vertebral artery location in relation to the vertebral body as determined by two-dimensional computed tomography evaluation. *Spine* 1994;19(23):2637.
9. Matas R. Traumatisms and traumatic aneurysms of the vertebral artery and their surgical treatment, with a report of a cured case. *Am Surg* 1893;18:477.
10. Smythe AW. A case of successful ligature of the innominate artery. *New Orleans J Med* 1869;22:464.
11. Berguer R. Vertebrobasilar ischemia: indications, techniques, and results of surgical repair. In: Cronenwett JL, Gloviczki P, Johnston et al., eds. *Vascular surgery.* Philadelphia: WB Saunders, 2000:1823.
12. Nagashima C. Surgical treatment of vertebral artery insufficiency caused by cervical spondylosis. *J Neurosurg* 1970;32:512.
13. Sullivan HG, Harbison JW, Vines FS, et al. Embolic posterior cerebral artery occlusion secondary to spondylitic vertebral artery compression, case report. *J Neurosurg* 1975;43:618.
14. Golueke P, Sclafani S, Phillips T, et al. Vertebral artery injury—diagnosis and management. *J Trauma* 1987;27:856.
15. Thomas GK, Anderson KN, Hain RF, et al. The significance of anomalous vertebral basilar artery communications in operations on the heart and great vessels. *Surgery* 1959;46:747.
16. Henry AK. Sternomastoid eversion giving an exposure extensile to the vertebral artery. In: Henry AK, ed. *Extensile exposure.* Edinburgh: Churchill Livingstone, 1973:58.
17. Berguer R. Distal vertebral artery bypass: technique, the "occipital connection," and potential uses. *J Vasc Surg* 1985;2:621.
18. Ausman JI, Diaz FG, Vacca DF, et al. Posterior fossa revascularization. In: Schmidck HH, Sweet WH, eds. *Operative neurosurgical techniques: indications, methods, and results,* 2nd ed. Orlando: Grune & Stratton, 1988:807.
19. Smith MD, Emery SE, Dudly A, et al. Vertebral artery injury during anterior decompression of the cervical spine. *J Bone Joint Surg Br* 1993;75:410.

ANTERIOR DECOMPRESSION FOR RADICULOPATHY

BRADFORD L. CURRIER
CHOLL W. KIM

INDICATIONS FOR SURGERY

Disk degeneration proceeds in an age-related fashion. In young and middle-aged adults, tears in the annulus may lead to "soft" disc herniations (1). With time, disk height loss, ligamentum flavum hypertrophy, and facet and uncovertebral joint osteophyte formation contribute to stenosis of the spinal canal and neural foramen (2). These "hard disks" are most common in persons older than 55. Together, these constitute the major causes of cervical radiculopathy.

Nonsteroidal antiinflammatory agents, epidural steroid injections, and activity modification constitute the mainstay of initial treatment (3–5). Nonoperative care is often successful and should be tried for at least 6 to 12 weeks before considering surgery, unless pain or weakness is debilitating (1,2,6–8). Surgery is generally indicated when there is progressive motor loss or persistent disabling arm pain. Approximately one-third of patients with cervical radiculopathy will have persistent symptoms and may be considered surgical candidates (8). It is important to correlate clinical findings with imaging studies prior to undertaking surgery, because many asymptomatic persons have abnormal imaging studies (9).

BENEFITS AND LIMITATIONS

The pros and cons of anterior and posterior decompressions have been discussed in Chapter 9. The anterior approach provides excellent visualization of the pathology, and decompression can be accomplished without retracting neural elements.

Anterior procedures are best suited for one- or two-level disease. When performed at one level, satisfaction rates are over 90%, whereas at three levels the satisfaction rates drop to 50% to 85% (2). Central lesions are more safely decompressed anteriorly, whereas lateral lesions can be approached either anteriorly or posteriorly. The main advantage of the posterior approach for radiculopathy is that a fusion is generally not required. Laminoforaminotomy is a good option for lateral soft cervical disc herniations occurring in stable, well-aligned spines (10). The procedure is discussed in detail in Chapter 9.

Adding a fusion to an anterior cervical discectomy (ACDF) provides additional benefits. The bone graft can indirectly decompress the foramen, stabilize a loose interspace, and correct a kyphotic deformity. The fusion prevents formation of additional osteophytes and allows spurs that were left behind to resorb.

Anterior cervical discectomy (ACD) without fusion avoids the problems associated with bone graft, immobilization, and instrumentation (11,12). The procedure has been shown to be efficacious, with spontaneous fusion rates as high as 72% (13,14). However, until long-term prospective studies demonstrate results that are better or equivalent to ACDF, a fusion is recommended to avoid progressive neck pain, kyphosis, buckling of the ligamentum flavum, and continued segmental motion leading to osteophyte regrowth and recurrent stenosis (15).

Microsurgical anterior foraminotomy can be performed without complete discectomy or fusion if the radicular symptoms are caused by uncovertebral joint osteophytes or lateral disc herniation and the patient has minimal neck pain. The procedure has not gained wide acceptance because it is an unfamiliar technique requiring retraction of the vertebral artery. Furthermore, only small series with short follow-up and technical notes have been reported (16–21).

RECOMMENDED APPROACH

The standard anterior approach following a dissection plane medial to the carotid sheath allows excellent exposure to all levels from C3 to T1. This approach is applicable to any of the anterior decompressive techniques, including ACD, ACDF, and microsurgical foraminotomy.

SPECIFIC PREOPERATIVE CONSIDERATIONS

If a fusion is planned (which is recommended), the options of autograft versus allograft (22) as well as bracing and instrumentation should be discussed with the patient preoperatively.

If possible, patients should refrain from taking aspirin or other antiinflammatory agents that impair hemostasis for 10 days before the operation to avoid bleeding and the risk of epidural hematoma. Patients should be advised to discontinue smoking and antiinflammatory agents postoperatively to avoid the risk of nonunion.

The risks of surgery should be discussed, including death, paralysis, nerve root injury, infection, pseudarthrosis, persistent pain, spinal fluid leak, bleeding, transfusion complications, hardware failure, hoarseness, dysphagia, esophageal injury, stroke, and the need for additional surgery.

OPERATING ROOM SETUP

The imaging studies and preoperative notes should be available in the operating room. Position the patient supine on the operating table with a small pad placed between the scapulae to extend the neck slightly. Plan the incision by palpating bony and soft tissue landmarks and visualizing Langer's lines on the anterior aspect of the neck. If electrophysiologic monitoring is desired, consult the anesthesiologist concerning the choice of anesthetic agents and place the electrodes before the patient is prepped and draped.

NEEDED INSTRUMENTS AND IMAGING

A moderate number of specialized instruments are required for an anterior cervical decompression. Self-retaining retractors that are held in place by the longus colli muscle are indispensable for adequate exposure. A distraction system, based on vertebral body screws, can help to open the interspace slightly and may also serve to maintain the cephalad/caudad exposure. A high-speed burr is essential for thinning out osteophytes and preparing the vertebral endplates for the fusion. Small Kerrison rongeurs (1 and 2 mm) can be used for the decompression as long as the footplate portion of the instrument is thin and does not protrude significantly into the spinal canal. Small curettes in a variety of sizes and angles will allow bone and soft tissue to be removed with minimal pressure on the neural elements. Bipolar cautery and topical hemostatic agents are needed for achieving hemostasis.

Adequate lighting and magnification can be achieved with an operating microscope or with loupes and a headlight. If the operating microscope is preferred, most surgeons expose the spine and position the retractors before bringing the microscope into the field. The surgical technician can drape the microscope while the surgeon exposes the spine.

During the exposure, it is mandatory to identify the correct level with an intraoperative radiograph after placing a marking needle in a disc space. Some surgeons prefer to use a C-arm fluoroscopic unit, whereas others use a portable radiograph. If a C-arm is chosen, it can be incorporated into the drapes.

SPECIFIC BIOMECHANICAL CONSIDERATIONS

Anterior cervical foraminotomy and partial discectomy increases the segmental motion at the operated level more than posterior keyhole foraminotomy (23). In a three-dimensional nonlinear finite element model, anterior unilateral foraminotomy and removal of the adjacent annulus (30%) and endplate resulted in a large increase in motion compared with the intact segment. The greatest increases in range of motion occurred in lateral bending to the side of the foraminotomy (125% increase) and extension (50% increase). Primary motion in the other planes increased by 15% to 25%. Adding an anterior bone graft decreased the motion (compared with the intact spine) by 50% to 87% in all planes. The authors concluded that keyhole foraminotomy (with resection of 50% of the facet joint) and anterior discectomy with fusion do not destabilize the motion segment, whereas anterior foraminotomy and discectomy significantly destabilizes the spine (23). The model has several limitations. The anterior decompression procedure analyzed may have been more extensive than unilateral microscopic foraminotomy in the amount of annulus removed and more extensive than anterior discectomy in the amount of uncinate process removed. In addition, the study only addressed the changes in spine flexibility at the operated segment. Adding a bone graft to the discectomy increased the stiffness of the motion segment more than the intact state. The deleterious long-term effect on the adjacent segments caused by segmentally increasing the stiffness was not addressed (24).

TECHNIQUE GUIDE

A transverse skin incision, starting at the midline and curving laterally along Langer's lines to the anterior border of the sternocleidomastoid muscle, provides excellent exposure. It is cosmetically superior to a longitudinal incision. The platysma may be incised longitudinally, in line with its fibers, or transversely, in line with the incision. The latter option is faster, but the exposure is more extensile if subcutaneous planes are developed and the muscle is split longitudinally. Incise the deep cervical fascia along the medial edge of the sternocleidomastoid muscle, and the pretracheal fascia along the medial border of the carotid sheath. Blunt dissection demarcates the fascial planes and allows the exposure to be performed safely and rapidly. Sweep the prevertebral fascia off the anterior longitudinal ligament with a Kitner sponge to expose the longus colli muscle. Place a marking needle in the disc and take an intraoperative radiograph to identify the correct level. The longus colli muscle allows an initial determination of the midline.

After marking the midline at the appropriate disc and the adjacent vertebral bodies, elevate the longus colli muscle to the anterolateral aspect of the disc. Limit the dissection to the lateral border of the vertebral body to avoid injury to the vertebral artery, located between the transverse processes. Electrocautery or a periosteal elevator can be used for this maneuver, with care to avoid injury to the esophagus, vertebral artery, and carotid sheath structures (Fig. 11.1A,B). A rubber catheter may be used to cover all but the tip of the electrocautery, thus avoiding inadvertent injury to nearby structures. Place self-retaining, toothed, or smooth-tipped retractors below the longus colli muscle. Toothed blades stay in place more reliably but can injure surrounding soft tissue if allowed to slip

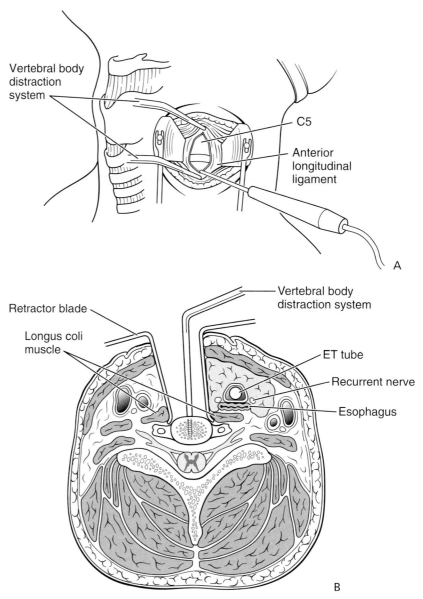

FIGURE 11.1. Cervical retractor. After deep dissection, self-retaining retractors are placed below the medial edges of the longus colli muscles to retract them laterally. The midline is carefully noted and marked with electrocautery. A vertebral body distraction system aids the decompression by opening the disc space **(A).** It is the author's preference to deflate and gently reinflate the endotracheal cuff once the retractors have been placed to decrease the risk of injury to the recurrent laryngeal nerve **(B).**

out from beneath the muscle. Blunt-tip blades are safer in this regard, but tend to slip out of position easily. The author's preference is to use toothed blades carefully placed below the longus colli muscle, with frequent monitoring of their position during the surgery. To decrease the pressure on the recurrent laryngeal nerve, lying between the trachea and the retracted longus colli muscle, the endotracheal tube cuff can be deflated and gently reinflated after the retractors are in place (25).

After placing the retractors, a vertebral body distraction system can be inserted by screwing midline posts into the vertebral bodies above and below the disc (Fig. 11.1). The system facilitates the decompression by gently distracting the interspace. If the screws are placed close to the endplates of the adjacent discs, there will be adequate room to perform the entire procedure, including fusion and instrumentation. The distraction screws also serve as soft tissue retractors and help keep the surgeon oriented relative to the midline.

ANTERIOR CERVICAL DISCECTOMY

An operating microscope or headlight and loupes are necessary to obtain adequate visibility. Remove the entire disk with curettes and a pituitary rongeur after first incising the annulus with a scalpel (Fig. 11.2). Avoid injury to the endplate, which may be soft in older individuals. Disrupting the endplate leads to unnecessary bleeding and may compromise the stability of a bone graft (26). The upward sloping uncinate processes of the caudal vertebrae clearly delineate the lateral borders of the disc space and are the most reliable landmark for identifying the midline. When treating radiculopathy by discectomy and fusion, it is generally not necessary to remove osteophytes, because they tend to resorb with time. If the nerve root is compressed by a bone spur, however, the osteophyte can be thinned out with a high-speed burr and then carefully pulled away from the dura with a small curette or thin foot plate Kerrison (Fig. 11.3).

The vertebral arteries lie just lateral to the uncinate processes and may be injured during foraminal decompression, particularly if the artery is tortuous (27). The distance between the lateral border of the uncinate process and the foramen transversarium is slightly greater in the lower cervical spine than at the upper levels (Table 11.1) (28,29).

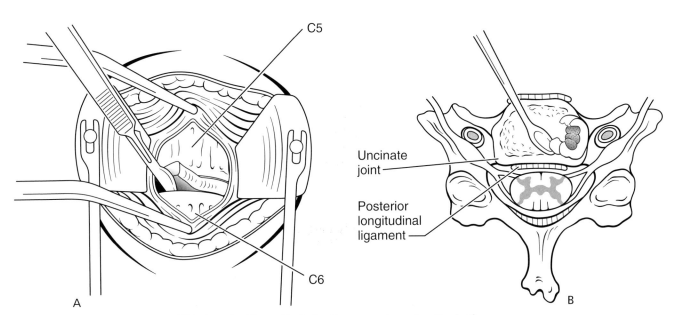

FIGURE 11.2. Discectomy. A no.15 blade scalpel is used to incise the exposed annulus. The knife blade should be directed away from the soft tissues laterally **(A).** The entire disc is excised using a pituitary rongeur, and the cartilaginous endplate is removed with a curette **(B).**

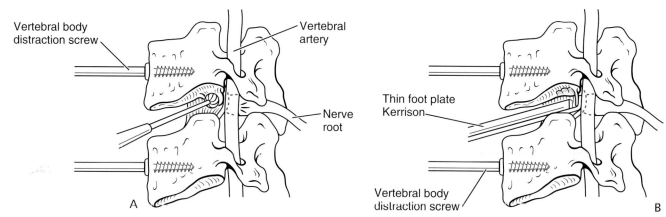

FIGURE 11.3. Osteophyte resection. If it is necessary to remove a bone spur compressing the nerve root, a high-speed burr may be used to thin the osteophyte. Avoid the vertebral artery, which lies just lateral to the midportion of the uncinate process **(A).** A thin-footplate Kerrison rongeur or curved curette may be used to complete the osteophyte removal **(B).**

The anterior/posterior location of the vertebral artery relative to the posterior corner of the vertebral body should be noted on the preoperative magnetic resonance imaging (MRI) or computed tomographic (CT) study. Consider this relationship when removing the posterior aspect of the uncinate process during foraminotomy. Use a small nerve hook to assess the foramen for stenosis or sequestered disc fragments. An epidural venous sinus surrounds the nerve root, and bleeding is often encountered when the foramen is explored. Bleeding can be controlled with a topical hemostatic agent and cottonoid patties. Avoid compressing the nerve root during foraminotomy by using instruments and techniques appropriate for the severity of stenosis. The pedicle of the vertebra below the disc space can be palpated with a small nerve hook and used as a guide to the foramen. It is not necessary to visualize the nerve root during the decompression, and it may be challenging to know when an adequate foraminotomy has been accomplished. Close scrutiny of the preoperative imaging studies and gentle palpation with the nerve hook guide the decision.

The posterior longitudinal ligament usually can be left intact unless a disc fragment is sequestered behind the ligament. Use a small nerve hook to palpate beneath the posterior longitudinal ligament; when necessary, use a thin-footplate Kerrison rongeur to excise the ligament.

Although some authors have reported good results with discectomy alone, we recommend fusing the interspace with bone graft and considering instrumentation as discussed earlier.

After the decompression and fusion have been completed, carefully remove the self-retaining retractors and inspect the esophagus and carotid sheath structures for evidence of injury. Obtain hemostasis, irrigate the wound, and close it in layers over a suction drain. Close the platysma and the subcutaneous tissue with 2–0 absorbable sutures and close the skin with a subcuticular suture.

TABLE 11.1. DISTANCE BETWEEN THE UNCINATE PROCESS AND THE FORAMEN TRANSVERSARIUM. IN MILLIMETERS (MM). ADAPTED FROM EBRAHEIM ET AL. (9).

	C3	C4	C5	C6	C7
Male	1.8	1.6	2.0	2.2	3.2
Female	1.6	1.2	1.6	2.2	3.4

UNCOFORAMINOTOMY

Approach the spine as described previously for an anterior discectomy. Elevate the longus colli muscle more extensively on the side of the neural compression. Expose the transverse processes above and below the affected disc space laterally and place a self-retaining retractor beneath the longus colli muscle (Fig. 11.4). Use a Penfield, curette, or Freer elevator to carefully dissect around the vertebral bodies, lateral to the uncinate process and between the transverse processes. Johnson and others place a table-mounted, malleable retractor lateral to the uncinate process to protect the vertebral artery and to maintain retraction of the ipsilateral longus colli muscle (19). They recommend lateral fluoroscopic imaging to place the retractor to the middle of the vertebral body to prevent compression of the nerve root posteriorly. Bring the operating microscope into the field and drill the lateral portion of the uncovertebral joint with a high-speed burr. Use a curette or thin-footplate Kerrison rongeur to remove the remaining posterior shell of bone and expose the lateral portion of the posterior longitudinal ligament. Excise all bone and soft tissue compressing the affected nerve root. A fusion is not routinely performed.

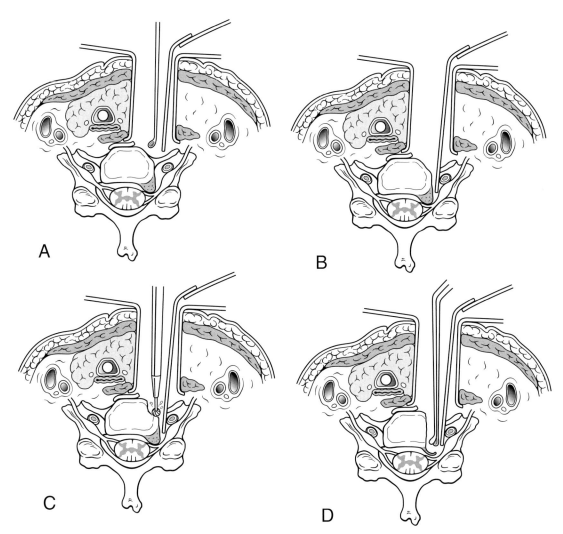

FIGURE 11.4. Uncoforaminotomy. The longus colli muscles are elevated and held in place with self-retaining anterior cervical retractors. The unilateral exposure is facilitated by a table-mounted malleable retractor system **(A).** The lateral aspect of the uncinate process is exposed. The malleable retractor protects the vertebral artery without compressing the nerve root **(B).** The lateral portion of the uncovertebral joint is drilled with a burr, leaving a thin posterior shell of bone over the nerve root **(C).** Disc, ligament, and bone are excised to decompress the nerve root **(D).** *Continued*

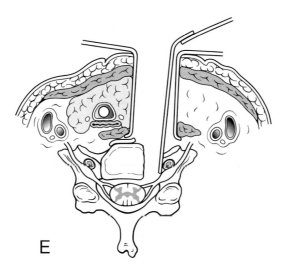

FIGURE 11.4. *(continued)* The remaining bone adjacent to the root is excised with a curette or thin-footplate Kerrison rongeur **(E)**. (Redrawn from Johnson JP, Filler AG, McBride DQ, et al. Anterior cervical foraminotomy for unilateral radicular disease. *Spine* 2000;25: 905–909, with permission.)

SPECIFIC POSTOPERATIVE MANAGEMENT ISSUES

One or two doses of antibiotics are recommended postoperatively to prevent infection. Drains are generally removed the day after surgery. Hoarseness and swallowing dysfunction may occur from neuropraxia of the recurrent laryngeal or superior laryngeal nerves and may necessitate consultation with an otolaryngologist. To prevent aspiration, the patient should be closely monitored for any swallowing difficulty when taking the first sip of water. Respiratory distress is uncommon but should alert the surgeon to the possibility of an expanding wound hematoma. Neurologic deterioration may occur secondary to intraoperative trauma, an epidural hematoma, or from migration of bone graft into the spinal canal. A plain radiograph and MRI or CT myelogram should be obtained promptly if there is any worsening of the patient's neurologic status.

Bracing with a hard or soft cervical collar is a matter of surgeon preference. The authors recommend a hard collar for 6 to 8 weeks when a single-level fusion is performed without instrumentation, and no immobilization when instrumentation is used. Isometric exercises can be instituted when the postoperative pain subsides, and range of motion exercises started when the graft has healed.

INTRAOPERATIVE COMPLICATIONS

Complications are uncommon during an anterior cervical decompression for radiculopathy. Neurologic deterioration, manifested by a decrease in amplitude or increase in latency on the somatosensory evoked potentials, can occur from bone graft compressing the spinal cord, overzealous segmental distraction, or direct trauma from instruments.

Injury to the vertebral artery is most likely to occur while using the burr laterally on the uncinate process (see Table 11.1). It is easy to become disoriented relative to the midline and stray too far to one side because of the lateral approach. The surgeon must identify the midline using the longus colli muscle and the uncinate processes and frequently reestablish orientation during the procedure. If the artery is injured, a topical hemostatic agent and direct pressure will stop the bleeding. It may be possible to repair or bypass the vessel, but ligation may be necessary.

The esophagus is a friable structure that can be easily damaged by a retractor, and an unrecognized esophageal tear can be disastrous. Always check the esophagus at the end of the procedure and primarily repair any defects that are identified. Consider asking a specialist for assistance, even for apparently simple esophageal repairs.

The carotid sheath encloses the carotid artery, internal jugular vein, and the vagus nerve. Although direct injury to any of these structures is very uncommon, prolonged or vigorous retraction of a plaque-filled carotid artery can lead to stroke.

The thoracic duct can be injured in left-sided approaches to the lower cervical spine. If a chyle leak is identified, the tear should be repaired.

The superior laryngeal and recurrent laryngeal nerves are at risk from excessive cephalad or caudal retraction, and the latter can also be compressed between the cervical retractors and the endotracheal tube cuff (discussed earlier). Injury to these structures, as well as the sympathetic chain (causing Horner's syndrome), will not be evident until the postoperative period.

Spinal fluid leakage is an uncommon problem during an anterior cervical decompression. Repair of a dural laceration is difficult because of the limited exposure afforded by the discectomy, but a watertight closure may be possible using microsurgical techniques (30). If a suture closure is not feasible, then fibrin glue placed posterior to the bone graft may suffice. The patient is placed on bed rest, with the head elevated, to decrease cerebrospinal fluid pressure on the repair.

Most intraoperative complications can be prevented by obtaining adequate exposure, insisting on excellent lighting, and using meticulous technique.

REFERENCES

1. Rothman R, Rashbaum R. Pathogenesis of signs and symptoms of cervical disc degeneration. *Instr Course Lect* 1978;27:203–215.
2. Truumees E, Herkowitz HN. Cervical spondylotic myelopathy and radiculopathy. *Instr Course Lect* 2000;49:339–360.
3. Bush K, Hillier S. Outcome of cervical radiculopathy treated with periradicular/epidural corticosteroid injections: a prospective study with independent clinical review. *Eur Spine J* 1996;5:319–325.
4. Heckman J, Lang CJ, Zobelein I, et al. Herniated cervical intervertebral discs with radiculopathy: an outcome study of conservatively or surgically treated patients. *J Spinal Disord* 1999;12:396–401.
5. Levine MJ, Albert TJ, Smith MD. Cervical radiculopathy: diagnosis and nonoperative management. *J Am Acad Orthop Surg* 1996;4:305–316.
6. DePalma AF, Rothman RH, Levitt RL, et al. The natural history of severe cervical disc degeneration. *Acta Orthop Scand* 1972;43:392–396.
7. Gore DR, Sepic SB, Gardner GM, et al. Neck pain: a long-term follow-up of 205 patients. *Spine* 1987;12:1–5.
8. Lees F, Turner J. Natural history and prognosis of cervical spondylosis. *Br Med J* 1963;11:1607–1610.
9. Boden SD, McCowin PR, Davis DO, et al. Abnormal magnetic-resonance scans of the cervical spine in asymptomatic subjects. A prospective investigation [see comments]. *J Bone Joint Surg Am* 1990;72:1178–1184.
10. Albert TJ, Murrell SE. Surgical management of cervical radiculopathy. *J Am Acad Orthop Surg* 1999;7:368–376.
11. Bertalanffy H, Eggert HR. Clinical long-term results of anterior discectomy without fusion for treatment of cervical radiculopathy and myelopathy: a follow-up of 164 cases. *Acta Neurochir* 1988;90:127–135.
12. Wirth FP, Dowd GC, Sanders HF, et al. Cervical discectomy: a prospective analysis of three operative techniques. *Surg Neurol* 2000;53:340–348.
13. Maurice-Williams RS, Dorward NL. Extended anterior cervical discectomy without fusion: a simple and sufficient operation for most cases of cervical degenerative disease. *Br J Neurosurg* 1996;10:261–266.
14. Murphy MG, Gado M. Anterior cervical discectomy without interbody bone graft. *J Neurosurg* 1972;37:71–74.
15. Yamamoto I, Ikeda A, Shibuya N, et al. Clinical long-term results of anterior discectomy without interbody fusion for cervical disc disease. *Spine* 1991;16:272–279.
16. Grundy PL, Germon TJ, Gill SS. Transpedicular approaches to cervical uncovertebral osteophytes causing radiculopathy. *J Neurosurg: Spine* 2000;93:21–27.
17. Hakuba A, Komiyama M, Tsujimoto T, et al. Transuncodiscal approach to dumbbell tumors of the cervical spinal canal. *J Neurosurg* 1984;61:1100–1106.

18. Jho HD. Decompression via microsurgical anterior foraminotomy for cervical spondylotic myelopathy. Technical note. *J Neurosurg* 1997;86:297–302.

19. Johnson JP, Filler AG, McBride DQ, et al. Anterior cervical foraminotomy for unilateral radicular disease. *Spine* 2000;25:905–909.

20. Kehr P, Lang G, Jung FM. Uncinectomy and uncoforaminectomy according to Jung. Technique, indications and results [in German]. *Langenbecks Arch Chir* 1976;341:111–125.

21. Kehr P, Lang G, Paternotte H, et al. Uncoforaminectomy of Jung in the management of osteoarthritis of the cervical spine and the post-traumatic cervical syndrome [in French]. *Int Orthop* 1979; 3:111–120.

22. Malloy KM, Hilibrand AS. Autograft versus allograft in degenerative cervical disease. *Clin Orthop* 2002;394:27–38.

23. Chen BH, Natarajan RN, An HS, et al. Comparison of biomechanical response to surgical procedures used for cervical radiculopathy: posterior keyhole foraminotomy versus anterior foraminotomy and discectomy versus anterior discectomy with fusion. *J Spinal Disord* 2001;14:17–20.

24. Hilibrand AS, Carlson GD, Palumbo MA, et al. Radiculopathy and myelopathy at segments adjacent to the site of a previous anterior cervical arthrodesis. *J Bone Joint Surgery Am* 1999;81: 519–528.

25. Apfelbaum RI, Kriskovich MD, Haller JR. On the incidence, cause, and prevention of recurrent laryngeal nerve palsies during anterior cervical spine surgery. *Spine* 2000;25:2906–2912.

26. Lim TH, Kwon H, Jeon CH, et al. Effect of endplate conditions and bone mineral density on the compressive strength of the graft-endplate interface in anterior cervical spine fusion. *Spine* 2001; 26:951–956.

27. Curylo LJ, Mason HC, Bohlman HH, et al. Tortuous course of the vertebral artery and anterior cervical decompression: a cadaveric and clinical case study. *Spine* 2000;25:2860–2864.

28. Ebraheim NA, Lu J, Brown JA, et al. Vulnerability of vertebral artery in anterolateral decompression for cervical spondylosis. *Clin Orthop* 1996:146–151.

29. Vaccaro AR, Ring D, Scuderi G, et al. Vertebral artery location in relation to the vertebral body as determined by two-dimensional computed tomography evaluation. *Spine* 1994;19:2637–2641.

30. McCulloch JA, Young PH. *Essentials of spinal microsurgery.* Philadelphia: Lippincott–Raven Publishers, 1998.

12

POSTERIOR DECOMPRESSION FOR RADICULOPATHY: LAMINOFORAMINOTOMY

NANCY E. EPSTEIN

The keyhole foraminotomy, a posterior approach to lateral or foraminal cervical disc disease and spondylostenosis, was originally introduced by Mixter and Barr and popularized by Scoville, Epstein, and Fager (1–3). Ducker later introduced the term *laminoforaminotomy* (4). This technique may be employed alone to remove soft disc herniations, degenerative spondylotic changes of the uncovertebral joints anteriorly or facet joints posteriorly, and root sleeve fibrosis, or in combination with laminectomy or laminoplasty to address coexistent myelopathy (1–7) (Fig. 12.1).

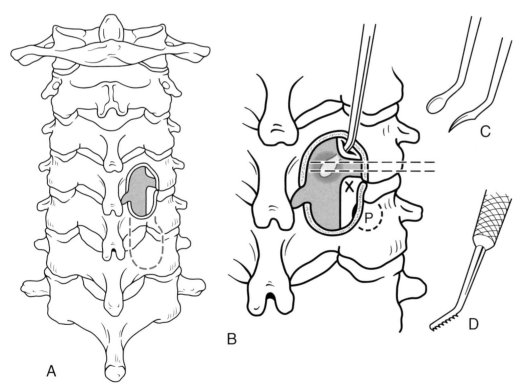

FIGURE 12.1. **A:** A keyhole foraminotomy is illustrated on the right at the C4-C5 level. The dotted line represents how an additional C5 hemilaminectomy and C6 laminotomy would allow for extension of the decompression to the subjacent C5-C6 level. **B:** The laminoforaminotomy at C4-C5 affords adequate visualization of the lateral aspect of the thecal sac and exiting C5 nerve root. Dissection may be performed using a small nerve hook, Penfield elevator, or down-biting curette *(C)* above or below the nerve root *(X)* and adjacent to the pedicle. **C:** Two small down-biting curettes are illustrated. **D:** A down-biting rasp facilitates spur excision.

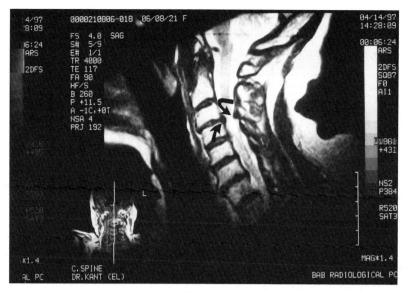

FIGURE 12.2. This midline sagittal magnetic resonance image demonstrated C3-C4 ventral cord compression due to spur formation (*mildly curved arrow*) and dorsolateral compression secondary to ossification of the yellow ligament (OYL) (*markedly curved arrow*) at the C2-C3, C3-C4 levels. The flexion and extension x-rays showed C3-C4 instability (active subluxation > 6 mm).

NEURODIAGNOSTIC STUDIES

Cervical radiculopathy and myelopathy should be evaluated with both magnetic resonance (MR) and computed tomographic (CT) examinations (4,5,8–12). While MR provides a soft tissue overview, CT (noncontrast CT, two-dimensional and three-dimensional reconstructions) and myelo-CT examinations better define calcified or

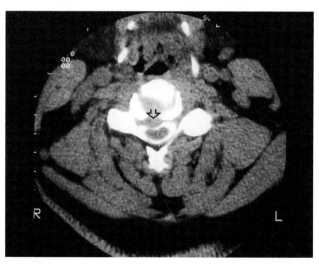

FIGURE 12.3 The transaxial myelo-CT scan demonstrated a right-sided anterolateral soft disc herniation (*open arrow*).

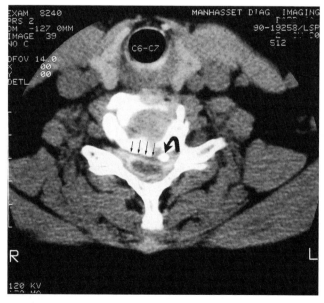

FIGURE 12.4 Myelo-CT demonstrating mild diffuse C5-C6 ventral cord compression and left lateral root compromise due to diffuse hypertrophy of the posterior longitudinal ligament (*double arrows*) containing punctate calcification and pearls (*single arrow*) of ossification. Ventral spur (*multiple arrows*) and early ossified posterior longitudinal ligament characterized by hypertrophied posterior longitudinal ligament (PLL) containing a pearl of ossification (*single curved arrow*) contributing to left-sided C7 root compression.

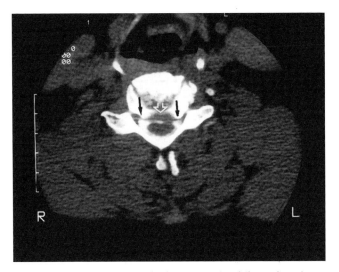

FIGURE 12.5 Myelo-CT study demonstrating bilateral uncinate hypertrophy (*black arrows*) resulting in compression of both nerve roots in the lateral and proximal neural foramina. Note the relative absence of midline cord compression (*single white arrow*). A fenestration procedure successfully addressed the pathology.

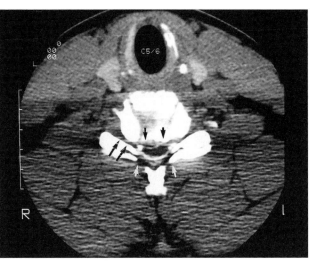

FIGURE 12.6 Myelo-CT scan demonstrating at the C5-C6 level significant ventral and dorsal cord compression secondary to congenital stenosis exacerbated by ventral spur formation (*black arrows*), dorsal laminar shingling (*white arrows*), and bilateral foraminal compromise attributed to hypertrophic changes of the facet joints (*double black arrows*).

ossified pathology (Figs. 12.2 to 12.6). The myelo-CT examination best defines the extent and locale of lateral and foraminal changes (8,9). Midline and paramedian pathology, such as large ossified lesions extending above or below an interspace, may be inaccessible through a laminoforaminotomy. It is therefore critical to document the fullest extent of the pathology on both the MR and CT studies prior to choosing this limited approach.

INDICATIONS FOR LAMINOFORAMINOTOMY

Unilateral, bilateral, and multilevel cervical radiculopathy may be approached through a laminoforaminotomy. The majority of patients undergoing these procedures should exhibit focal root deficits that correspond specifically to the level of disease. The roots most commonly compromised, in descending order, are the C7 root at the C6-C7 level, the C6 root at the C5-C6 level, the C5 root at the C4-C5 level, and the C8 root at the C7-T1 level (1,10). In the laminoforaminotomy series by Rodrigues et al. (10), lateral and foraminal disease was encountered at the C6-C7 level in 25 patients, the C5-C6 level in 19 patients, the C4-C5 level in 4 patients, and the C7-T1 level in 3 patients.

SURGICAL INDICATIONS

Anterolateral, lateral, or foraminal cervical pathology may be addressed anteriorly with an anterior discectomy with fusion, or posteriorly utilizing the laminoforaminotomy (1–15). Monoradicular syndromes may warrant a single-level laminoforaminotomy, whereas bilateral radicular complaints involving the same level may require a fenestration approach, that is, with adjacent laminoforaminotomies (Figs. 12.7–12.9). Multilevel unilateral radicular pathology may require ipsilateral hemilaminectomies with laminoforaminotomies, whereas myelopathy combined with radiculopathy may require laminectomy or laminoplasty (9,13,14,16).

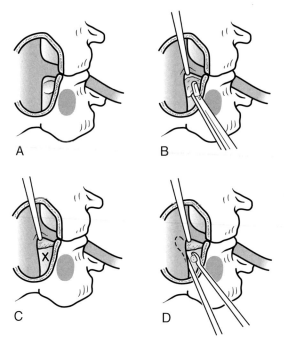

FIGURE 12.7 **A:** Illustration of a typical laminoforaminotomy, initiated with a typical one-level medial facetectomy with foraminotomy. **B:** Dissection of the nerve root with a blunt nerve hook, accompanied by gentle cephalad and dorsal retraction usually adequately exposes a soft sequestrated disc fragment, which can be removed with a small pituitary forceps. **C:** Lateral and foraminal discs are often accompanied by spurs, which are also readily exposed with gentle cephalad and dorsal nerve root retraction. **D:** Down-biting curettes, introduced medially, laterally, and foraminally, ventral to the nerve root and thecal sac, are employed to dissect, morcellate, and remove spur.

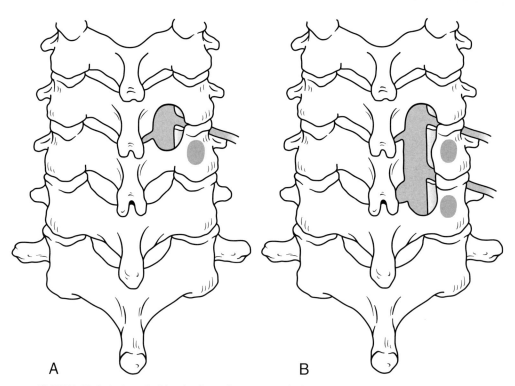

FIGURE 12.8 **A:** A typical laminoforaminotomy, including partial lateral and foraminal removal of the superior and inferior hemilaminae, is used to address unilateral and unisegmental root compression. **B:** Adjacent, two-level, dorsolateral cervical nerve root compromise requiring a two-level laminoforaminotomy completed using unilateral laminotomy, hemilaminectomy, and laminotomy.

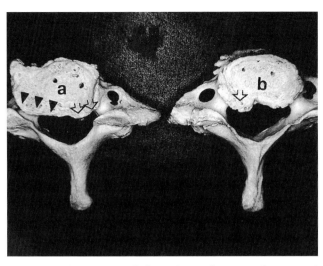

FIGURE 12.9 A: Anatomical specimen demonstrating ventral left-sided (*double open arrow*) and right-sided foraminal spurs (*triple closed arrows*) compressing the spinal cord and exiting nerve roots. **B:** A large right-sided lateral spur is visualized (*single open arrow*). The fenestration approach, consisting of bilateral adjacent laminoforaminotomy, allowed for extensive decompression of bilateral foraminal compromise.

POSITIVE ASPECTS OF THE LAMINOFORAMINOTOMY

The laminoforaminotomy allows for the removal of lateral or foraminal pathology without compromising stability (6,17–19) (Figs. 12.10 and 12.11). If less than 50% of the facet has been removed, no fusion and only transient bracing is required. Chen et al. (6) also found that the laminoforaminotomy had less of an effect on stability than anterior discectomy with fusion procedures, which routinely require several months of immobilization for fusion and are associated with a 1% to 7% pseudarthrosis rate. The laminoforaminotomy offers limited morbidity because the posterior approach is only through muscle. Anterior dissection encounters tracheal, esophageal, or carotid-related complications, tracheal swelling, respiratory compromise, swallowing difficulties, infection related to esophageal perforation, and stroke.

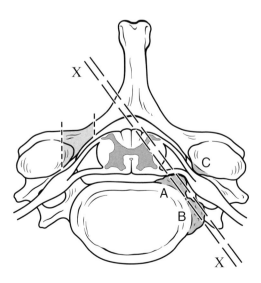

FIGURE 12.10 Transaxial image of the cervical spine illustrating proximal ventral foraminal **(A)** and distal ventral foraminal **(B)** spur intrusion on the exiting cervical nerve root. Spurs **(A and B)** ventrally compress the motor root, while dorsolateral arthrotic changes of the facet **(C)** result in sensory root compression.

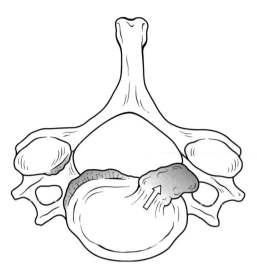

FIGURE 12.11 Ventral foraminal disc (*arrow*) intruding into the neural foramen resulting in focal ventral nerve root compression with contralateral spur formation.

AWAKE INTUBATION, AWAKE POSITIONING, AND INTRAOPERATIVE MONITORING

Awake fiberoptic nasotracheal or endotracheal intubation and positioning may be accompanied by somatosensory evoked potential (SEP) monitoring of the median/ulnar and posterior tibial nerves (14). During intubation, patients are placed in hard cervical collars that are left in place for the final positioning, prone or sitting. Electromyography (EMG), employing needle electrodes, may be performed during the short periods of root dissection when muscle relaxant has worn off. Prophylactic administration of 1 g methylprednisolone at the time of induction may be employed, along with the appropriate dose of an antistaphylococcal antibiotic.

Prone Position

Patients are placed in the prone position using bilateral chest rolls (smaller patients), a Wilson frame (medium-sized to large patients), or an extra-large Cloward saddle (largest patients). The three-pin head holder is applied using local anesthesia (0.5% lidocaine), and the patient is asked to turn over onto the operating table. Once the neck is in a neutral position, the head holder is affixed to the Mayfield headrest. When the patient is prone, the arms are held down with minor tension by the sides, paralleling the trunk. Placing the patient's arms on bilateral arm rests is not an option because this will preclude intraoperative lateral radiographs. After final positioning, SEP baselines are checked for stability; only then does induction follow. The prone position affords the surgeon a reduced risk of air embolism and hypotension and the facilitation of simultaneous fusion, although it may involve greater intraoperative blood loss (average 2 units), with a wet, more obscured operative field increasing the anatomic challenge of nerve root dissection.

Sitting Position

The sitting position offers its own unique requirements, benefits, and risks. These patients similarly undergo awake intubation and awake positioning under continuous SEP monitoring. However, these patients also require central venous lines and Doppler monitors should air embolism occur. Additionally, prior to raising the patient to the seated position, the patient must be fully hydrated, typically with 1 liter of normal saline, to avoid hypotension. Positioning of the arms and elbows in the seated patient is critical. The arms, elbows, and wrists must be supported by sheets or blankets so that they rest in a horizontal position, avoiding tension on the nerve roots and facilitating intraoperative dissection. Once the patient is placed in the seated position, blood pressure, pulse, SSEPs, and the neurologic examination are monitored for 5 to 10 minutes. When all parameters are stable, induction follows. A significant "drop out" of SSEPs in the presence of a normal blood pressure indicates relative hypotension or underperfusion of the cord; this should be managed with the immediate artificial induction of hypertension until the SEP changes resolve.

During the surgery, if air embolism should occur, open veins must be coagulated, the wound must be packed with a saline-soaked lap pad, and air must be aspirated from the central venous line. Only those patients in whom air persists should be turned into the left lateral decubitus position to trap the air in the right atrium and avoid cardiovascular compromise. The sitting position affords reduced operative blood loss and a clearer operative field, but includes a greater risk of cord ischemia or stroke and the possibility of death secondary to air embolism.

Intraoperative Radiography

Intraoperative radiographs confirming the level of surgery are essential and may include a routine lateral radiograph, fluoroscopy, fluoronavigation, or fluoronavigation combined with stereotactic guidance.

LAMINOFORAMINOTOMY

Localization

Once anesthesia has been induced, with the patient positioned supine or prone, the wound is then infiltrated with 30 cc of 0.5% bupivacaine hydrochloride and 1:200,000 epinephrine (30 cc). Percutaneously, a short needle must be carefully placed into the interspinous ligament at the presumed correct level; following radiographic confirmation of the correct level, 0.25 cc of methylene blue may be injected. Alternatively, the wound may be opened with a clamp placed on a spinous process or interspinous ligament for more direct localization. This latter maneuver is best when applied to the large or obese patient.

Incision and Exposure

Too short an incision and prolonged retraction can contribute to skin and muscle necrosis. Therefore, the wound must be long enough to allow minimal tension on the skin, while the retractors on the muscles should be prophylactically released every 20 minutes. After identifying the correct surgical level by using operating loupes or an operating microscope, an up-biting curette (360-degree rotating) should be employed to dissect the ligamentum flavum away from the laminar margins. A 2-mm Kerrison rongeur (360-degree rotating) is then used to remove one-third to one-half of the cephalad and one-third of the caudad hemilaminae. More extensive removal may be warranted based on the underlying pathology and the patient's size. The dorsal bony cortex should be initially removed with a 4-mm medium- to low-speed diamond burr. The 2-mm rotating Kerrison rongeur is then used to remove the thin residual rim of ventral cortical bone, while a 2-mm up-biting curette (2 mm) and Kerrison rongeur combined aid dissection and removal of residual hypertrophied or ossified yellow ligament, exposing the underlying dura.

Extent of Exposure

The severity of foraminal pathology dictates how much of the cephalad and caudad lamina needs to be removed. Foraminal lesions often require greater cephalad than caudad exposure. Ebraheim et al. (20) noted that a semicircular laminotomy involving the cephalad lamina may be all that is needed to remove a lateral soft disc herniation because the disc space itself is located above the leading edge of the caudad lamina. However, for lesions demonstrating greater cephalad and caudad extension, more extensive laminotomy, hemilaminectomy, or laminectomy may be required to avoid excessive traction for exposure.

Fenestration Procedure

Bilateral lateral, foraminal, and dorsolateral disease (e.g., ossification of the yellow ligament) involving a single segment may require the fenestration technique or adjacent, bilateral laminoforaminotomies. Benefits include enhanced stability provided by preservation of a portion of the cephalad and caudad hemilaminae, the spinous processes, and the interspinous and supraspinous ligaments. However, significant multilevel spinal stenosis, or surgery in the massively obese patient where exposure is difficult, may be safer if a full laminectomy is performed.

Facet Resection

Laminoforaminotomy involving 25% resection of the facet joint affords adequate visualization of 4 mm of the proximal neural foramen, an exposure sufficient for performing most laminoforaminotomies (6,10,17–19). In Baba and colleagues' series (16), 16 patients required less than 25% resection of the facet joint, while 8 patients required 25% to 50% facet joint excision to address their pathology. When Zdeblick et al. (19) performed 25%, 50%, 75%, and 100% facetectomy in an *in vitro* model, 25% facet resection was nearly comparable to the stability of the intact specimen, while significant segmental hypermobility correlated with resection of more than 50% of the facet joint. Technically, removal of the medial facet is accomplished using a 4-mm diamond burr, 2-mm rotating rongeur, and 1- to 2-mm rotating curette. For moderate foraminal compromise, the rongeur may be used to remove the residual "shelf" of anterior cortical bone, while more severe compression may be relieved with the 1- to 2-mm up-biting curette.

Foraminal Root Dissection

When the bony exposure is complete, the dorsal sensory and ventral motor roots should be readily identified. They may exit the thecal sac through a single dural sleeve or, occasionally, the ventral motor root may have separate, thinner, grayish ventral dural investment. Differentiating the ventral motor root from the foraminal disc herniation is crucial to avoid inadvertent injury to the involved motor root. Epidural bleeding may be controlled with direct coagulation of the venous plexus or by the application of microfibrillar collagen, or both.

Once the nerve root is skeletonized superiorly and inferiorly as it exits the foramen, and after veins and other adhesions are lysed, the root should be gently mobilized with a small Penfield dissector. It is then gently retracted superiorly under continuous EMG monitoring. The Penfield dissector is replaced by a small nerve hook, which allows the root to be freed and elevated away from the underlying disc or spur. Fibers of the underlying posterior longitudinal ligament may have to be incised with an 11 blade knife, allowing for the introduction of a 2-mm down-biting curette below the ligament. Careful dissection with this curette is performed using a downward and outward rotating maneuver. If a soft sequestrated disc is present, retraction of the root may adequately expose the disc herniation, allowing it to spontaneously extrude. More typically, the disc fragment has to be delivered using both the Penfield dissector and down-biting curette. Multiple disc and spur fragments are usually small, measured in millimeters. Spurs in particular may also be removed in a piecemeal fashion, yielding seemingly tiny ossific particles. It must be remembered that the endpoint is a free nerve root, and that overdissection risks root or cord injury and should be avoided at all cost.

Once dissection is complete, microfibrillar collagen may be placed over the dura, followed by a pledget of Gelfoam and an epidural drain. After routine closure, the anesthetic is reversed and the patient is placed in a hard or soft collar; full neurologic assessment follows. The patient is then extubated and returned to the recovery room. If the patient fails to awaken normally or exhibits a new deficit, the nasotracheal or endotracheal tube should be left in place and an immediate CT scan obtained. Factors that may delay extubation include morbid obesity, asthma, prolonged operative time, and blood loss. Postoperatively, the collar is worn for comfort for 1 to 2 weeks.

Laminoforaminotomy with Laminectomy or Laminoplasty

Laminoforaminotomy may be combined with laminoforaminotomy or laminoplasty where cervical radiculopathy coexists with myelopathy. In Baba and colleagues' (16) series of 17 patients, the laminoforaminotomy and laminoplasty successfully addressed these two concurrent pathologies. Frequently, in older individuals, diffuse cervical stenosis in conjunction with foraminal compression requires laminectomy (9,13,14).

OUTCOMES

Good to excellent outcomes are reported in up to 96% of patients following laminoforaminotomy performed for radiculopathy (1–5,7–16). Poor prognostic factors include long-term preoperative complaints and long-standing preoperative neurologic deficits (10,12). Additionally, patients appear to exhibit continued good long-term outcomes, as documented in Davis's study (8), in which 86% of patients were still doing well 15 years later. However, in cases in which myelopathy is combined with radiculopathy, success rates drop to 76% (16).

Complication and Reoperation Rates

Following laminoforaminotomy, the complication rate is 2%, attributed to cord or root injury, postoperative hematomas, cerebrospinal fistulas, and infection; the reoperation rate is 6%, which predominantly addresses recurrent disc disease (2,5,7,8,20).

REFERENCES

1. Epstein JA, Lavine LS, Aronson HA, et al. Cervical spondylotic radiculopathy: the syndrome of foraminal constriction treated by foraminotomy and the removal of osteophytes. *Clin Orthop* 1965;40:113–122.
2. Fager CA. Posterolateral approach to ruptured median and paramedian cervical disk. *Surg Neurol* 1983;20:443–452.
3. Scoville WB. Cervical disc: classifications, indication and approaches with special reference to posterior keyhole operation. In: Dunsker S, ed. *Cervical spondylosis.* New York: Raven Press, 1981:155–167.
4. Zeidman SM, Ducker TB. Posterior cervical laminoforaminotomy for radiculopathy: review of 172 cases. *Neurosurgery (US)* 1993;33(3):356–162.
5. Aldrich F. Posterolateral microdiskectomy for cervical monoradiculopathy caused by posterolateral soft cervical disc sequestration. *J Neurosurg* 1990;72:370–377.
6. Chen BH, Natarajan RN, An HS, et al. Comparison of biomechanical response to surgical procedures used for cervical radiculopathy: posterior keyhole foraminotomy versus anterior foraminotomy and discectomy versus anterior discectomy with fusion. *J Spinal Disord* 2001;14:17–20.
7. Henderson CM, Hennessey RG, Shuey HM Jr, et al. Posterior-lateral foraminotomy as an exclusive operative technique for cervical radiculopathy: a review of 846 consecutively operated cases. *Neurosurgery* 1983;13:504–512.
8. Davis RA. A long-term outcome study of 170 surgically treated patients with compressive cervical radiculopathy. *Surg Neurol (US)* 1996;46(6):523–530.

9. Malone DG, Benzel EC. Laminotomy and laminectomy for spinal stenosis causing radiculopathy or myelopathy. In: Clark CR, Ducker TB, eds. *The cervical spine,* 3rd ed. Philadelphia: Lippincott–Raven Publishers, 1998:817–823.

10. Rodrigues MA, Hanel RA, Serrat DM, et al. Posterior approach for soft cervical disc herniation: a neglected technique? *Spine* 2001;55:17–22.

11. Simeone FA. Posterior discectomy for soft cervical disc herniation. In: Al-Mefty O, Origitano TC, Harkey HL eds. *Controversies in neurosurgery.* New York: Thieme, 1996:227–228.

12. Woertgen C, Holzschuh M, Rothoerl RD, et al. Prognostic factors of posterior cervical disc surgery: a prospective, consecutive study of 54 patients. *Neurosurgery* 1997;40(4):724–728.

13. Epstein NE, Epstein JA, Carras R. Cervical spondylosis, stenosis, and myeloradiculopathy in patients over 65: diagnostic techniques and management. *Neuro-Orthopedics* 1988;6(1):13–32.

14. Epstein NE. Myelopathy: laminectomy. In: Herkowitz H, Clark C, eds. *The cervical spine.* Philadelphia: Lippincott–Raven Publishers, 2001.

15. Herkowitz HN, Kurz LT, Overholt DP. Surgical management of cervical soft disc herniation. A comparison between the anterior and posterior approach. *Spine* 1990;15(10):1026–1030.

16. Baba H, Chen Q, Uchida K, et al. Laminoplasty with foraminotomy for coexisting cervical myelopathy and unilateral radiculopathy: a preliminary report. *Spine* 1996;21(2):196–202.

17. Panjabi MM, Duranceau J, Goel V, et al. Cervical anatomy of the middle and lower regions. *Spine* 1991;16:861–869.

18. Raynor RB, Pugh J, Shapiro I. Cervical facetectomy and its effect on spine strength. *J Neurosurg* 1985;63:278–282.

19. Zdeblick TA, Zou D, Warden KE, et al. Cervical stability after foraminotomy. A biomechanical *in vitro* analysis. *J Bone Joint Surg Am* 1992;74(1):22–27.

20. Ebraheim NA, Xu R, Bhatti RA, et al. The projection of the cervical disc and uncinate process on the posterior aspect of the cervical spine. *Surg Neurol* 1999;51(4):363–367.

13

ANTERIOR DECOMPRESSION FOR MYELOPATHY: MULTILEVEL DISCECTOMY

PAUL A. HOUSE
RONALD I. APFELBAUM

Cervical myelopathy results from a wide variety of conditions in which the cervical spinal cord is compressed. Common causes for myelopathy include degenerative cervical spondylosis, intrinsic and extrinsic spinal cord tumors, and ossification of the posterior longitudinal ligament (OPLL). Degenerative cervical spondylosis is by far the most common condition leading to myelopathy, except in the Asian population, where OPLL is most common. In degenerative spondylosis, spinal cord compression occurs from a combination of herniated or protruding cervical discs accompanied by posterior osteophytes and hypertrophied soft tissue.

Physical decompression of the cervical spinal canal is required to halt progression of the disabling effects associated with myelopathy. Decompression can be accomplished posteriorly by a decompressive laminectomy or by a variety of laminoplasty techniques. Decompression can also be accomplished anteriorly by either corpectomy or interbody approaches. This chapter discusses the benefits and limitations of anterior decompression for myelopathy using multilevel intervertebral discectomy with bony fusion and complete removal of the intrusions into the spinal canal for treatment of multisegmental degenerative cervical spondylosis.

Once the decision has been made to perform cervical decompression via an anterior approach, the clinician must decide whether to perform multilevel discectomies or a vertebral corpectomy with strut graft fusion. The published literature to date does not answer the question of which operation may be most appropriate in which circumstances. In the opinion of the authors, multilevel anterior cervical discectomies with fusions for spondylosis have several advantages over corpectomy and may be preferable in many cases.

One of the advantages of multilevel anterior discectomy, as described below, is multipoint fixation for distraction. Multipoint fixation allows cervical lordosis to be more easily restored than corpectomy procedures, which of necessity only allow two-point distraction. The success of any cervical fusion depends on bony incorporation and fusion through the graft material. Since shorter pieces of graft bone are needed for multilevel discectomy and fusion than for strut grafting after corpectomy, the graft bone may be more quickly incorporated into a solid fusion mass than with the longer strut grafts used for corpectomy approaches. Additionally, shorter pieces of graft material are more readily available, either from commercial preparations or from the patients themselves.

Because long bone grafts are needed to perform cervical corpectomy, the fibula is often used as grafting material. However, fibula grafting material is too straight to accurately recreate normal cervical lordosis. Fibula bone is also much more dense than iliac crest bone; denser bone is incorporated more slowly and is more prone to cause telescoping or pistoning of the graft into adjacent vertebral bodies.

Thus, while expansion of the cervical spinal canal to normal dimensions can be accomplished by either operative procedure, long-term operative success also ultimately depends on bony fusion and restoration of lordotic posture. For these reasons, multilevel anterior cervical discectomy with fusion is the authors' preferred technique for treatment of degenerative cervical spondylosis.

In this chapter, we describe the multilevel anterior cervical discectomy approach in detail, including the special instrumentation we use to facilitate the procedure.

INDICATIONS AND CONTRAINDICATIONS

Multilevel degenerative cervical spondylosis is the predominant condition amenable to treatment using this technique. Although this condition is often approached using a posterior decompression, when the canal is straight or kyphotic the results are poor, mandating an anterior approach. As noted, we feel that an intervertebral discectomy approach facilitates better lordosis restoration and spine stabilization than a corpectomy approach. Cases of segmental OPLL in which ligamentous ossification is confined to the regions behind the intervertebral disc and does not extend for a significant distance behind the adjacent vertebral bodies can also be treated with this technique.

In patients with continuous multisegmental OPLL, however, vertebrectomy is more likely to provide the exposure necessary for complete anterior canal decompression. Similarly, in some cases of severe cervical spondylosis, bony overgrowth may extend completely behind the vertebral bodies. In these cases it may be necessary to remove the entire vertebral body to restore the vertebral canal to normal dimensions.

OPERATIVE PREPARATIONS

The patient is positioned supine. Care must be taken to avoid neck hyperextension. Intubation, therefore, is often best performed with the patient awake and locally anesthetized, using a fiberoptic endoscope to guide the endotracheal tube. The patient's ability to move all extremities can then be assessed before the patient is fully anesthetized to assure neurologic integrity. The endotracheal tube is positioned to the left side of the patient's mouth for a right-sided approach.

The table is flexed to elevate the patient's back, placing the neck above the level of the heart to reduce venous congestion. The legs are also slightly flexed, creating a chaise lounge position that limits further inferior settling of the patient. Halter head traction is placed to provide direct axial traction with 10 pounds of weight. The head is not turned. A small towel roll can be placed between the scapulae to allow the shoulders to fall posteriorly to improve fluoroscopic visualization. Caudally directed shoulder traction is created by placing stockinette sleeves over the arms and securing them with wide tape spirally wrapped in a loose pattern from the shoulders to the hands. The stockinette is extended to the foot of the table, and 5-pound weights are hung from the stockinette to provide constant traction. This maneuver facilitates visualization of the lowest cervical levels as the shoulders are gradually pulled down. This setup is preferable to using tape to retract the shoulders. Although taping results in the best exposure initially, visualization gets progressively worse as the patient settles inferiorly in the bed.

The operative microscope is positioned with the base above the patient's head and to the patient's right. A portable fluoroscope is positioned with the base to the patient's left to provide real-time lateral fluoroscopy during the procedure. The fluoroscope unit must be aligned precisely to provide true lateral images. Alignment is accomplished by superimposing the facets. Aligning the facets in the anterior-posterior direction controls for rotation, and aligning them in the cranial-caudal direction controls for tilt. Once the fluoroscopic image is optimized, the entire unit can be rolled cranially to increase access to the patient's neck, if needed. More commonly, we leave it in position and can operate without interference, with the surgical approach from about 45 degrees to the patient rather than directly perpendicular to the long axis of the neck.

APPROACHING AND EXPOSING THE SPINE

Although external landmarks can be used to approximate the appropriate level of the incision, we prefer a quick fluoroscopic image with an external radiopaque reference to precisely plan the incision in the upper third of the levels to be decompressed, because it is almost always easier to access the lower vertebrae than the upper. A transverse incision beginning near the midline and extending past the medial border of the sternocleidomastoid muscle is planned in a Langer's line (Fig. 13.1). Some surgeons advocate the use of a vertical incision when more than two levels are to be decompressed. In our experience, a transverse incision is all that is required with multilevel decompressions or vertebrectomy. Transverse skin crease incisions are cosmetically superior since they blend with the natural skin creases. Also, these incisions heal better because they are not under tension.

The skin and soft tissue of the neck stretch easily and do not limit vertical access, even if four or five levels need treatment. The key to obtaining vertical access is a wide opening, superiorly and inferiorly, of the sternocleidomastoid muscle fascia along the medial border of this muscle. If this is done well beyond what initially seems necessary, vertical access should not be a problem.

After injection of a local anesthetic that contains epinephrine to enhance hemostasis, a skin incision is created to the level of the platysma and hemostasis is completed with bipolar cautery (Fig. 13.2). The platysma muscle is then elevated by placing a curved tonsil clamp beneath it, starting in the midline. The muscle is then sharply incised with electrocautery (Fig. 13.3). Large veins may be encountered below the platysma and can usually be mobilized but may be ligated if necessary. The superficial cervical fascia is then sharply incised along the medial border of the sternocleidomastoid muscle (Fig. 13.4). It is important to note that this step is the key to adequate exposure. Cephalad and caudad exposure is increased by further opening the investing fascia along the sternocleidomastoid rather than performing an extensive subplatysmal dissection.

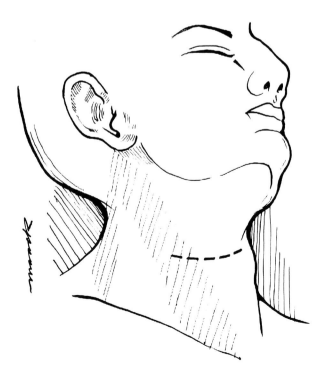

FIGURE 13.1. A horizontal skin crease incision is used, extending from the midline to just lateral of the medial border of the sternocleidomastoid muscle (*shaded area*).

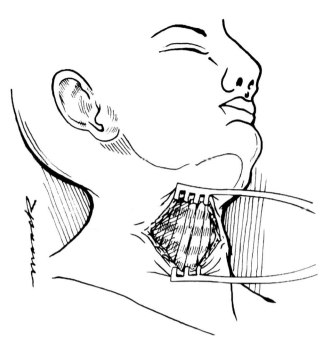

FIGURE 13.2. The skin is incised and retracted to expose the platysma muscle.

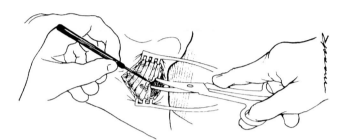

FIGURE 13.3. The platysma muscle is elevated with a curved clamp and incised with electrocautery.

Soft tissue dissection is then carried out bluntly with the index finger until the prevertebral fascia is reached (Fig. 13.5).

The natural tissue planes will open with minimal pressure. The carotid artery is palpated through its sheath as the planes are opened. The path of dissection is medial to the carotid sheath and turns further medially after accessing the space deep to the larynx. Cloward handheld retractors are used for retraction, primarily medially, as the plane of

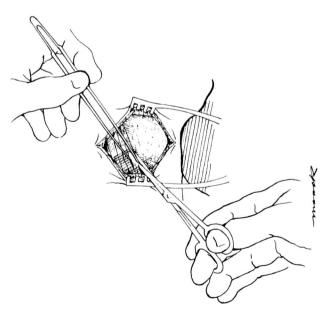

FIGURE 13.4. The sternocleidomastoid muscle fascia is opened sharply along the medial edge of the muscle.

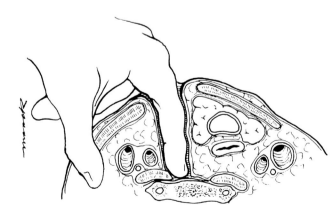

FIGURE 13.5. Blunt dissection opens the natural tissue plane medial to the carotid sheath and lateral to the trachea and esophagus to the level of the prevertebral fascia.

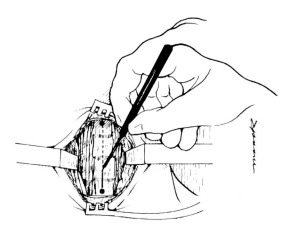

FIGURE 13.6. Exposure of the anterior surface of the vertebrae. The midline is marked (*dots*) above and below the incision in the anterior longitudinal ligament.

dissection is deepened (Fig. 13.6). The larynx, esophagus, and strap muscles are identified and carefully retracted medially. The omohyoid muscle may cross this access pathway. If so, the muscle can usually be sufficiently mobilized by working above and below it, so that multilevel discectomies can be performed without sacrificing it. However, the retraction system may need to be repositioned when transitioning between levels if it is necessary to segmentally work on either side of the omohyoid muscle. Once the prevertebral space is entered, several loose layers of tissue may need to be incised to reach the level of the anterior longitudinal ligament (ALL). Usually, a small incision with scissors will allow the tissue to spread apart, providing clear access to the anterior spine.

Lateral fluoroscopy is used to positively identify the vertebral and disc levels to be treated. Soft tissue dissection is continued cranially and caudally until the entire anterior surface of the vertebral bodies above and below the disc levels to be treated, as well as all the intervening vertebrae, is visualized. The midline is then marked by making a small electrocautery incision in the ALL and marking it with indelible ink above and below the extent of the eventual final position of the anterior plate (Fig. 13.6) before sharp dissection is begun. This maneuver later facilitates true midline plate alignment.

The ALL is then incised in the midline over the entire extent of the desired exposure. The ALL and longus colli muscle are elevated off the vertebral bodies subperiosteally to expose the anterior surface of the spine (Fig. 13.7). At each intervertebral disc level, there are often significant anterior osteophytes (to which the muscles may be adherent). Carefully elevating the longus colli muscle subperiosteally, without shredding, facilitates placement of the retractor. We use a small (8-mm) Key periosteal elevator and work from the midline laterally over the vertebral body. At the disc space, it may be easier to work from inferior to superior to separate the ALL and longus colli from the marginal osteophyte and annulus. Once the longus colli muscle has been elevated, toothed self-retaining retractor

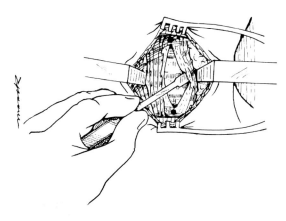

FIGURE 13.7. The incised anterior longitudinal ligament and longus coli muscle bellies are elevated from the anterior surface of the spine with a small periosteal elevator.

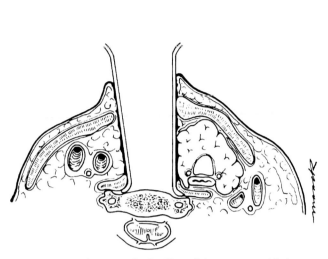

FIGURE 13.8. Sharp-toothed self-retaining retractor blades are placed beneath the longus coli muscles.

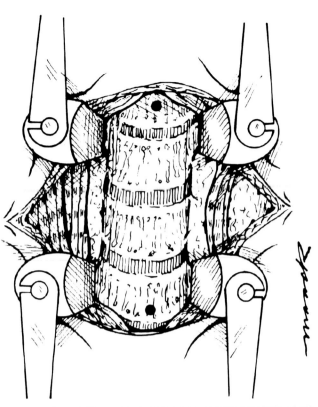

FIGURE 13.9. Self-retaining retractors are placed under the longus colli muscles. Two retractors may be used in long exposures, or one may be placed and repositioned to expose the various levels.

blades are placed under the elevated muscle (Figs. 13.8 and 13.9). Toothed blades are used because they hold their position better than smooth blades, thus avoiding slippage, which could compress the carotid laterally and the esophagus medially. We usually do not use cranial caudal self-retaining retractors because sufficient exposure can usually be obtained using only the lateral self-retaining retractor system and the distracting pins.

The anesthesiologist is asked to temporarily deflate the endotracheal tube cuff once the lateral retractor blades are set. The cuff is fully deflated and then reinflated to the

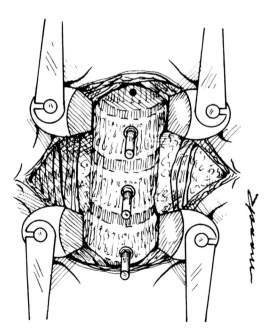

FIGURE 13.10. Caspar retractor posts are placed in each vertebra in the midline.

172

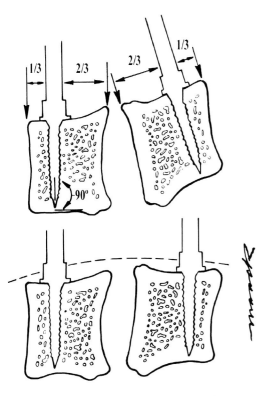

FIGURE 13.11. Schema of retractor post placement. The upper and lower posts are placed one-third of the way from the upper and lower ends of their respective vertebrae, and all posts are placed perpendicular to the posterior wall of the vertebrae and close to full depth. This placement allows correction of kyphosis (*upper vs. lower figures*) after disk excision as distraction occurs.

point where a seal is again achieved. The cuff deflation allows the endotracheal tube to recenter in the larynx after traction. This maneuver has been shown to significantly reduce the incidence of recurrent laryngeal nerve injury (1).

Large anterior osteophytes will commonly be present and are most easily removed before distraction pins are placed. The osteophytes can be removed with Leksell rongeurs (see Fig. 13.16B) or an acorn-shaped high-speed drill bit (see Fig. 13.16C). Osteophyte removal at this stage also greatly facilitates subsequent anterior plating.

Caspar distraction posts (Aesculap Instrument Corp., Center Valley, PA) are then placed (Fig. 13.10). Each post should be placed under fluoroscopic guidance so that it is perpendicular to the posterior wall of the vertebral body (Fig. 13.11). This placement allows the restoration of cervical lordosis as distraction is applied (Figs. 13.11 and 13.12). The distraction posts will most often not be parallel to one another at their initial placement due to cervical degeneration. The most superior and inferior posts need to be placed with the plating system in mind. Placing the uppermost post in the upper third of

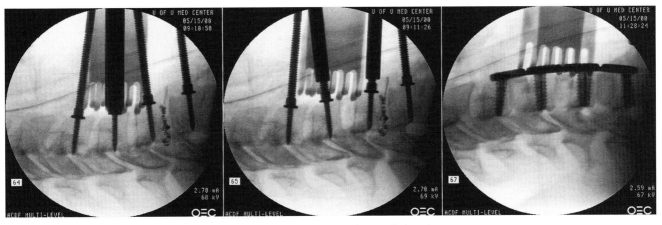

FIGURE 13.12. The distractor posts are placed under fluoroscopic guidance. If placed perpendicular to the posterior vertebral cortex, they will restore lordosis as well as open the disc space (compare the second and third images).

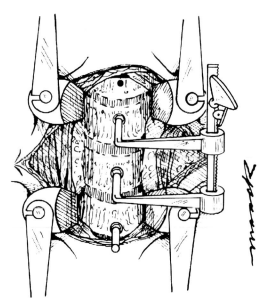

FIGURE 13.13. Distractor in place at upper level.

the vertebral body and the lowermost post in the lower third of the involved vertebral body (Fig. 13.11) will avoid conflict with the future screw holes or plate fixation pins. Distraction is sequentially applied to each level as individual discs are resected (Fig. 13.13).

DISCECTOMY

The procedure usually begins on the most superior disc and proceeds inferiorly. The distractor is placed on the posts at this level, and the anterior aspect of the disc annulus is sharply incised with a no. 15 blade. The disc should be opened widely for full access to the disc space. An initial discectomy is performed using pituitary rongeurs (Fig. 13.14) and angled curettes. The majority of the intervertebral disc is easily removed with the

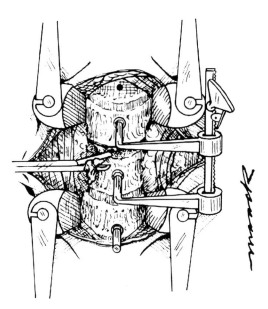

FIGURE 13.14. Discectomy in progress.

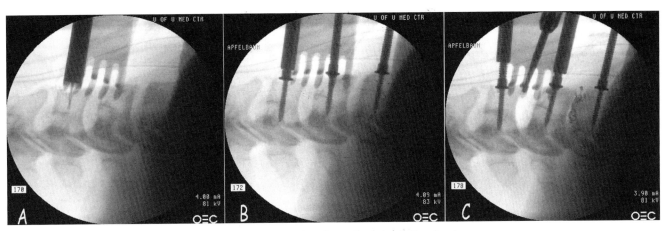

FIGURE 13.15. Fluoroscopic sequence. **A:** Drilling pilot hole for distraction post. **B:** Post in place. **C:** Dissection of upper level; disc removed; beginning flattening of upper endplate of this level.

rongeurs once the anterior annulus has been opened. Angled curettes are then used to remove the remaining disc material and cartilaginous endplates. Full removal is critical to future fusion. As the annulus is opened and the disc removed, distraction is increased to optimize the spinal alignment and maximize the height of the disc space (Fig. 13.15).

The operative microscope is brought into the field as the posterior longitudinal ligament (PLL) is approached and is then used for the remainder of the decompression. To accept a graft well, the endplates of the vertebrectomy need to be flattened from side to side and front to back. A parallel-sided graft should have maximum contact with the vertebrae to both facilitate fusion and maintain the alignment. Our goal is to prepare the endplates to achieve a "gapless" fusion as we enlarge the intervertebral space to gain access to the spinal canal, allowing us to decompress the neural elements.

Typically, the upper vertebral surface of a disc space has an inverted cup-shaped contour when viewed from the side. The lower vertebral body at a disc space will typically slope upward from anterior to posterior on the lateral view (Figs. 13.15 and 13.16A). From the anterior perspective, the contour of the upper vertebral bodies is often fairly straight from side to side, while the lower one is closer to the upper body laterally than at the midline.

To create the flat surfaces desired, we usually start by removing the anterior portion of the upper vertebrae to the level of the central decompression (Figs. 13.15C and 13.16C). This is done with a high-speed air drill and a small acorn-shaped bit, such as the Midas AM8 or the Midas II GS 130 (Medtronic Sofamor Danek, Memphis, TN). Using gentle stroking actions and moving the drill in a side-to-side motion across the whole disc space will result in a uniform surface (Fig. 13.16D). Such removal may or may not breach the cortex, depending on its thickness. The cortex at the center of the vertebral endplate is not violated but can be shaved down to a uniform contour. One must ensure that all cartilage has been removed. Repositioning the microscope at this point so that the surgeon's line of sight is straight down the face of the bone is very helpful in identifying any small surface irregularities and allowing removal of the posterior bone in a flat plane (Fig. 13.16H). If the surface being worked on is viewed tangentially, the surface preparation is more difficult and may be less precise. Again, side-to-side uniform stroking motions with the drill are best to achieve a flat endplate.

The lower surface of the intervertebral disc space is prepared with the drill, using the upper surface as an alignment guide. A greater amount of bone is sequentially removed as the resection proceeds posteriorly (Fig. 13.16E). The uncinate processes and the portion of the posterior osteophytes at the disc space will come into view as the bone resection is deepened to the level of the spinal canal. Bony prominences are sequentially thinned down and resected using a light touch with the drill.

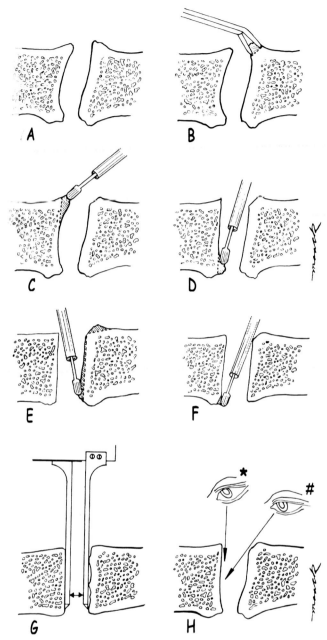

FIGURE 13.16. Schema of sequential steps of interspace preparation and grafting. **A:** Initial view. **B:** Removing surface osteophytes with rongeurs. **C:** Removing anterior portion of superior vertebrae to level of central depression (*shaded area*). **D:** Removing posterior portion of superior vertebra from central depression to level of posterior longitudinal ligament. **E:** Contouring inferior aspect of the interspace with burr, making it parallel with upper one. **F:** Undercutting marginal osteophyte accessible from interspace. **G:** Use of calipers to assist in assessing parallelism of endplates. **H:** By moving microscope to the position marked by the asterisk (*), in the axis of the endplate, the surgeon can easily detect small surface irregularities and perfect the endplate preparation. If it is viewed obliquely *(#),* this is more difficult to do with precision. *Continued*

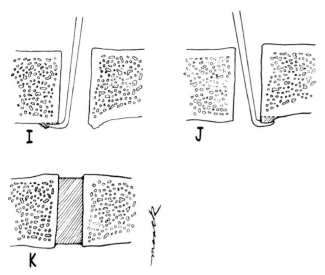

FIGURE 13.16. *(continued)* I: Small right-angle curettes are used to remove the remaining superior osteophytes. **J:** Similarly, the inferior osteophytes are removed. **K:** Final graft position with parallel endplates and gapless fit.

As the posterior osteophytic lips are encountered, the angle of drilling can be modified to place the cutting surface of the drill between the PLL and the posterior osteophyte (Fig. 13.16F). The osteophytic lips can be resected without drilling through the PLL by using a light touch and moving the drill from side to side. The drill bit should always be kept moving to avoid cutting or burning through the PLL and exposing the dura.

To ensure that the endplates have been left truly parallel, the Caspar adjustable calipers are placed into the disc space (Fig. 13.16G). The endplate–caliper interface is examined visually and with lateral fluoroscopy by placing the calipers in the prepared interspace and moving them from side to side. No lucency should be visible at any endplate–caliper interface. The dimensions should be equal. When satisfactorily parallel endplates have been fashioned, neural decompression begins.

CANAL DECOMPRESSION

Central canal decompression is the primary goal when performing discectomies for myelopathy. Therefore, meticulous attention to posterior osteophyte removal is vital for success. As previously mentioned, the high-speed drill can be used to partially undercut the posterior osteophytic lips.

Further osteophyte removal is performed with curettes. This is initiated using a 5–0 bone curette with a 45-degree up-angled cutting surface. The small curette allows the PLL to be safely stripped while also permitting some bone removal. The curette is gently slipped behind the vertebral body. While pulling upward, a smooth turning motion is used to cut the osteophytic material up toward the surgeon and into the disc space (Fig. 13.17). We then switch to a 4–0, 45-degree curette with a 12-inch handle introduced under the inferior edge of the superior vertebrae and used in a similar fashion to remove the osteophytes and to create a smooth posterior vertebral body surface. Care must be taken prior to the introduction of larger curettes to first remove enough bone so that posteriorly directed pressure on the PLL and dura are avoided.

Standard up-angled bone curettes are somewhat limited in their ability to reach behind the vertebral body, and the 40-degree angulation is not optimal at the inferior edge of disc space. We therefore use specially designed 90-degree curettes with a 4–0 cup (R&B Surgical Solutions, Cleveland, OH) to extend the osteophyte removal behind the

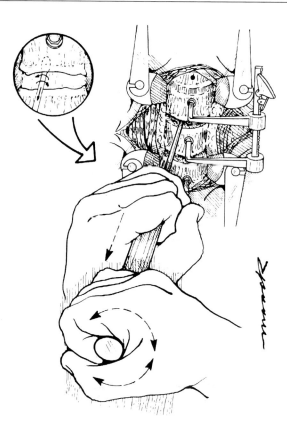

FIGURE 13.17. Technique to remove osteophytes behind vertebrae with small right-angled curettes. While pulling firmly upward to keep the curette in contact with the bone (left hand), it is rotated (right hand) to cut the bone away.

vertebral bodies as needed (Figs. 13.16I,J). These curettes have 12-inch handles for improved leverage and are available in three sizes, each with a progressively longer reach behind the vertebrae. Using these curettes sequentially, one-half of the posterior vertebral surface adjacent to the interspace can be accessed (Fig. 13.18). In this manner, extensive posterior bony pathology can be removed while providing canal decompression and avoiding the need for vertebrectomy. We do not consider canal decompression complete until a right-angled nerve hook can be placed behind the superior and then the inferior vertebral body, slid from side to side, and imaged at each side and in the midline (Fig. 13.18E). We want to see the hook flat on the posterior cortex, which assures that no residual canal compression remains.

The PLL may be thickened in cervical spondylosis and, if so, should be thinned or removed for complete canal decompression. A 5–0, up-angled curette can be gently insinuated through the fibers of the PLL to create a working space. The PLL is removed in a medial to lateral fashion with a 2-mm Kerrison punch. Any herniated disc fragments

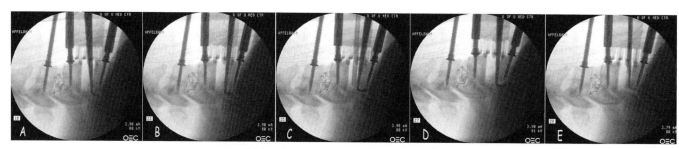

FIGURE 13.18. A large osteophyte is palpated by the Caspar periosteal elevator **(A)**, and sequentially removed using progressively longer 4–0 right-angle curettes **(B** through **D)** until fully removed. This is confirmed with a right-angle nerve hook, which lies flat against the posterior vertebral cortex **(E)**.

are removed, with special attention paid to finding fragments that may have migrated behind the vertebral body. In some patients, the PLL may be attenuated and a small nerve hook can be gently inserted through a rent to lift the PLL, creating a working space for its resection or through which to palpate to ascertain the completeness of the decompression.

NERVE ROOT DECOMPRESSION

Radiculopathy will often be present concurrently in the patient with myelopathy due to cervical spondylosis. Neuroforaminal compression is caused by both protruding disc fragments and hypertrophied bone. Adequate neuroforaminal decompression is vital to ensure excellent symptomatic relief from multilevel cervical discectomy procedures.

Neuroforaminal decompression is initiated with the high-speed drill bit. Drilling is performed in a light, quick manner at the edge of the intervertebral disc space using a **U**-shaped motion. All pressure on the drill is directed laterally during this maneuver. Particular vigilance is necessary to avoid posterior pressure that could compromise the nerve root sheath. The majority of the foraminotomy is completed using the drill. A lip of posterior osteophyte from the superior endplate is often present in the neuroforamina. The up-angled 5–0 or 4–0 curette is used with a smooth, turning, circular motion to remove these residual bone protrusions.

HEMOSTASIS

Bleeding may ensue from the bone and from epidural areas. Bone bleeding may occur behind the vertebral body. In such instances, wax may be applied with angled Caspar periosteal elevators, and the excess removed with the same tool or a nerve hook.

Gelfoam slurry made by mixing powdered Gelfoam (Pharmacia & Upjohn Co., Kalamazoo, MI) and thrombin is very effective for all types of bleeding in this area. It is applied and then pressed into the bleeding site with gentle pressure on a cottonoid patty. The excess can be removed with suction or irrigation. It works very fast. Regular Gelfoam pledgets can also be used. Bipolar cautery may be helpful in controlling bleeding from epidural vessels or cut edges of the PLL. Angled-tip forceps and low power settings work best.

GRAFT SELECTION AND HARVESTING

With the introduction of loadsharing anterior cervical plating systems, high fusion rates are now routinely obtained using allograft tricortical iliac crest bone. Commercially prepared allograft bone is selected to match the size of the prepared interspace. Graft bone for each disc space is individually cut from the piece of donor crest using a parallel-bit reciprocating saw blade. The gap between the parallel blades is chosen to match the measured height of the previously created distracted disc space. Using a parallel-bladed saw ensures that the graft surface is true and planar with a minimal amount of time and effort.

In the authors' experience, autologous bone is rarely needed for multilevel fusion procedures. The use of autologous bone may be considered for patients who are prone to poor bone fusion, such as smokers or diabetics. Tricortical iliac bone grafts are used when autologous bone is desired. To harvest the graft, a linear skin incision is created several centimeters lateral to the anterior superior iliac spine to avoid injury to the lateral femoral cutaneous nerve. The incision is placed directly over the iliac crest. Soft tissue dissection is carried out to the iliac crest, exposing the fibrous insertions of the attached muscles. The muscle insertions are initially stripped using monopolar electrocautery and then using a periosteal elevator, exposing only the minimal amount of crest necessary.

Graft harvest is conducted with a parallel-bit reciprocating saw. Because multiple grafts are needed, the parallel-bit blade minimizes the amount of crest taken for each graft. The Caspar graft harvesting tool is then used to make the inferior cut at the precise depth needed.

Whether allograft or autograft bone is used, the graft may be further fashioned *ex vivo,* if needed, with an acorn-shaped bit to gently smooth any rough cortical edges. The depth of the interspace is measured with the calipers, and the exact depth is verified from the fluoroscopic images to provide several millimeters of clearance between the thecal sac and the posterior aspect of the graft. We place the largest graft that will fill the interspace, cutting the graft 1 to 2 mm shorter than the measured depth for safety. The interspace usually has a prepared width of 16 to 20 mm, depending on the patient's anatomy and the levels that were operated.

GRAFT INSERTION

The tricortical graft is inserted with the noncorticated surface facing the dura. The graft is gently tapped into place with the anterior edge either flush with or countersunk approximately 1 mm below the anterior aspect of the vertebral body (Fig. 13.16K). Final position of the graft is confirmed with fluoroscopy. A nerve hook is placed alongside the graft, with the hook touching the posterior aspect of the graft edge. This is done to confirm that the graft has not rotated and that neural elements are not compressed (Fig. 13.19).

The Caspar distractor is gently released. The entire procedure is repeated at each involved level as detailed previously. Again, it is important that at each level the endplates and graft are fashioned as previously described. By placing the distractor pins perpendicular to the posterior cortex, fashioning parallel endplates, and using a parallel graft, normal cervical lordosis is restored and maintained when cervical distraction is removed. It is neither necessary nor desirable to use wedge-shaped grafts. The distractor posts are removed after satisfactory graft placement, and the post holes are waxed for hemostasis.

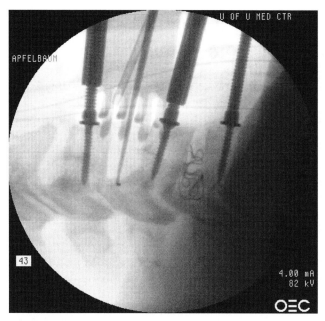

FIGURE 13.19. A nerve hook placed lateral to the graft confirms its depth, assuring no canal intrusion.

PLATING

Many cervical plating systems have been developed. The latest generation of dynamic plating systems allows true load sharing by the bone graft, because the graft is exposed to axial loading from the weight of the head and cervical muscle forces. Axial loading of the graft encourages faster bone incorporation and consequently higher rates of fusion than have previously been possible. The following describes placement of the ABC (Aesculap) dynamic plating system.

When using a loadsharing system, the plate chosen is typically shorter than the earlier-generation plate used for the same fusion. Loadsharing systems allow a greater degree of settling to initially occur across each disc space than nonloadsharing plating systems. Therefore, it is important to use a plate that will not encroach upon the adjoining disc spaces as settling occurs.

Plate alignment is performed with the aid of fluoroscopy to ensure that the plate lies flush against all vertebral bodies. Any residual anterior osteophytes are removed with rongeurs or with an air drill. The plate contour is then adjusted as needed to match the achieved cervical curvature so that the plate lies flush on the entire anterior spine surface and does not move when digital pressure is alternately applied to each end. The indelible ink midline marks placed initially on the vertebral bodies now aid in plate centering (Fig. 13.20). A temporary pin is applied at each end of the plate to fix the plate in an optimal position prior to screw placement.

Under fluoroscopic guidance, a double-barreled drill guide is used to create converging screw holes in one vertebral body at a time. At the most cranial and caudal vertebral bodies, the drill holes are angled up and down, respectively, increasing holding power. If using bicortical screws, an adjustable drill guide allows drilling to progress millimeter by millimeter until the posterior cortex is engaged. If using unicortical screws, a 14-mm, fixed-depth drill guide can usually be used. Bicortical screws may have a stronger purchase than unicortical screws when bone density is poor. Otherwise, unicortical screws are equivalent when using this loadsharing system.

Screws are placed at each vertebral body level. Although the hole is drilled to 14 mm for unicortical screws, we choose a screw length that will extend to 75% to 80% of the

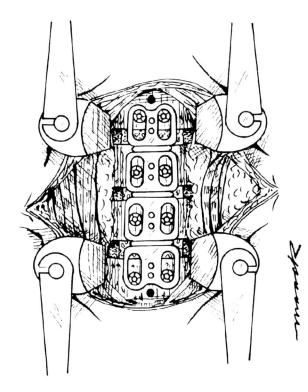

FIGURE 13.20. ABC dynamic plate. Note midline marks to aid in vertical alignment. Also note placement of screws at the distal ends of the superior and inferior slots and centrally at intermediate levels to allow the desired dynamic settling.

vertebral body depth for improved purchase. Once all screws have been placed, the internal locking mechanism of each screw is engaged. This mechanism ensures that screws are unable to back out of the body or plate, while still allowing axial settling to occur. The temporary pins are removed, and bone wax is inserted into the temporary pin sites to tamponade any bone bleeding, if needed.

CLOSURE

The wound is gently irrigated with saline to remove any devitalized tissue fragments, blood, and debris. The longus colli muscles are brought up over the lateral plate edges to normal anatomic position. The muscles can be sutured to one another with two or three interrupted 3–0 absorbable sutures, if desired. Using handheld Cloward retractors, each layer of the neck is examined for points of bleeding as the strap muscles are allowed to fall back into normal position. We do not routinely use drains. After additional gentle irrigation, the sternocleidomastoid muscle fascia is reapproximated with interrupted absorbable sutures. Similarly, the platysma is reapproximated and sutured. Finally, the skin is closed with buried, interrupted absorbable sutures and secured with sterile tape strips.

COMPLICATIONS

Intraoperative complications may accompany multilevel cervical discectomies but are generally rare. Dural tears can occur during the procedure. In cases of spondylosis, dural tears are rare, but tears are more common in cases of OPLL where the dura becomes calcified. Some dural tears can be closed primarily. If not, covering the tear with a suitable material such as fascia lata augmented with fibrin glue and then placing a lumbar drain will usually allow the area to heal.

Vertebral artery injury can also rarely occur. Curylo (2) describes the possibility of an ectatic vertebral artery injury from cervical corpectomy. Importantly, in cases in which vertebral artery injury with cervical corpectomy is a concern, discectomy becomes the procedure of choice.

Recurrent laryngeal nerve injury and swallowing dysfunction are the most common postoperative problems. Injury to the recurrent laryngeal nerve has been shown to occur primarily from endolaryngeal injury to the nerve by traction (1). The incidence can be reduced to about 1% by deflating and then reinflating the endotracheal tube cuff after retractor placement or repositioning. Most cases of nerve injury that occur are transient but can last several months.

Dysphagia is also common. Its incidence increases with the duration of surgery and when higher levels are treated. Usually, solid or dry foods are difficult to swallow initially. Most patients have some symptoms of dysphagia but recover spontaneously. Dietary modification usually suffices, but, if the difficulty is severe, a feeding tube can be used until dysphagia resolves to assure adequate nutrition.

POSTOPERATIVE BRACING

With dynamic loadsharing plating, the graft is maintained under compression and remains an integral part of the construct along with the plate and screws. Even when some graft absorption occurs, which always happens as part of the normal biology of bone healing, the construct's integrity and strength remain. The patient's neck therefore remains stable, and postoperative bracing is generally not needed. We feel it is important for patients to regain neck mobility and strength. By avoiding postoperative bracing and encouraging patients to use their neck muscles, patients are able to regain motion and experience less neck pain. If, however, quality of the vertebral bone is a concern, a rigid external collar may be used for 6 to 8 weeks.

CONCLUSION

This anterior cervical discectomy technique has allowed us to achieve canal decompression, and hence cord decompression, reliably in multilevel spondylotic myelopathy; such full decompression is critical if the patient is myelopathic. We feel that reconstruction of the spine is superior with this approach because lordosis can be restored and multiple points of fixation exist for anterior plate fixation. The grafts are shorter and can therefore incorporate quicker and more fully. Consequently, construct failure has been rare.

This approach is more labor intensive and therefore more time-consuming than other approaches, but it has proven very effective in decompressing and stabilizing the spine. We often can avoid the use of external arthrosis, and only in rare cases have we needed to augment the anterior construct with posterior instrumentation. For these reasons, it is our anterior technique of choice for multilevel cervical spondylosis myelopathy.

REFERENCES

1. Apfelbaum RI, Kriskovich MD, Haller JR. On the incidence, cause, and prevention of recurrent laryngeal nerve palsies during anterior cervical spine surgery. *Spine* 2000;25(22):2906–2912.
2. Curylo LJ, et al. Tortuous course of the vertebral artery and anterior cervical decompression: a cadaveric and clinical case study. *Spine* 2000;25(22):2860–2864.

14

ANTERIOR DECOMPRESSION FOR MYELOPATHY: CORPECTOMY

THEODORE A. BELANGER
SANFORD E. EMERY

INDICATIONS AND CONTRAINDICATIONS

The technique of cervical corpectomy has many applications, but by far the most common is for neurologic decompression in the degenerative spine. The focus of this chapter is on cervical corpectomy to treat patients with cervical spondylotic myelopathy. With some variations, many of the concepts and techniques described are also applicable for certain congenital, infectious, neoplastic, or traumatic conditions.

Patients with spinal cord compression, clinical evidence of myelopathy, and appropriate medical status to withstand general anesthesia are appropriate candidates for surgical intervention (Fig. 14.1). The natural history of cervical myelopathy is one of stepwise

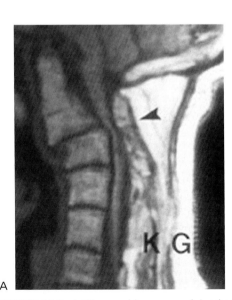
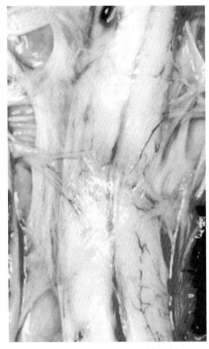

A   B

FIGURE 14.1. A 40-year-old man complained of gait difficulty with upper and lower extremity weakness of 1 year's duration. He was ambulatory but required a walker. Examination showed obvious long tract signs with bilateral upper and lower extremity weakness. **A:** Sagittal magnetic resonance image showing severe spinal cord compression from a degenerative subluxation of the cervical spine. The patient was treated with C4 corpectomy and strut grafting. The immediate postoperative period was uneventful, but 1 week postoperatively the patient died of a myocardial infarction. **B:** Gross pathology specimen from the same patient showing spinal cord deformation. *Continued.*

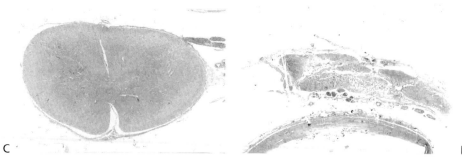

C

D

FIGURE 14.1. *(continued)* **C:** Histology of a normal spinal cord. **D:** Histology from the patient, showing severe spinal cord atrophy from chronic compression. (From Emery SE. Cervical spondylotic radiculopathy and myelopathy: anterior approach and pathology. In: White AH, Schofferman JA, eds. *Spine care.* St. Louis: Mosby, 1995, p. 178, with permission.)

progression over time; therefore, an early surgical treatment approach is recommended for these patients (1–6). Most patients can be treated on an elective basis, but the occasional patient with severe involvement or rapid progression should be treated more urgently.

Once a patient has been deemed an appropriate surgical candidate, the surgeon must decide on the surgical approach that is to be used. Various methods exist for treatment of myelopathy, including anterior (discectomy vs. corpectomy with fusion) and posterior (laminectomy or laminoplasty) techniques. The decision regarding the specific surgical approach to take is largely based on the pathoanatomy of the disease process, as well as the preferences and experience of the treating physician. Most patients can be treated safely and effectively via an anterior decompression and fusion (7–17). Patients whose neurologic compression is largely from soft disc encroachment can be treated with discectomy and fusion. Patients whose spinal cord impingement extends above or below the disc space by either bony protrusions, migrated disc fragments, or ossification of the posterior longitudinal ligament are better treated via corpectomy and strut grafting (18–20).

Contraindications are infrequently encountered, but include previous radiation to the anterior neck, aberrant vertebral artery anatomy, or medical contraindications to general anesthesia. "Chin on chest" deformity may make an anterior approach impossible until a posterior osteotomy is carried out. Tobacco abuse has been shown to increase the rate of fusion failure in patients undergoing anterior arthrodesis (21).

BENEFITS AND LIMITATIONS

Most of the neurologic compression in patients with cervical spondylotic myelopathy occurs anterior to the spinal cord and nerve roots and is most directly addressed via corpectomy (1,2). The surgical approach is identical to that used for anterior cervical discectomy and fusion. Axial, radicular, and myelopathic symptoms can all be addressed with a high degree of satisfaction using this technique. The incidence of serious complications—such as injury to the trachea, esophagus, spinal cord, or vertebral artery—is extremely low with careful technique (22,23). The rates of fusion and neurologic improvement are high (6–8,10–15,24–27).

The limitations of anterior corpectomy and strut grafting are important to recognize. There are several situations in which an anterior corpectomy and strut grafting may be inadequate to prevent postoperative kyphosis, graft settling, or nonunion. In the face of poor bone quality or postlaminectomy kyphosis, a combined posterior procedure may be added to achieve posterior stability (28,29). A combined approach will also be necessary to carry out an osteotomy in a patient with rigid, severe cervical kyphosis. A circumferential approach could be used when a patient's biology predisposes him or her to a higher nonunion rate because of osteoporosis, tobacco abuse, diabetes, rheumatoid disease, cancer, or infection. When to perform a combined approach for circumferential fusion is largely based on surgeon judgment (29).

RECOMMENDED APPROACH

The preferred surgical approach for cervical corpectomy is an anterior Smith-Robinson approach. The authors prefer a left-sided approach under most circumstances. The recurrent laryngeal nerve is protected in the tracheoesophageal groove on the left, whereas it has a variable course on the right, most commonly crossing the operative field at the sixth cervical vertebral level. The Smith-Robinson approach has application throughout the cervical spine, often providing access as cranial as the base of the first cervical vertebra and as caudally as the upper one or two thoracic vertebrae, depending on the specific anatomy and habitus of a particular patient.

SPECIFIC PREOPERATIVE CONSIDERATIONS

Once the diagnosis of cervical myelopathy has been established by a thorough history and physical examination, the area of neurologic compression should be determined by magnetic resonance imaging (MRI). This radiologic modality will also help determine if alternate pathology, such as tumor or demyelinating disease, is present. In addition to standard radiographs and MRI, the authors recommend liberal use of myelograms, with postmyelogram computed tomography (CT) scans. The myelogram can often clarify the extent of decompression that is required, as well as demonstrate which neuroforamina are compromised. The CT scan most clearly demonstrates the bony pathoanatomy. The CT scan also shows the relationship between the vertebral arteries and the spinal canal, which has some variations that can occasionally affect the surgical plan. The vertebral foramina occur quite medially in a minority of patients (2% to 3%), placing the arteries at risk when performing a wide decompression (30). This situation is best appreciated preoperatively so that adjustments may be made.

A frequently encountered situation is the patient with cervical myelopathy who has had a previous anterior cervical spine surgery. It is not always certain whether a given patient sustained a recurrent laryngeal nerve palsy from the previous surgery, because many patients will describe a hoarse voice and sore throat postoperatively. The previous surgical approach may be contralateral to your preferred side, and it is tempting to perform the current surgery on your favored side through previously untouched tissue planes. If surgery is undertaken contralateral to the previous surgery, the surgeon risks the possibility of a bilateral recurrent laryngeal nerve palsy, which could be a devastating problem. Therefore, in patients who have had previous anterior cervical spine surgery, the authors recommend proceeding ipsilateral to the previous approach. An alternative precaution would be otolaryngologic examination preoperatively to check vocal cord motion. Adequate exposure is typically achieved without significant difficulty or risk.

OPERATING ROOM SETUP

The patient is carefully positioned supine on the operating table (Fig. 14.2) after general endotracheal anesthesia and spinal cord monitoring are established. Preferably, esophageal stethoscopes, temperature probes, and gastric tubes are omitted to allow unimpeded retraction of the esophagus intraoperatively. A Mayfield (horseshoe) headrest can be used to allow precise positioning of the head and neck. A roll is placed behind the scapulae to allow the shoulders to drop back. The neck is kept in neutral to slight extension to allow space for the surgical approach. Further neck extension is strictly avoided because this

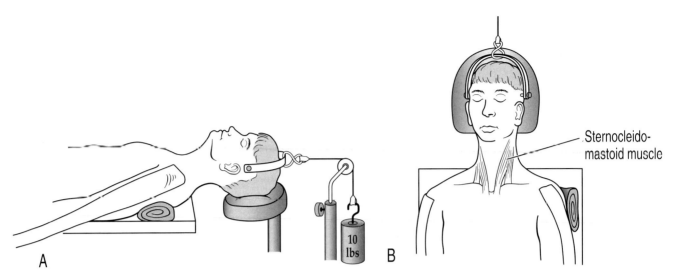

FIGURE 14.2. A: Patient positioning for a multilevel anterior cervical corpectomy. Spinal cord monitoring should be initiated prior to positioning the patient. Note that a roll is placed under the scapulae to allow the shoulders to drop back and the neck to extend slightly. The shoulders are taped to pull them distally without undue force to allow for a lateral cervical radiograph intraoperatively. The head rests upon a horseshoe headrest for precise positioning in slight extension. Excessive extension is avoided. Skull tong traction is in place. Skull tong traction may be omitted in favor of using the Caspar screw-post distracter for intraoperative distraction of a one-level corpectomy. **B:** Frontal view shows the skull tong traction in place, the shoulders taped with distal traction, and the chin tipped up and rotated slightly away from the side of the operative approach.

position can result in further spinal cord impingement and injury. The chin is turned slightly away from the operative side.

No skull traction is necessary when performing a single-level corpectomy. When performing a multilevel corpectomy, 5 pounds of traction is applied using skull tongs. Additional traction up to 25 pounds is applied only after the decompression is completed. Gentle traction is applied to the shoulders with tape to pull them distally, allowing for radiographic imaging of the lower cervical spine. Excessive traction is avoided to prevent injury to the brachial plexus. The table is placed in a slight reverse Trendelenburg position to level the operative field and to reduce venous engorgement in the neck. This may also reduce postoperative airway edema.

NEEDED INSTRUMENTS AND IMAGING

The specific instruments needed for an anterior Smith-Robinson approach and a cervical corpectomy are fairly standard. Scalpel, dissecting scissors, blunt handheld retractors, blunt dissection tools such as Kitner dissectors, and electrocautery are needed for exposure. Much of the blunt dissection can be performed by the surgeon's finger. A spinal needle can be used as a radiographic marker to confirm the levels to be decompressed. The corpectomy requires Leksell, pituitary, and Kerrison punch rongeurs, as well as a power burr. Straight and angled curettes, along with hemostatic aids such as thrombin, Gelfoam, patties, bone wax, and cautery, will be needed to carefully pull bone and disc material away from the posterior longitudinal ligament and the foramina. Disc space distraction, when necessary, can be aided with the use of a Cloward lamina spreader or a Caspar screw-post distracter. This should be avoided in patients with severe spinal cord impingement because distraction may create further spinal cord injury when performed prior to decompression. Instruments for bone graft harvest will be needed, including osteotomes, an oscillating saw, and appropriate retractors. High-quality spinal cord monitoring is important. A localizing radiograph is necessary early in the case, and a second radiograph should be taken after the strut graft is in place to confirm its position.

SPECIFIC BIOMECHANICAL CONSIDERATIONS

Biomechanically speaking, the technique of cervical corpectomy and strut grafting is very straightforward. The graft is held firmly in place by the tensile force created by the posterior ligaments and the lateral annulus and soft tissues that remain after decompression (28,31). The posterior longitudinal ligament, when left intact, also contributes. This tensile force, coupled with the endplate preparation and application of anterior instrumentation, helps prevent extrusion of the graft. Ideally, the graft is held securely enough to prevent motion at the interface between the native vertebral bodies and the strut graft so that fusion can readily occur. Because of the reliance on predominantly posteriorly generated tensile forces, patients with compromised posterior ligamentous structures, either from previous surgery or severe kyphotic deformity, may be predisposed to graft extrusion or fusion failure. In a situation of attenuated or absent posterior structures, consideration should be given to performing posterior instrumentation (i.e., lateral mass plating) to restore the posterior tension band effect. Application of an anterior plate may be insufficient to compensate for the absence of a posterior tension band effect.

The same tensile forces that secure the graft in place may also result in some subsidence of the graft into the vertebral bodies above and below it (32). A few millimeters of settling are generally not clinically significant. Application of an anterior plate may prevent some settling. Some plates are specifically designed to allow for some subsidence, and the surgeon should be aware of these design differences when selecting an anterior cervical plate system. Excessive graft settling is more likely in osteoporotic bone; this may be another indication for combined posterior instrumentation.

TECHNIQUE GUIDE

A transverse incision is made at the appropriate level from just across the midline to the medial border of the sternocleidomastoid muscle. This incision is carried out through skin, subcutaneous fat, and platysma muscle. The superficial layer of the deep cervical fascia is then encountered, with several large branches of the external jugular vein often present. These branches can generally be preserved, but their ligation is without serious consequence. The deep cervical fascia is divided with scissors longitudinally along the medial border of the underlying sternocleidomastoid muscle. A longitudinal fascia incision is favored, because this permits easy exposure of the multiple spinal segments necessary for a corpectomy and strut graft procedure. This fascia layer should be carefully developed with blunt scissor dissection prior to dividing it, because numerous small vessels are found within this layer.

Next, the carotid sheath is palpated to clearly identify its location. Blunt dissection proceeds between the carotid sheath and the pharynx, trachea, and esophagus, identifying the anterior cervical spine. This can usually be accomplished with the surgeon's finger. Blunt handheld retractors are used to maintain visualization of the spine and to protect the carotid sheath, trachea, and esophagus. The visceral and prevertebral fascia layers are divided with a scissors between the underlying longus colli muscles, which should be visible on each side of the spine. The fascia is then gently elevated off the levels of interest out to the longus colli muscles. Electrocautery is used along the edges of the longus colli bilaterally to minimize venous bleeding while exposing the vertebrae of interest out to their lateral margins. Excessively wide dissection will eventually lead the surgeon to the vertebral arteries, and is to be avoided. At this point, an intraoperative radiograph is taken with a marker in place to confirm the levels of decompression.

Once exposure of the levels of interest is accomplished, the decompression can be carried out (Fig. 14.3). A single-level corpectomy is specifically discussed here, but a multilevel decompression can be performed using an identical technique at each vertebral level. First, discectomies are performed above and below the vertebral body to be removed. The posterior longitudinal ligament should be visible posteriorly, with the uncovertebral joints at each lateral margin clearly visible to the surgeon. This provides orientation to the midline, spinal canal, neuroforamina, and vertebral arteries. The disc space can gently be distracted with a Cloward lamina spreader or a Caspar screw-post distracter. Aggressive distraction should be avoided when spinal cord impingement is present. The anterior portion of the vertebral body can be resected with rongeurs or a burr. The posterior portion is resected with a burr. Various burr tips can be used, including round carbide burrs, side-cutting burrs, and diamond-tip burrs, depending on the preference of the surgeon. Burring proceeds down to the thin posterior shell of cortical bone. This thin layer of bone is outlined by the disc spaces above and below, and by a gutter on each side made by the burr and curettes down to the posterior longitudinal ligament. The remaining central wafer can then be removed en bloc with curettes. At this point, the width of the decompression should generally be about 15 to 16 mm, with the uncovertebral joints determining the widest safe extent of bony resection. There is, of course, variation among patients with respect to vertebral size and the location of the vertebral arteries, and adjustments should be made to accommodate these differences.

The posterior longitudinal ligament is not routinely excised, though it can be done when disc fragments are found extruding posteriorly, between the ligament and the dura. When ossification of the posterior longitudinal ligament is present, the dura and ossified ligament may be intimately adherent, making thorough decompression treacherous. In that circumstance, the surgeon can either carefully remove the ossified ligament and deal with any resulting dural defect or free the central posterior longitudinal ligament on either side, leaving it freely floating anterior to the spinal cord (i.e., the anterior floating method). Disc material and osteophytes can also be removed from the neuroforamina using curettes, pituitary rongeurs, Kerrison rongeurs, or a 3-mm diamond burr, if necessary. The surgeon must be aware of the proximity of the vertebral arteries to the uncovertebral joints when decompressing the neuroforamina.

Once decompression is complete, the endplates are prepared for graft insertion (Fig. 14.4). The endplates should be burred down to bleeding cancellous bone (33). Flat surfaces should be developed to accept a graft with flat ends, thereby maximizing contact between the graft and host bone. A small posterior lip (2 or 3 mm) should remain to prevent graft intrusion into the spinal canal. Similarly, a small anterior lip should remain to prevent anterior graft extrusion. Distraction of the corpectomy site can than be performed with a screw-post distracter (for a single-level corpectomy) or by increasing skull tong traction to 20 to 25 pounds (for a multilevel corpectomy). The length of the graft needed is then measured with a malleable needle probe. The probe should snap into place snugly, without undue force. This probe is then used to obtain a graft of appropriate length. The authors prefer iliac crest for a one-level corpectomy, and fibula for two or more levels. We generally use autograft fibula for standalone anterior procedures and allograft for circumferential arthrodesis.

The flattest side of the graft is inserted facing the spinal canal. With the traction at 20 to 25 pounds, the upper end of the graft is held manually with a Kocher, while the inferior end is gently tamped into place. It should fit snugly in the corpectomy defect, much like the malleable probe. If the graft is too long, it can be revised. A graft that is too short is more difficult to deal with, often necessitating the use of a second, longer graft. Once the graft has been fully seated, the screw-post distracter is removed, or the traction

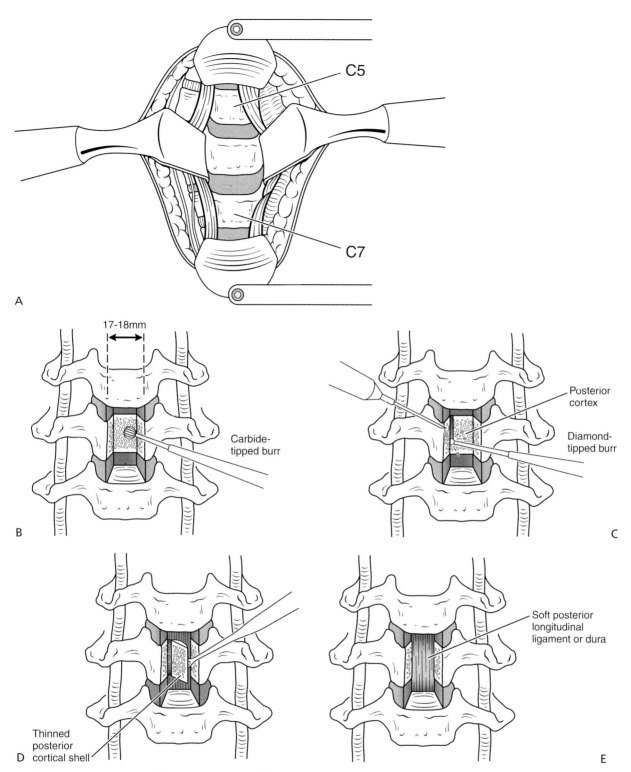

FIGURE 14.3. A: Exposure of the anterior aspect of the cervical spine is performed, clearly visualizing the disc spaces to be included in the decompression. Exposure should be a few millimeters lateral to the medial edge of the longus colli. Handheld blunt retractors should be used to maintain exposure and protect the trachea, esophagus, and carotid sheath. Once the levels are confirmed by radiography, discectomies can be performed above and below the vertebral body that is to be resected. **B:** The anterior half of the vertebra to be resected is then removed with rongeurs or a power burr or both. The lateral walls of the vertebral body should not be resected. **C:** A burr is used to remove the posterior half of the vertebral body as far laterally as the uncovertebral joints bilaterally (typically about 14 or 15 mm wide), leaving a thin shell of cortical bone lying over the posterior longitudinal ligament. A central cortical wafer of bone is outlined with a burr and curettes on each side, being mindful of the uncovertebral joints as a lateral boundary line for decompression. Patients with abnormal vertebral artery anatomy will be occasionally encountered, requiring a modification of the decompression width. This is best discovered on preoperative computed tomography scan. **D:** The thin, central, posterior wafer of bone is then removed en bloc with curettes and pituitary rongeurs. **E:** The posterior longitudinal ligament is thus exposed. It need not routinely be excised. If disc material is believed to have extruded posterior to this ligament, it can be carefully taken down, visualizing the dura mater. The decompression is thereby complete.

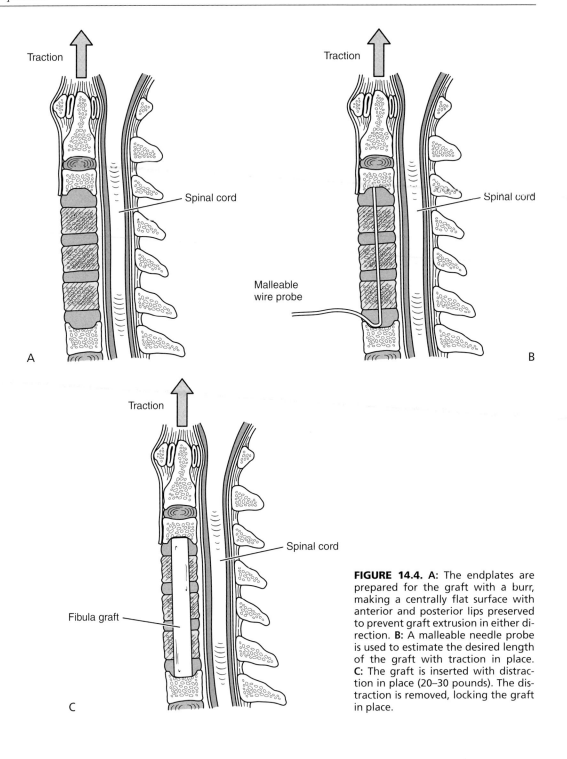

FIGURE 14.4. A: The endplates are prepared for the graft with a burr, making a centrally flat surface with anterior and posterior lips preserved to prevent graft extrusion in either direction. **B:** A malleable needle probe is used to estimate the desired length of the graft with traction in place. **C:** The graft is inserted with distraction in place (20–30 pounds). The distraction is removed, locking the graft in place.

is reduced to 5 to 10 pounds, locking the graft in place. If instrumentation is used, it should be applied once the distraction is removed. Screws should not be placed into the graft, because the screw holes weaken the graft. An intraoperative radiograph is obtained to confirm the position of the graft relative to the spinal canal and endplates (Fig. 14.5). Distraction of the facet joints should be visible at the levels spanned by the graft. If improperly positioned, the graft should be reseated. The wound is irrigated and closed over a Penrose drain, which is left in place for about 24 hours. It is not necessary to close the various fascia layers, but reapproximation of the platysma muscle is paramount for achieving a good cosmetic result.

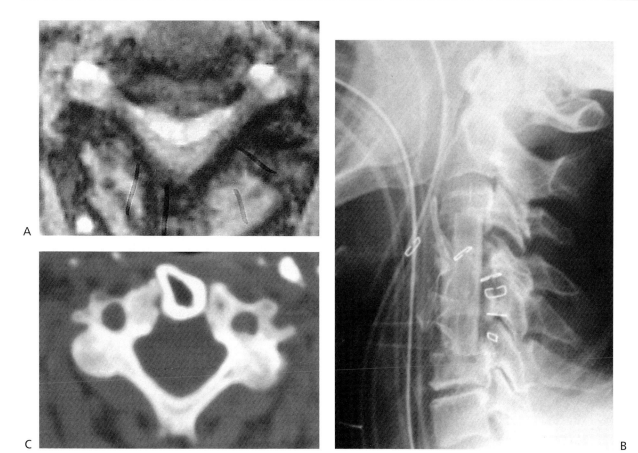

FIGURE 14.5. A: Preoperative magnetic resonance image showing cervical spinal cord deformation from anterior disc and spondylosis. **B:** Intraoperative radiograph showing strut graft in place. Note the mild facet distraction, the endplate preparation with anterior and posterior lips, and the position of the graft relative to the anterior vertebral cortices and the spinal canal. **C:** Postoperative computed tomography scan showing the position of the graft and the extent of the decompression.

SPECIFIC POSTOPERATIVE MANAGEMENT ISSUES

Postoperative immobilization should be initiated in the operating room, prior to transfer off the operating table. The type of immobilization necessary is dependent on several factors, including the number of levels involved, the presence or absence of internal fixation, bone quality, quality of graft fit, and surgeon preference. If a one-level corpectomy is performed with a well-fitting strut graft, good bone quality, and an anterior plate, then a soft collar may be all that is necessary. A noninstrumented one-level corpectomy or the average two-level corpectomy (with or without a plate) can be kept in a hard collar. Corpectomies of three or more levels (with or without a plate) are best immobilized with a cervicothoracic orthosis. A halo vest would only be necessary as a salvage measure in an unusual situation such as an osteotomy, severely osteoporotic bone, graft instability, or absence of posterior elements from previous surgery. Rigid immobilization is used for 6 to 8 weeks and is then replaced by a soft collar for a few days or weeks, as guided by the patient's comfort. Adjustments in the type or duration of immobilization can be made according to the surgeon's judgment on a case by case basis.

An important issue to be concerned with after any major anterior cervical spine procedure is postoperative airway edema (34). Patients who undergo surgery of short duration, without prolonged retraction of their upper airway, generally do well postoperatively with regard to airway concerns. However, patients who have undergone multilevel procedures or combined anterior and posterior surgeries often have significant postoperative airway edema. If they are extubated immediately after surgery, these patients can occasionally experience serious respiratory problems. The authors recommend a very low threshold for leaving such patients intubated in a critical care setting. They should then be extubated only after meeting strict criteria, such as passing a leak test. Most patients are extubated within 24 to 48 hours, with few regrets on the part of the surgeon.

In addition to wound monitoring, airway management, and neck immobilization, patients need to be evaluated for evidence of neurologic compromise in the immediate postoperative period (23). Radiographic visualization of the graft and implant position should take place prior to leaving the operating room. Despite this reassurance, if a patient develops evidence of spinal cord dysfunction beyond the patient's preoperative status, urgent imaging should be performed. Radiographs may not be adequate to show spinal cord impingement from graft malposition or epidural hematoma; therefore, computed tomography or magnetic resonance imaging may be required. If instrumentation or the graft is found to be impinging on the spinal canal, the patient must be brought back to the operating room on an urgent basis to correct the problem.

Consideration should be given to treating the patient with a steroid protocol if spinal cord dysfunction is present. If this is to be done, it should be initiated as early as possible, using a similar protocol to that outlined for use in traumatic spinal cord injury (30 mg/kg methylprednisolone IV bolus over 1 hour, followed by 5.4 mg/kg/hr for the next 23 hours). Steroid treatment should not be considered a substitute for timely reoperation, but rather as a helpful adjunct.

INTRAOPERATIVE COMPLICATIONS

Many serious intraoperative complications related to anterior cervical spine surgery are described in the literature. Most of these can be avoided through careful preoperative planning and intraoperative execution. Recurrent laryngeal nerve palsy is a well-known complication, avoided by choosing a left-sided approach and using careful retraction of the trachea and esophagus with blunt handheld retractors. If a self-retaining retractor is used, the endotracheal cuff should be deflated and reinflated to a lower pressure to reduce compression of the recurrent laryngeal nerve in the tracheoesophageal groove after setting the retractor.

Injury to the carotid sheath contents, trachea, esophagus, spinal cord, vertebral artery, or other nerves in the anterior neck can be minimized through careful dissection, accurate identification, and thoughtful protection of these structures during surgery. Injury to the esophagus carries a high risk of morbidity and mortality, especially if unrecognized at the time of surgery. Blunt retractors should be used to protect the esophagus throughout the procedure. Knowledge of the course of the vertebral arteries and constant accurate orientation of the surgeon to the uncovertebral joints will prevent injury to these vessels. If vertebral artery injury occurs, hemorrhage can be difficult to control. If simple hemostatic efforts are unsuccessful, it may be necessary to elicit the help of a vascular surgeon and achieve exposure of the involved vertebral artery to gain control of bleeding. Repair or ligation of the vessel can then be accomplished, with some potential for neurologic injury to the patient. Dural tears should be rare in spondylotic patients, but can be problematic in patients with long-standing ossification of the posterior longitudinal ligament (35).

Injury to the spinal cord is likewise prevented by careful surgical technique and constant orientation to the location of the spinal canal. Direct manipulation of the delicate spinal cord is to be strictly avoided because permanent neurologic injury can result. Similarly, distraction of the spine or vigorous manipulation of the vertebrae should be avoided until the decompression is completed. Use of high-quality spinal cord monitoring during surgery is mandatory for patients with myelopathy. Intraoperative signal reduction that is determined to be due to surgical disturbance of the spinal cord should be addressed immediately. Any distraction should be removed, surgical manipulation near the spinal cord should cease, and intravenous steroids should be administered. A wake-up test can be performed if the accuracy of the neurodiagnostic information is in question. In general, the decompression and strut grafting should be completed once these interventions have taken place. Although such surgical complications can be disastrous, they are fortunately very uncommon in the setting of careful planning and surgical technique.

REFERENCES

1. Bohlman HH, Emery SE. The pathophysiology of cervical spondylosis and myelopathy. *Spine* 1988;13:843–846.
2. Clarke E, Robinson PK. Cervical myelopathy: a complication of cervical spondylosis. *Brain* 1956; 79:483–510.
3. Cloward RB. The anterior approach for removal of ruptured cervical disks. *J Neurosurg* 1958;15: 602–617.
4. Gregorius FK, Estrin T, Crandall PH. Cervical spondylotic radiculopathy and myelopathy: a long-term follow-up study. *Arch Neurol* 1976;33:618–625.
5. Lees F, Turner JWA. Natural history and prognosis of cervical spondylosis. *Br Med J* 1963;2: 1607–1610.
6. Nurick S. The natural history and the results of surgical treatment of the spinal cord disorder associated with cervical spondylosis. *Brain* 1972;95:101–108.
7. Emery SE. Cervical spondylotic myelopathy: diagnosis and treatment. *J Am Acad Orthop Surg* 2001;9:376–388.
8. Emery SE. Surgical management of cervical myelopathy. *Instr Course Lect* 1999;48:423–426.
9. Epstein JA, Janin Y, Carras R, et al. A comparative study of the treatment of cervical spondylotic myeloradiculopathy. Experience with 50 cases treated by means of extensive laminectomy, foraminotomy, and excision of osteophytes during the past 10 years. *Acta Neurochir* 1982;61:89–104.
10. Fujiwara K, Yonenobu K, Ebara S, et al. The prognosis of surgery for cervical compression myelopathy: an analysis of the factors involved. *J Bone Joint Surg Br* 1989;71:393–398.
11. Hanai K, Fujiyoshi F, Kamei K. Subtotal vertebrectomy and spinal fusion for cervical spondylotic myelopathy. *Spine* 1986;11:310–315.
12. Macdonald RL, Fehlings MG, Tator CH, et al. Multilevel anterior cervical corpectomy and fibular allograft fusion for cervical myelopathy. *J Neurosurg* 1997;86:990–997.
13. Okada K, Shirasaki N, Hayashi H, et al. Treatment of cervical spondylotic myelopathy by enlargement of the spinal canal anteriorly, followed by arthrodesis. *J Bone Joint Surg Am* 1991;73:352–364.
14. Orr RD, Zdeblick TA. Cervical spondylotic myelopathy: approaches to surgical treatment. *Clin Orthop* 1999;359:58–66.
15. Saunders RL, Bernini PM, Shirreffs TG Jr, et al. Central corpectomy for cervical spondylotic myelopathy: a consecutive series with long-term follow-up evaluation. *J Neurosurg* 1991;74:163–170.
16. Yonenobu K, Fuji T, Ono K, et al. Choice of surgical treatment for multisegmental cervical spondylotic myelopathy. *Spine* 1985;10:710–716.
17. Zdeblick TA, Bohlman HH. Cervical kyphosis and myelopathy: treatment by anterior corpectomy and strut-grafting. *J Bone Joint Surg Am* 1989;71:170–182.
18. Abe H, Tsuru M, Ito T, et al. Anterior decompression for ossification of the posterior longitudinal ligament of the cervical spine. *J Neurosurg* 1981;55:108–116.
19. Hanai K, Inouye Y, Kawai K, et al. Anterior decompression for myelopathy resulting from ossification of the posterior longitudinal ligament. *J Bone Joint Surg Br* 1982;64:561–564.
20. Onari K, Akiyama N, Kondo S, et al. Long-term follow-up results of anterior interbody fusion applied for cervical myelopathy due to ossification of the posterior longitudinal ligament. *Spine* 2001;26:488–493.
21. Hilibrand AS, Fye MA, Emery SE, et al. Impact of smoking on the outcome of anterior cervical arthrodesis with interbody or strut-grafting. *J Bone Joint Surg Am* 2001;83:668–673.
22. Smith MD, Emery SE, Dudley A, et al. Vertebral artery injury during anterior decompression of the cervical spine: a retrospective review of ten patients. *J Bone Joint Surg Br* 1993;75(3):410–415.
23. Yonenobu K, Hosono N, Iwasaki M, et al. Neurologic complications of surgery for cervical compression myelopathy. *Spine* 1991;16:1277–1282.
24. Emery SE, Bohlman HH, Bolesta MJ, et al. Anterior cervical decompression and arthrodesis for the treatment of cervical spondylotic myelopathy: two to seventeen-year follow-up. *J Bone Joint Surg Am* 1998;80:941–951.
25. Emery SE, Fisher JR, Bohlman HH. Three-level anterior cervical discectomy and fusion: radiographic and clinical results. *Spine* 1997;22:2622–2624.
26. Hilibrand AS, Fye MA, Emery SE, et al. Increased rate of arthrodesis with strut grafting after multilevel anterior cervical decompression. *Spine* 2002;27(2):146–151.

27. White AA III, Southwick WO, Deponte RJ, et al. Relief of pain by anterior cervical-spine fusion for spondylosis: a report of sixty-five patients. *J Bone Joint Surg Am* 1973;55:525–534.
28. Albert TJ, Vacarro A. Postlaminectomy kyphosis. *Spine* 1998;23:2738–2745.
29. McAfee PC, Bohlman HH, Ducker TB, et al. One-stage anterior cervical decompression and posterior stabilization: a study of one hundred patients with a minimum of two years of follow-up. *J Bone Joint Surg Am* 1995;77(12):1791–1800.
30. Curylo LJ, Mason HC, Bohlman HH, et al. Tortuous course of the vertebral artery and anterior cervical decompression: a cadaveric and clinical case study. *Spine* 2000;25:2860–2864.
31. Riew KD, Hilibrand AS, Palumbo MA, et al. Anterior cervical corpectomy in patients previously managed with a laminectomy: short-term complications. *J Bone Joint Surg Am* 1999;81(7):950–957.
32. Hughes SS, Pringle S, Phillips F, et al. Multilevel cervical corpectomy and fibular strut grafting: immediate clinical and radiographic follow-up. Unpublished data.
33. Emery SE, Bolesta MJ, Banks MA, et al. Robinson anterior cervical fusion: comparison of the standard and modified techniques. *Spine* 1994;19:660–663.
34. Emery SE, Smith MD, Bohlman HH. Upper-airway obstruction after multilevel cervical corpectomy for myelopathy. *J Bone Joint Surg Am* 1991;73:544–551.
35. Smith MD, Bolesta MJ, Leventhal M, et al. Postoperative cerebrospinal-fluid fistula associated with erosion of the dura. Findings after anterior resection of ossification of the posterior longitudinal ligament in the cervical spine. *J Bone Joint Surg Am* 1992;74:270–277.

CERVICAL LAMINECTOMY

PAUL R. COOPER
JOHN K. RATLIFF

Cervical laminectomy is most commonly performed to obtain access to the spinal canal for the removal of intradural tumors or for the relief of spinal cord compression caused by degenerative disease such as spondylosis or ossification of the posterior longitudinal ligament (OPLL). Because the spinal canal is narrowed, meticulous care in performing laminectomy is essential to avoid injury to the spinal cord. Although a variety of techniques may be used successfully, the description that follows is one that has proven successful and safe in avoiding complications and improving neurologic function.

INTUBATION

When the spinal canal is narrowed by spondylosis or tumor, abrupt movements or manipulation of the spine at or beyond normal physiologic range is potentially dangerous. We therefore use awake fiberoptic intubation with minimal manipulation of the neck. After intubation is achieved with the patient on a stretcher or hospital bed, an abbreviated motor examination is performed to confirm that the spinal cord has not been injured; general anesthesia is then induced. The surgeon must be present and involved in all aspects of anesthesia monitoring and positioning.

EVOKED POTENTIAL MONITORING

We utilize somatosensory and motor evoked potential monitoring in all patients. However, the evidence that their use improves outcome is lacking. Motor evoked potentials provide nearly instantaneous feedback of corticospinal tract injury. Unfortunately, they are frequently unobtainable in patients with neurologic compromise. Somatosensory evoked potentials are more likely to be elicited than motor evoked potentials; however, there is a longer time interval between injury and changes in potentials, and irreversible injury may occur before perturbation of potentials. In short, although both motor and somatosensory evoked potentials may be predictive of increased neurologic dysfunction, it is not clear that they are preventive.

PATIENT POSITIONING

Patients are placed in a cervical collar, and a three-pin head holder is fixed to the skull. The patient is rotated to the prone position on the operating table from the hospital bed, and the head holder is fixed to a Mayfield attachment on the operating table. The table is then placed in reverse Trendelenburg position so that the cervical spine is parallel to the floor. The body position should be adjusted so that the chin is at least 6 inches above the

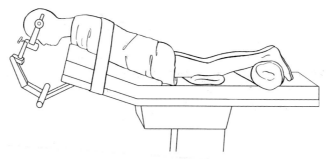

FIGURE 15.1. Positioning. The patient's head is immobilized in the Mayfield head holder. The neck is maintained in neutral position. In cases adding fusion, the neck is extended. The arms, legs, and all pressure points are padded.

end of the table because the body tends to slide caudally while in a reverse Trendelenburg position (Fig. 15.1).

The cervical spine is maintained in a neutral position, confirmed by fluoroscopy or lateral x-ray. The shoulders are taped down to a footboard or to the foot of the bed to facilitate the operative exposure. Excessive distraction on the shoulders may produce a stretch injury of the brachial plexus, affecting either the C5 root or the upper trunk, and should be avoided.

Although a horseshoe headrest may be used instead of the three-pin head holder, maintenance of head position is less secure and skin breakdown over the malar eminence may occur. Furthermore, if the globe rests on the head rest, blindness may result.

SOFT TISSUE DISSECTION

The length and location of the vertical midline incision may be determined with x-ray or fluoroscopy. The skin and subcutaneous tissues are incised, exposing the cervical fascia. The fascia is incised in the midline, and a subperiosteal dissection of the muscle is carried out on either side of the midline using the electrocautery. Muscle is retracted to expose the lateral masses, and, if lateral mass plates are to be used, the lateral border of the lateral masses are exposed (Fig. 15.2).

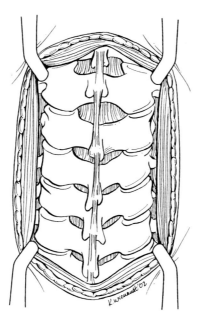

FIGURE 15.2. Exposure. The cervical fascia is divided in the midline and dissected off the spinous processes, laminae, and facets bilaterally.

If the arch of the atlas is to be removed, at this level the electrocautery should not be used more than 1 centimeter from the midline to avoid injuring the vertebral artery. Rather, a small periosteal elevator is used to dissect the soft tissues off the arch of the atlas. As dissection proceeds laterally, the pulsation of the vertebral artery may be palpated with a finger.

After muscle dissection is complete, exposure is maintained with cerebellar retractors. During the course of the procedure, the retractors should be relaxed every 45 minutes to minimize muscle ischemia.

BONE REMOVAL

Before bone removal is carried out, an x-ray is taken to confirm the correct bone levels. We use a high-speed, extra-rough diamond drill bit to fashion two troughs in the laminae just medial to the facet joints. Because diamond bits will not snag soft tissue, the possibility of injury to the underlying dura or spinal cord is minimized. Constant irrigation is carried out to minimize thermal injury to the underlying cord and roots. Drilling is frequently stopped, and a small curette or a nerve hook is used to feel for remaining bone without entering the spinal canal. We cannot emphasize too strongly that instruments such as rongeurs should never be introduced into the spinal canal (Fig. 15.3).

After drilling is complete, the most caudal lamina is elevated slightly to expose the ligamentum flavum, which is cut progressively more rostrally on either side of the midline to expose the dura (Fig. 15.4). In this fashion the laminae are removed en bloc (Fig. 15.5). At the rostral end of the laminectomy, care must be taken not to rotate the uppermost lamina against the dura as it is removed.

In patients with cervical spondylotic myelopathy or OPLL, foraminotomies are unnecessary because the sensory symptoms of the hands and upper extremity weakness are due to spinal cord compression rather than root dysfunction.

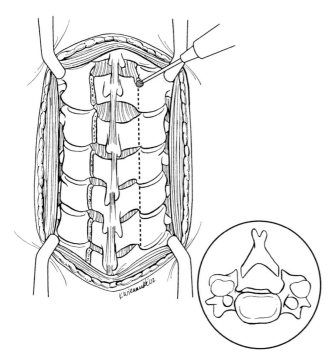

FIGURE 15.3. Bone removal. Troughs are created using a high-speed drill bilaterally at the junction of the lamina and the facet over the length of the decompression.

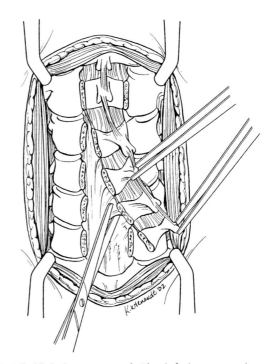

FIGURE 15.4. Bone removal. The inferior supraspinous and interspinous ligaments are divided. The laminae are elevated en bloc, and the underlying ligamentum flavum is sectioned under direct vision.

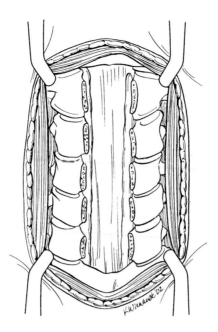

FIGURE 15.5. Bone removal. After the superior supraspinous and interspinous ligaments are sectioned, the laminae specimen is removed. Gelfoam is used to control epidural bleeding.

Epidural veins may be torn when the ligamentum flavum is cut. Although bleeding may be profuse, it is usually easily controlled with strips of thrombin-soaked Gelfoam. Bone bleeding is controlled with bone wax.

SOFT TISSUE CLOSURE

After removal of self-retaining retractors, meticulous hemostasis of muscle is obtained using the bipolar cautery. A drain is not placed. The muscle and fascia are closed in separate layers using heavy (zero or 1–0) interrupted absorbable sutures. The subcutaneous tissue is closed with interrupted sutures of 3–0 absorbable material. The skin may be closed with a subcuticular suture or skin staples. A cervical collar is used for a week for patient comfort. If the incision is carried into the upper thoracic region, as may be necessary to obtain exposure of C7, a figure-of-eight brace is used to minimize the chance of the caudal end of the wound being pulled apart.

CAVEATS

Cervical laminectomy may result in progressive deformity in patients with preexisting kyphosis. In adult patients, development of postlaminectomy spinal deformity clearly correlates with facet disruption or resection (1,2). Furthermore, in patients with compression from spondylosis and a straightened or kyphotic alignment, the spinal cord is less likely to move posteriorly and laminectomy may not lead to satisfactory decompression, unlike in patients with a lordotic spine. In the former cases, an anterior decompressive operation may be preferable (3). However, stabilization of the spine and prevention of late deformity may be achieved by placement of lateral mass plates and screws at the time of laminectomy.

Development of postlaminectomy kyphosis is a significant risk in younger patients (4). In patients with intraspinal tumors, laminectomy may be unavoidable and facet removal may be extensive in order to obtain the lateral exposure needed for anteriorly placed intradural tumors. In such patients (and particularly in pediatric patients), lateral mass plates should be placed at the time of laminectomy. In all patients, lateral cervical spine films should be obtained several weeks after surgery and every 1 to 2 months for the first year to make certain that alignment is maintained.

REFERENCES

1. Zdeblick T, Abitbol JJ, Kunz DN, et al. Cervical stability after sequential capsule resection. *Spine* 1993;18:2005–2008.
2. Zdeblick T, Zou D, Warden KE, et al. Cervical stability after foraminotomy. *J Bone Joint Surg Am* 1992;74:22–27.
3. Chiles B, Leonard MA, Choudhri HF, et al. Cervical spondylotic myelopathy: patterns of neurological deficit and recovery after anterior cervical decompression. *Neurosurgery* 1999;44:762–769.
4. Cattell H, Clark GL. Cervical kyphosis and instability following multiple laminectomies in children. *J Bone Joint Surg Am* 1967;49:713–720.

POSTERIOR DECOMPRESSION FOR MYELOPATHY: LAMINOPLASTY

KAZUO YONENOBU
JOHN G. HELLER
TAKENORI ODA

Laminectomy has long been a standard procedure to decompress the spinal cord for cervical myelopathy secondary to multisegmental spondylosis and ossification of the posterior longitudinal ligament (OPLL), with or without developmental spinal canal stenosis. However, subsequent neurologic deterioration has been observed due to postoperative malalignment such as swan-neck deformity, instability of the cervical spine, and the so-called laminectomy membrane (1).

Because of the unfavorable results of laminectomy, several Japanese spine surgeons developed posterior procedures in which decompression of the spinal cord could

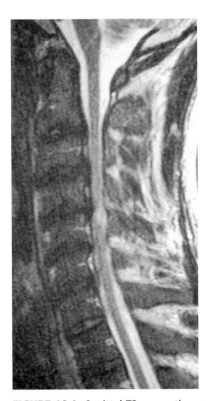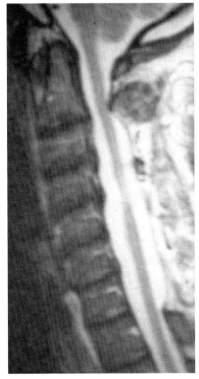

FIGURE 16.1. Sagittal T2 magnetic resonance image showing multilevel spinal cord compression due to spondylosis combined with congenital stenosis before **(left)** and after **(right)** an open-door laminoplasty from C3 to C7. Note that the space available for the spinal cord has increased substantially and that the spinal cord is well decompressed.

be achieved while preserving the posterior elements of the cervical spine that were thought to be important contributors to alignment and stability. In 1973, Oyama and colleagues (2) introduced the expansive Z-shaped laminoplasty in which the posterior wall of the spinal canal was preserved by Z-plasty of the thinned laminae. In 1978, Hirabayashi (3) reported his expansive open-door laminoplasty, which gained wide acceptance. Over time, various modifications and supplementary procedures were devised for posterior decompression of the spinal cord and for preservation of stability of the cervical spine. Each has proved effective in providing indirect decompression of the cervical spinal cord via a posterior approach (Fig. 16.1). Essentially all of the laminoplasty variants effectively expand the cross-sectional area of the spinal canal while preserving alignment, stability, and motion.

INDICATIONS AND CONTRAINDICATIONS

The indications for laminoplasty are similar to those for conventional cervical laminectomy. Generally, cervical laminoplasty is indicated for myelopathy secondary to developmental canal stenosis, multisegmental spondylosis, continuous or mixed type of OPLL, and multilevel segmental type of OPLL. Laminoplasty is also indicated for the distal type of cervical spondylotic amyotrophy with spinal canal stenosis.

Some believe that laminoplasty is well suited to the treatment of myelopathy secondary to soft disc herniations, or one- or two-level spondylosis associated with developmental spinal canal stenosis. This school of thought reserves anterior decompression and fusion for those with disc herniations causing radiculopathy. The role of laminoplasty in treating multilevel spondylosis with radiculopathy or radiculomyelopathy is less well defined.

Spinal cord tumors can also be extirpated by laminoplasty. This is especially true for skeletally immature patients because the risk of postoperative kyphosis and instability is lower than with laminectomy. Laminoplasty and fusion has also been recommended for myelopathy secondary to multilevel subaxial subluxation in patients with rheumatoid arthritis. For myelopathy secondary to multisegmental spondylosis associated with athetoid cerebral palsy or other movement disorders, laminoplasty with segmental instrumentation and fusion can be successful in managing a difficult clinical circumstance, provided that the athetoid movements of the neck can be properly controlled with a halo vest during the postoperative period.

A fixed kyphotic cervical spine is an absolute contraindication for laminoplasty, because spinal cord decompression cannot be achieved in this circumstance. In this situation, if a posterior procedure must be employed, one should consider segmental instrumentation and fusion to maintain the desired alignment, or consider an anterior decompression and fusion procedure. The age of the patient does not place a limit on laminoplasty, since the surgical invasiveness of this procedure is similar to that of laminectomy. Other contraindications to laminoplasty include spinal cord compression due to ossification of the ligamentum flavum, primary epidural fibrosis, and previous laminectomies.

BENEFITS AND LIMITATIONS

The essential benefit of laminoplasty is the ability to indirectly decompress the spinal cord without the technical difficulty of a multilevel anterior decompression or the need to sacrifice motion, as with anterior fusion-based procedures. This avoids the need for postoperative restriction of motion and most complications related to anterior grafts. An early active range of motion is encouraged rather than restricted. Problems with dysphonia and dysphagia are not an issue either. Also, expansion of the spinal canal can be obtained with little risk of losing spinal stability. Finally, some types of laminoplasty allow the opportunity to pursue individual nerve root decompression, especially on the "open" side of an open-door procedure via foraminotomies. This can also be done on the "hinge" side prior to opening the laminoplasty, but it is technically more difficult.

The limitations of laminoplasty are similar to those for other posterior decompressive procedures: It is not possible to expose or directly remove the anterior pathology affecting the spinal cord or nerve roots, and it is not applicable to those with significant cervical kyphosis. There are two additional disadvantages of laminoplasty. First, cervical range of motion may be reduced to varying degrees by stiffening or inadvertent fusion of the facet joints. Some believe that the effect is more likely if the hinges are placed too far laterally into the apophyseal joints. Second, axial discomfort of varying degrees may result after laminoplasty.

RECOMMENDED APPROACH

Laminoplasty employs a midline posterior approach to the subaxial cervical spine. Typically, in cervical spondylotic myelopathy, the extent of decompression is from C3 through C7. In this situation, the exposure of laminae is sufficient from the caudal side of C2 to the cranial side of T1. It is easy to expand the decompression to the upper cervical or upper thoracic spine by extension of the posterior approach cranially or caudally.

SPECIFIC PREOPERATIVE CONSIDERATIONS

It is important to evaluate the sagittal alignment of the cervical spine with lateral radiographs. Sagittal magnetic resonance images (MRI) can also be helpful in this regard. A fixed kyphotic deformity is an absolute contraindication. A preoperative computed tomography (CT) scan or CT-myelogram is useful for defining the pertinent bone anatomy. Pertinent CT information includes the width of the spinal canal, the relative position of the junction of the articular processes and the laminae, and the thickness of each lamina. One should also assess the patient's comfortable active range of motion in flexion and extension, which may facilitate intraoperative positioning. If the patient can comfortably flex his or her cervical spine without provoking any symptoms, then one may wish to position the patient in slight cervical flexion intraoperatively, which can facilitate preparation of the troughs and hinges.

OPERATING ROOM SETUP

The surgeon's usual setup for a posterior approach to the cervical spine is sufficient for laminoplasty. The authors prefer that the patient be placed in prone position on a laminectomy frame to decrease abdominal pressure. A three-point pin fixation device such as a Mayfield three-pin head holder is recommended to secure the head and to maintain the desired cervical alignment. Elevating the head (i.e., reverse Trendelenburg) is also desirable to reduce the epidural venous pressure and thus intraoperative bleeding.

NEEDED INSTRUMENTS AND IMAGING

The basic instruments for decompression are similar to those in a cervical laminectomy. High-speed burrs are essential for efficient and safe preparation of the troughs and hinges. There are several special instruments that may facilitate the procedure. These are described later in this chapter in the sections on techniques for each procedure. An image intensifier is usually not necessary.

SPECIFIC BIOMECHANICAL CONSIDERATIONS

The genesis of laminoplasty was the need to achieve indirect spinal cord decompression via a posterior approach without sacrificing segmental stability or spinal alignment. Because the cervical soft tissues are believed to contribute significantly to both alignment and stability, steps may be taken during exposure and wound closure to preserve their function. The important structures helping to stabilize the cervical spine in lordosis are believed to be the nuchal muscles and ligaments, especially the muscles inserting on the spinous process of the axis. The soft tissue exposure or reconstruction methods described here may be used alone or in combination as an alternative to the surgeon's standard midline posterior exposure and repair.

Reattachment of the Nuchal Muscles to the Spinous Process of the Axis

The rectus major, inferior oblique, and semispinalis cervicis muscles may be detached from the spinous process of the axis along with a thin piece of bone (Fig. 16.2). After completing the laminoplasty, these muscles are reattached by suturing the bony fragments through a hole in the spinous process of the axis. The other nuchal muscles are also repositioned and sutured to each other to reconstruct a suspensory nuchal ligament.

Preservation of the Spinous Process, Ligament, and Muscles Complex

In this method of exposure, the laminae on one side are exposed by conventional subperiosteal means, while the nuchal, supraspinous, and interspinous ligaments are preserved (Fig. 16.3). The spinous processes are then cut at their bases, and the laminae on the opposite side are exposed by retracting the nuchal muscles with the resected spinous processes laterally. After the laminoplasty, the nuchal muscles with spinous processes are repositioned and sutured to the nuchal muscles on the opposite side. This precludes the use of local spinous process autografts to prop open the laminoplasty. However, this exposure is well suited to the use of plate fixation, allograft, or synthetic props.

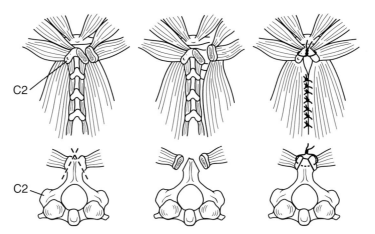

FIGURE 16.2. The rectus major, inferior oblique, and semispinalis cervicis muscles may be detached from the spinous process of the axis along with a thin piece of bone **(left** and **center).** After completing the laminoplasty, these muscles are reattached by suturing the bony fragments through a hole in the spinous process of the axis. The other nuchal muscles are also repositioned and sutured to each other to reconstruct a suspensory nuchal ligament **(right).**

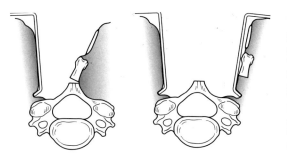

FIGURE 16.3. The laminae on one side are exposed by conventional subperiosteal means, while the nuchal, supraspinous, and interspinous ligaments are preserved. The spinous processes are then cut at their bases **(left)**, and the laminae on the opposite side are exposed by retracting the nuchal muscles with the resected spinous processes laterally **(right)**.

TECHNIQUE GUIDE

There are two fundamental types of laminoplasty: the unilateral hinge (open-door) and the bilateral hinge (French-door) types. The principal variations of each laminoplasty from C3 to C7 are described in this section. The basic concept of each surgical procedure is similar to that of the expansive open-door laminoplasty (4). No single laminoplasty procedure has been proved to be superior to any other with statistical evidence. As to incidence of surgical complications, no difference between the two procedures has been reported, although some claim that midline laminotomy during the French-door variants carries a slightly higher risk of dural or spinal cord injury or both. On the other hand, the paucity of epidural veins in the midline makes hemostasis less problematic with the French-door methods.

Theoretically, the maximum expansion of the canal is obtained at its central part in the bilateral hinge type of laminoplasty, and at its opening side in the unilateral hinge type. Whether this is of clinical importance is unknown. In the latter procedure, decompression can be extended along the nerve roots on the open side by foraminotomy. Spinal fusion with bone graft from the ilium can be added to either type of laminoplasty, with or without segmental instrumentation. This is not often necessary, but when a surgeon judges that a posterior decompression and fusion of this extent is required, the authors recommend against merely doing a laminectomy for the decompressive portion of the procedure. By preserving the laminae, one maintains a much larger host bone surface onto which the fusion can heal, thus creating a lower likelihood of failure.

Unilateral Hinge (Open-Door) Laminoplasty

Classic Expansive Open-Door Laminoplasty of Hirabayashi (3–5)

A midline approach is made along the nuchal ligament to the line of the spinous processes. The spinous processes and laminae are exposed subperiosteally from the caudal end of C2 to the cranial half of T1, with care taken not to damage the supraspinous and interspinous ligaments. When the subperiosteal dissection reaches the midportion of the lateral masses, self-retaining retractors are applied. Then, the base of the spinous process of T1 undergoes osteotomy and is folded toward the hinge side. Generally speaking, the open side is created on the more symptomatic side, particularly if a foraminotomy is intended as part of the decompression.

A trough is then created at the junction of the articular processes (lateral masses) and the laminae using a high-speed cutting burr followed by a diamond-tip burr (Fig. 16.4). The more aggressive burr is used to remove the outer cortex and cancellous bone of the lamina–lateral mass junction. A 4.0- to 4.5-mm round or oval burr or its equivalent is recommended. A diamond-tip burr (3.0 to 4.0 mm) is then used to thin the inner cortex of the laminae without penetrating the facet capsular tissue or injuring the epidural veins. Bear in mind that the cranial part of the lamina will require more attention with the burr because the cranial part is thicker than the caudal part and is covered by the caudal portion of the adjacent lamina above. While thinning the inner cortex, the pressure

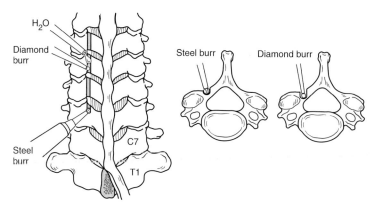

FIGURE 16.4. Left: This schematic illustrates the initial use of a cutting burr to prepare the open-side trough at the junction of the laminae and lateral masses. The appearance of the second burr above it suggests that it may be desirable to perform the final phase of bone removal with a diamond-tip burr to minimize injury to the underlying epidural veins. The axial schematic views **(center** and **right)** demonstrate more effectively where the trough is to be placed with respect to the laminae and lateral masses.

applied with the burr is directed medially. There is no need to penetrate any further ventral than the diameter of the initial cutting burr.

Bleeding from the cancellous surface of the lateral masses may be readily controlled with sparing use of bone wax, Avitene, or a viscous slurry of powdered Gelfoam and thrombin solution. Avoiding venous injury at this stage is strongly advised due to the epidural venous hypertension created by the stenosis. Once the laminoplasty is opened and the canal has been decompressed, such bleeding is both more accessible and more easily controlled.

In the original Hirabayashi technique, the bottom of the trough on the open side is resected with a thin-bladed (1.0- or 1.5-mm) Kerrison rongeur. For cutting of the laminae along the trough, one might also use a scalp clip holder instead of a Kerrison rongeur (Fig. 16.5). That is, a scalp clip holder is inserted into the trough and then opened to separate both edges of the trough by cracking any remaining sliver of inner cortex. With this technique, no instruments need be inserted into the spinal canal, which avoids neural tissue injury and may prevent bleeding from the epidural space.

Once the open side is completed, another trough is created on the opposite side, which functions as the hinge. The same cutting burr is used to remove outer cortex and

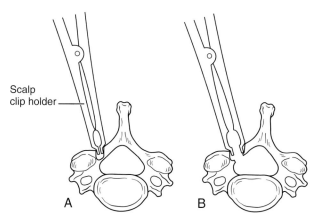

FIGURE 16.5. An alternative to removing any remaining bone bridges with a Kerrison punch is illustrated here. A scalp clip holder is employed to crack any remaining thin bone spicules by applying a local distraction force.

cancellous bone. This trough is set slightly more laterally (perhaps by 1 to 2 mm) than the trough on the open side. Above all else, the surgeon should avoid fashioning the hinge through the laminae, as this tends to result in a floppy hinge and a higher risk of displacement into the canal. If cancellous bone is not encountered beneath the outer cortex, stop and reevaluate the location of the trough before proceeding. It is important to preserve just enough of the inner cortex of the laminae on the hinge side. The objective is a stiff hinge that will actually bend open. If the cortex is too thick, it will break. If it is too thin, the hinge will be floppy. At the correct thickness, the hinge is somewhat stiff. Remember that the cranial edges of the laminae are always thicker; thus, more work will be required with the burr cranially at each level in order to uniformly thin the inner cortex. Pause frequently to test the stiffness of each lamina. If you have correctly detached the open side, you will be looking for the laminae to yield a little to firm pressure. If no motion is observed, first check to be sure that the open side is fully detached. Then proceed further with the diamond-tip burr. If anything, the tendency is to remove too much bone and to be too medial early in one's experience.

After creation of the troughs on the both sides, the ligamenta flava at C2-3 and C7-T1 are removed (Fig. 16.6). Usually, the extradural cavity is spacious at the region of the ligamentum flavum, so there is no serious danger when this ligament is cut transversely with Kerrison rongeurs or a no. 15 blade.

If the caudal edge of the C2 level contributes to the stenosis, one may decompress this level by removing the ventral cortex and cancellous bone with a burr, while preserving the dorsal arch of C2 (6). If such a dome laminectomy is needed, the authors recommend that it be done before making either of the troughs. However, the ligamentum flavum should be left in place as a protective barrier for the dura until the troughs have been completed.

The laminae are raised little by little from C7 to C3 by bending open the hinges. If the hinge thickness was prepared correctly, it should bend open in a greenstick fashion (Fig. 16.7). The door opening may be facilitated by simultaneously applying a force to the spinous process as well as the cut edge of the lamina. During this process, the tissues that resist opening are carefully coagulated with bipolar cautery and then divided. These include the yellow ligaments on the open side and any fibrous adhesions between the ventral side of the laminae and the dura, as well as numerous epidural venous branches. One should coagulate and divide the latter as far dorsal as possible. Hemostasis is more easily managed if one avoids the longitudinal veins running along the lateral margins of the spinal canal (Fig. 16.8). Bleeding from the epidural venous plexus is controlled with bipolar coagulation or by soft compression with Avitene. If the veins are initially inaccessible, they will be more easily managed once the hinge is fully opened and the venous pressure is reduced. Given the proximity of the spinal cord and nerve roots, indiscriminate or blind use of electrocautery is ill-advised.

In the classic Hirabayashi procedure, the sutures are placed through the articular capsules or paravertebral muscle or both on the hinge side, then passed through the interspinous ligaments or transspinous drill holes of the opened laminae, and then tied to prevent the lifted laminae from closing (Fig. 16.9). Held in this position for 3 to 6 months, the hinge will heal and the position of the laminae will remain secure

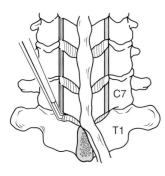

FIGURE 16.6. A 2.0- or 3.0-mm Kerrison punch is employed to excise the ligamenta flava at C2-3 and C7-T1 as one prepares to open the laminoplasty.

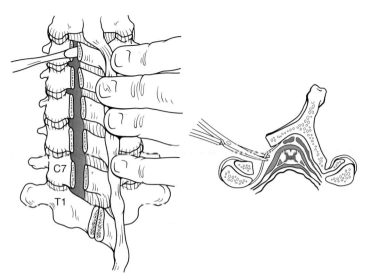

FIGURE 16.7. The laminoplasty is opened along its entire length gradually. The greenstick hinges are slowly and repeatedly bent open by simultaneously applying forces at the cut edge of the laminae and the spinous processes, if the latter have been left intact. **Left:** As the laminoplasty begins to open, the surgeon gains access to the underlying epidural veins. These are coagulated with bipolar forceps and then divided with scissors **(right).** Alternatively, one may accomplish both tasks simultaneously with the bipolar forceps.

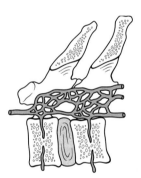

FIGURE 16.8. The cervical epidural veins (viewed from inside the spinal canal) encountered on the open side of an open-door laminoplasty. When coagulating and dividing these veins, staying more dorsal will minimize the need to deal with the more troublesome longitudinal veins along the lateral gutters.

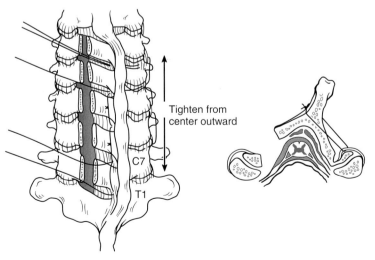

FIGURE 16.9. In the classic Hirabayashi procedure, the laminoplasty door is tethered open via sutures between the spinous processes and the facet capsules and/or paravertebral muscles.

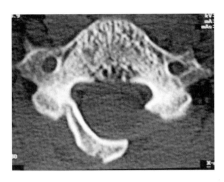

FIGURE 16.10. Axial computed tomography image made 1 year after a Hirabayashi-style laminoplasty. Note that the hinge has healed and that any risk of restenosis due to hinge closure has been eliminated.

(Fig. 16.10). Alternatively, arthroscopic suture anchors have been employed to suture open the laminae (Fig. 16.11).

More secure fixation may be achieved by bridging the open-side gap with miniplates and screws (Fig. 16.12). Originally described by O'Brien et al. (7), this method has been proven *in vitro* to resist closure more effectively than suture methods. More recently, specially designed plates have become available to facilitate this fixation technique (Fig. 16.13). The plates may be applied to each of the levels as described by O'Brien et al., or they may be alternated with local bone grafts as described later in this chapter, according to surgeon preference.

Prior to closure, check carefully for paravertebral bleeding points that may have been tamponaded by the self-retaining retractors. The wound is then closed in layers over a closed suction drain by the surgeon's preferred method.

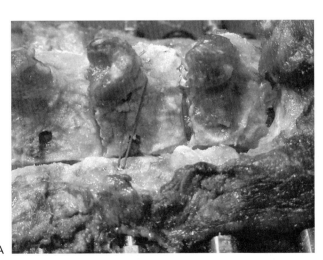
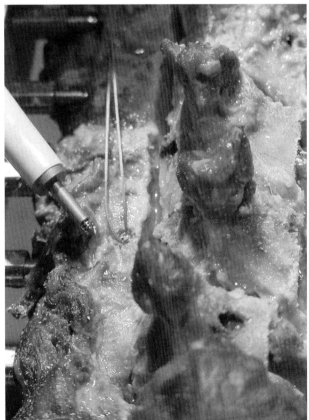

FIGURE 16.11. Left: Photograph of an *in vitro* specimen prior to biomechanical testing, wherein an arthroscopic suture anchor has been used to hold the lamina open. **Right:** An example of such a device and how the anchor is positioned within the lateral mass.

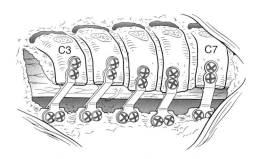

FIGURE 16.12. An intraoperative diagram demonstrating the use of segmental plating to prop open the laminoplasty via secure fixation at each level.

En Bloc Laminoplasty Procedure of Itoh and Tsuji (8)

The decompressive portion of this laminoplasty variant is the same as that of the Hirabayashi open-door laminoplasty described earlier. The essential difference is in how the door is kept open to avoid restenosis. After a conventional posterior midline approach, each spinous process is carefully removed en bloc by a Stille bone-cutting forceps, rib cutter, or similar instrument. They are cut to preserve maximum length and kept to be used as prop bone grafts on the open side. When the C6 or C7 spinous processes are either too small or dysplastic, one can harvest the T1 spinous process, employ spacers fashioned from synthetic materials (e.g., polyethylene or ceramics), or use an iliac crest graft. Sections of allograft rib also function well in this capacity. Typically, the creation of bilateral troughs and the procedure for unilateral opening are the same as those of expansive open-door laminoplasty.

The grafts are used to bridge the space between the cut edge of the laminae and the corresponding lateral mass. At a minimum, grafts are required at the C4 and C6 levels. It is not necessary to place them at each level. How to secure their position is a matter of surgeon preference and experience.

Classically, Itoh and Tsuji employed fine stainless steel wires passed sequentially through drill holes in the laminae, grafts, and lateral masses (Fig. 16.14). They also employed a similarly configured wire to suture the hinge side. Bone chips from the remaining removed spinous processes are put in the trough on the hinge side of the laminae.

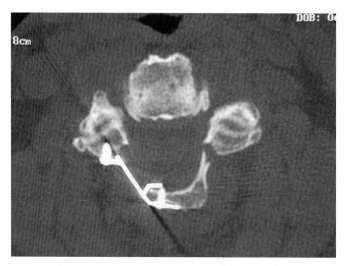

FIGURE 16.13. A postoperative axial computed tomography image through a level fixed with a novel plate design intended to facilitate miniplate fixation for open-door laminoplasties.

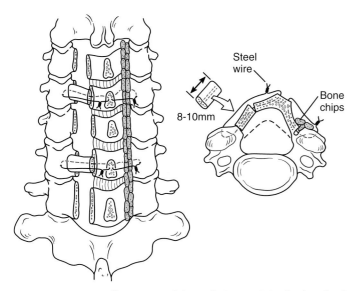

FIGURE 16.14. An illustration of the technique originally described by Itoh and Tsuji to prop open the laminoplasty via autogenous local spinous process grafts secured in place with thin wires. Their original procedure also included bone grafting the trough, but this is done less often today in an attempt to reduce spontaneous fusions and preserve range of motion.

Nonabsorbable sutures may also be used, though it can be cumbersome to tie them within the depth of the wound (Fig. 16.15). Nonetheless, conventional suture materials avoid the postoperative imaging artifacts inherent to stainless steel. In our current practice, the stability of the lifted laminae is made sufficient by securing the laminae and grafts in position only on the opening side. Therefore, the tunnels at the graft level are created only on the opening side of the lamina and inferior articular process. We now create the tunnel within the lamina by using a small diamond-tip burr as follows. First, the lamina is lifted like an open door. Second, the raspatory is inserted between the lamina and the dural tube for protection of the spinal cord. Finally, a perforating hole is created from the outer side of the lamina to the inner side by a small diamond–tip burr.

If the hinges are suitably stiff, one may fashion the grafts into a self-locking configuration, relying upon precise carpentry, the recoil of the hinges, and the force of the overlying musculature to secure the interlocking bone edges (Fig. 16.16). This method has proved

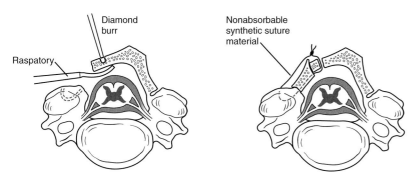

FIGURE 16.15. Securing the spinous process grafts may be simplified by using a burr hole through the laminae. Nonabsorbable sutures may also be used in order to reduce postoperative imaging artifact.

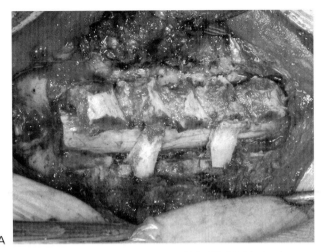
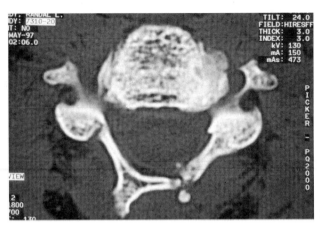

FIGURE 16.16. An intraoperative photograph **(A)** depicting two self-locking notched spinous process autografts placed at the C4 and C6 levels. An axial computed tomography image **(B)** demonstrating the shape and position of such grafts. Note that the graft–lateral mass junction has now healed.

quite satisfactory, but it requires careful craftsmanship to achieve the optimal graft size and shape.

The authors no longer put bone chips on the hinge side, because the hinges will heal on their own, and the presence of the graft fragments is believed to promote unintended fusion between adjacent laminae on the hinge side.

Bilateral Hinge (French Door) Laminoplasty

Spinous Process–Splitting Laminoplasty of Kurokawa et al. (9)

After exposure of the spinous processes and laminae, the dorsal part of each spinous process is removed. These resected fragments are saved to be used as bone grafts later in the procedure. Troughs for the hinges are created at the transitional area between the articu-

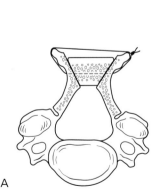
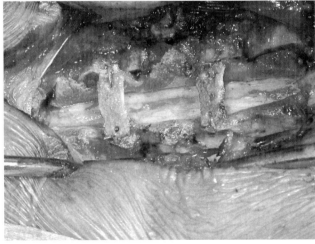

FIGURE 16.17. A: A schematic illustration of how a suture or steel wire may be passed through drill holes in the hemi-laminae and a bone graft (local spinous process, iliac autograft, or allograft rib). One may also employ ceramic spacers when commercially available. **B:** An intraoperative photograph of a French-door procedure performed with a T-saw, then fixed with split spinous process autografts sutured at C4 and C6.

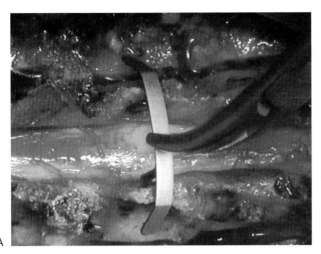
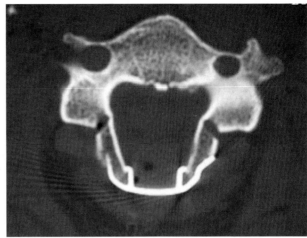

A   B

FIGURE 16.18. A: In addition to grafts and spacers, one may also employ a fixation staple to secure the position of the French doors until the hinges heal. **B:** Postoperative axial computed tomography scan following the use of such a staple during a midline laminoplasty procedure.

lar processes and laminae on both sides. The laminae are then cut in the midline with a diamond-tip burr (2.0 to 3.0 mm) and opened bilaterally like a French door. Some surgeons prefer to reverse the sequence of fashioning the troughs and dividing the midline in order to control the stiffness of the hinges more precisely. Care must be taken to avoid direct injury to either the dura or the spinal cord. The French-door method tends not to have much trouble with bleeding, since there are few significant epidural veins crossing the dorsal midline.

To fill the defects between the separated laminae, bone grafts from the spinous processes or ilium are fashioned and secured through drill holes with wires or sutures (Fig. 16.17).

Ceramic (10) or hydroxyapatite (11) spacers or pieces of allograft can also be substituted for an autogenous graft. When spacers made of ceramics or hydroxyapatite are used, absorption of the tip of the spinous process may occur and the spacer may separate from the base of the spinous process. Healing between the spanning graft or prop and the host laminae is not crucial to long-term success. Once the hinges heal, the hemilaminae will remain securely in place. For this reason, it is also possible to employ a special clip to rapidly secure the French door in the open position (Fig. 16.18).

SPECIFIC POSTOPERATIVE MANAGEMENT ISSUES

Postoperative immobilization of the cervical spine is optional, and possibly to be discouraged. One of the authors (JGH) employs soft cervical collars primarily to discourage inadvertent use of the neck as a lever arm to help patients out of bed. The collar can actually be used as a tool in their resistive muscle-strengthening exercises. Patients are encouraged to ambulate as soon as feasible after surgery, which may be strongly influenced by the severity of their myelopathy. Active range of motion of the cervical spine is encouraged as comfort allows. Some evidence exists to support this approach to reduce the likelihood of significant postoperative neck pain. By 6 weeks after surgery, patients should start active resistive exercises to rehabilitate their neck and upper extremity muscles.

Unless a supplemental fusion has been added to the laminoplasty, immobilization is unnecessary, and probably counterproductive. Because most laminoplasties seek to spare motion, neither surgeon nor patient need be concerned with the postoperative restrictions inherent to healing multilevel fusions. This includes any theoretical restriction on medications, such as antiinflammatory agents.

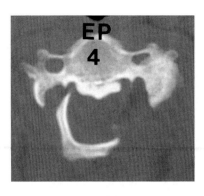

FIGURE 16.19. An axial computed tomography scan revealing a displaced hinge. This resulted from excessive thinning of the inner cortex during the hinge preparation. To avoid this pitfall, be sure to thin the laminar cortex uniformly, especially noting the thickness at the cranial side, and check the stiffness of the hinge frequently.

COMPLICATIONS

Intraoperative complications unique to laminoplasty may be grouped into technical issues related to the laminoplasty, such as hinge displacement (Fig. 16.19), restenosis, and graft displacement (Fig. 16.20), or complications from direct injury to structures during execution of the procedure (Fig. 16.21). The technical complications are primarily technique dependent and become less likely with increased surgeon experience. For example, a characteristic intraoperative complication of laminoplasty is fracture or displacement of a hinge, which may encroach upon the spinal canal and lead to either a spinal cord injury or nerve root palsy. The possibility of this occurring can be kept to a minimum if the inner cortex of the lamina destined to be the hinge is thinned step by step while its mobility is assessed until the surgeon is very familiar with this procedure. If a fractured lamina is difficult to maintain in a proper position by suturing or other means, removal of the lamina is recommended.

Two principal postoperative complications are characteristic of laminoplasty: motor root palsy and axial (neck and shoulder) pain. Nerve root palsy usually occurs on postoperative day 1, 2, or 3. The initial symptom can be severe pain in the unilateral shoulder or upper arm, followed by motor-dominant paralysis such as weakness of deltoid and biceps brachii muscles. The onset may also be insidious and pain free. The fifth cervical nerve root is more frequently involved, followed by the sixth and seventh in order. The prevalence of nerve root palsy varies among surgeons and procedures, but it is now estimated to be from 5% to 10%, regardless of the method. Although the mechanism of this complication has not yet been fully clarified, nerve root tethering due to posterior migration of the spinal cord has been suggested to be the major cause (12). The prognosis of this nerve root palsy is fairly good. The motor paralysis usually recovers to normal grade within 12 months. Therefore, we just do close observation and recommend physical therapy, although some surgeons advocate early nerve root decompression by additional facetectomy. However, one must bear in mind that this complication is not unique

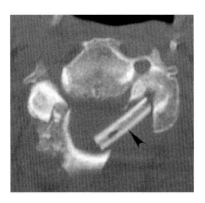

FIGURE 16.20. An axial computed tomography scan revealing a displaced piece of rib allograft. In this instance, technical errors included excessive resection of the lateral masses when preparing the open side and failing to secure the graft properly. The self-locking method failed in this case. The likelihood of graft dislocation would have been far less if sutures, wires, or plates and/or screws had been employed.

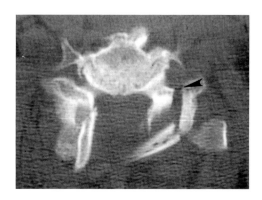

FIGURE 16.21. This computed tomography scan demonstrates the potential for injury if the surgeon is not properly oriented to the margins of the laminae and lateral masses as well as the depth of penetration. The arrowhead points to a violation of the foramen transversarium, which fortunately did not lead to vascular injury.

to laminoplasty. For reasons that remain unclear, similar root lesions can occur during multilevel anterior corpectomies with fusion (13).

Postoperatively, patients undergoing laminoplasty will experience varying degrees of neck complaints, such as nuchal pain and stiffness of the neck and shoulder muscles (14). However, most of these symptoms usually resolve by 1 year after surgery. They also appear to be less likely in the face of an early active range of motion. The causes of these symptoms have yet to be clarified. However, changes in and around the facet joints by surgical intervention may be one of the causes. Damage to the paravertebral muscles may also be associated with these symptoms. However, as with motor root palsies, it is a misconception to believe that axial complaints are unique to laminoplasty. A recent study of patients with multilevel cervical cord compression treated by either corpectomy and fusion or laminoplasty revealed an equal incidence of such complaints in both treatment groups (15). The authors recommend conservative treatment, which includes active range of motion, muscle training, antiinflammatory agents, muscle relaxants, and possibly passive treatment modalities (e.g., heat, ice, ultrasound). Passive manipulation and local tissue massage are contraindicated until one has proved that the hinges are firmly healed and there is no risk of inducing restenosis.

REFERENCES

1. Cybulski GR, D'Angelo CM. Neurological deterioration after laminectomy for spondylotic cervical myeloradiculopathy: the putative role of spinal cord ischemia. *J Neurol Neurosurg Psychiatry* 1988;51:717–718.
2. Oyama M, Hattori S, Moriwaki N. A new method of posterior decompression [in Japanese]. *Centr Jpn J Orthop Traumatol Surg (Chubuseisaisi)* 1973;16:792–794.
3. Hirabayashi K. Expansive open-door laminoplasty for cervical spondylotic myelopathy [in Japanese]. *Operation* 1978;32:1159–1163.
4. Hirabayashi K, Watanabe K, Wakano K, et al. Expansive open-door laminoplasty for cervical spinal stenotic myelopathy. *Spine* 1983;8:693–699.
5. Hirabayashi K. Expansive open-door laminoplasty. In: The Cervical Spine Research Society Editorial Committee, eds. *The cervical spine: an atlas of surgical procedures.* Philadelphia: JB Lippincott Co, 1994:233–250.
6. Matsuzaki H, Hoshino M, Kikuchi T, et al. Dome-like expansive laminoplasty for second cervical vertebra. *Spine* 1989;14:1198–1203.
7. O'Brien MF, Peterson DP, Casey ATH, et al. A novel technique for laminoplasty augmentation of spinal canal area using titanium mini-plate stabilization: a computerized morphometric analysis. *Spine* 1996;21:474–484.
8. Itoh T, Tsuji H. Technical improvements and results of laminoplasty for compressive myelopathy in the cervical spine. *Spine* 1985;10:729–736.
9. Kurokawa T, Tsuyama N, Tanaka H, et al. Enlargement of spinal canal by the sagittal splitting of the spinous process [in Japanese]. *Bessatsu Seikeigeka* 1982;2:234–240.
10. Hase H, Watanabe T, Hirasawa Y, et al. Bilateral open laminoplasty using ceramic laminas for cervical myelopathy. *Spine* 1991;16:1269–1276.
11. Nakano K, Harata S, Suetsuna F, et al. Spinous process-splitting laminoplasty using hydroxyapatite spinous process spacer. *Spine* 1992;17:S41–S43.

12. Tsuzuki N, Abe R, Saiki K, et al. Extradural tethering effect as one mechanism of radiculopathy complicating posterior decompression of the cervical spinal cord. *Spine* 1996;21:203–211.
13. Saunders RL, Pikus HJ, Ball P. Four-level cervical corpectomy. *Spine* 1998;23:2455–2461.
14. Hosono N, Yonenobu K, Ono K. Neck and shoulder pain after laminoplasty: a noticeable complication. *Spine* 1996;21:1969–1973.
15. Edwards CC, Heller JG, Murakami H. Corpectomy versus laminoplasty for multilevel cervical myelopathy: an independent matched cohort analysis. *Spine* 2002;27:1168–1175.

BIBLIOGRAPHY

Baba H, Chen Q, Uchida K, et al. Laminoplasty with foraminotomy for coexisting cervical myelopathy and unilateral radiculopathy: a preliminary report. *Spine* 1996;21:196–202.

Baba H, Uchida K, Maezawa Y, et al. Lordotic alignment and posterior migration of the spinal cord following en bloc open-door laminoplasty for cervical myelopathy: a magnetic resonance imaging study. *J Neurol* 1996;243:626–632.

Edwards CC, Heller JG, Hal SD III. T-saw laminoplasty for the management of cervical spondylotic myelopathy: clinical and radiographic outcome. *Spine* 2000;25:1788–1794.

Edwards CC, Heller JG, Murakami H. Corpectomy versus laminoplasty for multilevel cervical myelopathy: an independent matched cohort analysis. *Spine* 2002;27:1168–1175.

Heller JG, Edwards CC, Murakami H, et al. Laminoplasty versus laminectomy and fusion for multilevel cervical myelopathy: an independent matched cohort analysis. *Spine* 2001;26:1330–1336.

Heller JG, Qureshi AA, Marik G. Maintaining the laminar position after "open door" laminoplasty: biomechanical comparison of three methods, including a novel laminoplasty fixation plate. *Spine* (in press).

Herkowitz HN. A comparison of anterior cervical fusion, cervical laminectomy, and cervical laminoplasty for the surgical management of multiple level spondylotic radiculopathy. *Spine* 1988;13:774–780.

Hirabayashi K, Satomi K. Operative procedure and results of expansive open-door laminoplasty. *Spine* 1988;13:870–876.

Kawai S, Sugano K, Doi K, et al. Cervical laminoplasty (Hattori's method): procedure and follow-up results. *Spine* 1988;13:1245–1250.

Nowinski G, Visarius H, Nolte LP, et al. A biomechanical comparison of cervical laminoplasty and cervical laminectomy with progressive facetectomy. *Spine* 1993;18:1995–2004.

Tomita K, Kawahara N, Toribatake Y, et al. Expansive midline T-saw laminoplasty (modified spinous process-splitting) for the management of cervical myelopathy. *Spine* 1998;23:32–37.

Yonenobu K, Hosono N, Iwasaki M, et al. Laminoplasty versus subtotal corpectomy: a comparative study of results in multisegmental cervical spondylotic myelopathy. *Spine* 1992;17:1281–1284.

Yonenobu K Yamamoto T, Ono K. Laminoplasty for myelopathy: indications, results, outcome, and complications. In: The Cervical Spine Research Society Editorial Committee, eds. *The cervical spine,* 3rd ed. Philadelphia: Lippincott–Raven Publishers, 1998:849–864.

17

DECOMPRESSION OF THE FORAMEN MAGNUM FOR CHIARI MALFORMATIONS

RANDALL R. MCCAFFERTY
PETER J. LENNARSON
VINCENT C. TRAYNELIS

A German professor of pathological anatomy, Hans Chiari, first described pegged cerebellar tonsils in the upper cervical region in 1891 (1). Chiari proposed that the hindbrain herniation resulted from hydrocephalus. Although this may occasionally occur, more recent studies suggest that the Chiari I malformation arises from underdevelopment of the posterior fossa (2–4). Milhorat et al. (3) reported that 100% of 364 patients had substantial hindbrain overcrowding, and 91% of these patients were found to have tonsillar herniation greater than or equal to 5 mm below the foramen magnum.

A Chiari I malformation may be frequently associated with hydromyelia or syringomyelia (3,5–7). Semantically, *syringomyelia* refers to a cystic cavitation of the spinal cord. In contrast, *hydromyelia* is a dilation of the central canal and is lined by ependyma. Controversy exists in the literature as to the etiology and pathophysiology of syringomyelia (8). The original proposals by Gardner and Williams have been disproved largely because they rely on a direct connection to the syrinx via the obex. More recent authors have argued that

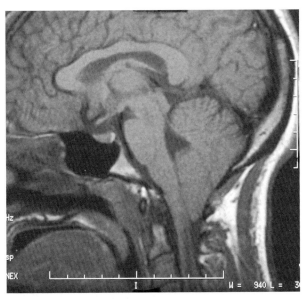
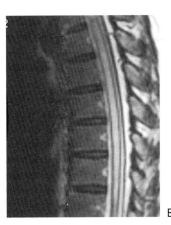

A   B

FIGURE 17.1. **A:** Preoperative craniovertebral junction (CVJ) magnetic resonance (MR) image of a Chiari I malformation with an associated syrinx. **B:** Preoperative thoracic MR scan. Note extensive syrinx. *Continued*

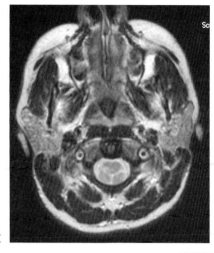
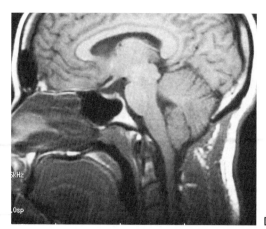
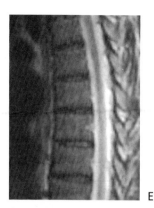

C   D   E

FIGURE 17.1. *(continued)* **C:** Preoperative axial view showing the cerebellar tonsils below the foramen magnum. **D:** Postoperative CVJ MR of the same patient following a decompression, duraplasty, and tonsillar resection. **E:** Postoperative thoracic MR scan of the same patient. The syrinx has resolved.

cerebrospinal fluid (CSF) enters the spinal cord via Virchow-Robin spaces to create a syrinx (9,10). Oldfield et al. (8) suggested that occlusion of the subarachnoid space at the foramen magnum resulted in progression of a syringomyelia. These investigators theorized that occlusion at the foramen magnum by the cerebellar tonsils creates a pistonlike force with each systolic pressure wave, which in normal patients drives CSF into the spinal canal from the basal cisterns. Oldfield et al. (8) proposed that this pistonlike force is what causes and propagates a syrinx in patients with a Chiari I malformation.

Regardless of the precise etiology of a Chiari malformation and its associated syringomyelia, all current theories typically incorporate craniocephalic disproportion and altered CSF flow dynamics (11). As a result, procedures for therapeutic intervention are designed to alter these variables (Fig. 17.1).

INDICATIONS

The clinical presentation of the symptomatic patient with a Chiari I malformation with or without syringomyelia can be wide and variable. Frequently, the diagnosis is made 5 years after the onset of symptoms. The average age of diagnosis is 25 ± 15 years; the condition occurs with a female to male ratio of 2–3:1 (3). The most common symptom is that of headache. The headaches typically are of pounding quality and radiate to the vertex, retroorbital area, and shoulders. They may occur with or be accentuated by physical exertion or a Valsalva maneuver. Signs associated with Chiari malformation may involve any major function of the central nervous system. A careful history and complete neurologic examination may reveal numerous findings.

Although a number of cranial nerves may be affected in the patient with a Chiari malformation, ocular disturbance is most common. A patient may complain of blurred or double vision or, less commonly, photophobia or visual field cuts. On examination, there may be evidence of decreased visual acuity or extraocular muscle palsy or palsies. Although rare, the patient may develop papilledema. Because the ocular disturbances frequently occur in young females, patients are commonly initially misdiagnosed with multiple sclerosis.

Many patients may experience otoneurologic symptoms. Dizziness, vertigo, tinnitus, or decreased hearing may all be associated with Chiari malformations. Clinical examination may reveal nystagmus. Abnormalities on audiometric or vestibular function testing may be found.

Family members may notice increased snoring. The patient may complain of dysphagia or dysarthria. Examination may disclose an impaired gag reflex, vocal cord paralysis, facial palsy, or hypoglossal palsy. Some patients may have abnormalities documented on a 24-hour sleep study.

Cerebellar symptoms also occur but manifest less frequently than ocular and otoneurologic disturbances. Lack of coordination, an unsteady gait, or tremors may be symptomatic complaints. On examination, the patient may reveal dysmetria or ataxia.

Although any patient with Chiari malformation may have symptoms referable to the spinal cord, such symptoms occur much more commonly when the hindbrain compression is associated with syringomyelia. The sensory disturbances may be intermittent and sparse and include paresthesias, hyperesthesias, dysesthesias, impaired temperature perception, and poor proprioception. As a result, the diagnosis may be difficult to make strictly on the history and examination. Examination findings may demonstrate dissociated sensory loss and decreased proprioception. Additionally, patients may have weakness, spasticity, and hyporeflexia or hyperflexia.

Chiari malformations and any associated syringohydromyelia are best visualized with magnetic resonance imaging (MRI). Although a postmyelogram computed tomographic (CT) scan can demonstrate both the descended cerebellar tonsils and associated syrinxes, currently these studies are best reserved for patients who cannot undergo MRI. Plain films of the skull and cervical spine may reveal osseous abnormalities or other abnormalities that may be important in the patient's evaluation or surgical planning. Flexion and extension views of the cervical spine may identify the rare patient with instability. Complete spinal imaging is of limited value but may be helpful in identifying scoliosis or additional bony abnormalities.

Surgical treatment is the mainstay of management of Chiari malformation, but not all patients require intervention. With the advent of MRI, low-lying tonsils have been found in numerous asymptomatic patients (12). In the adult population, a Chiari malformation may be diagnosed when the tonsils rest greater than 5 mm below the foramen magnum (13). Descent of tonsils less than 3 mm below the foramen magnum is considered normal. Most believe that decompression of the foramen magnum in asymptomatic patients in the pediatric population is not indicated (14,15). A survey of pediatric neurosurgeons in the United States demonstrated that fewer than 10% of respondents decompressed asymptomatic patients at the time of their initial presentation (14).

The broad constellation of symptoms may allow the surgeon to attribute any vague complaint to the presence of a Chiari malformation; however, it should always be remembered that treatment of descended cerebellar tonsils is not without risk. When evaluating the patient for surgical decompression, the surgeon needs to thoroughly consider the severity of symptoms, their impact on quality of life, concurrent medical conditions, progression of symptoms or radiographic findings, and the presence or absence of syringomyelia or syringobulbia. The decision to intervene surgically should be clearly reflective of the risks and benefits of observation.

Although the phenomenon is rare, there have been several case reports of the spontaneous resolution of a Chiari malformation and syringomyelia (16,17). A survey of neurosurgeons in the Japanese literature suggests that for the majority of patients, the symptomatic Chiari malformation is a chronic and progressive condition, but perhaps as many as 2% of patients have spontaneous resolution of symptoms (18). The proposed theories for this phenomenon are varied but essentially involve recanalization of CSF flow through arachnoid tears or reduced intracranial pressure by mechanisms such as improved venous flow. Additionally, in the pediatric population there is a tendency toward tonsillar ascent with increasing age. This occurs secondary to growth of the cranial vault as well as enlargement of the foramen magnum. Mikulis et al. (19) have reported that cerebellar tonsils 6 mm below the foramen magnum may be normal findings in a young child.

An additional study that may allow the surgeon to adequately select the patient with Chiari malformation for operative intervention is the cardiac gated cine MRI (20). This study documents the CSF flow profile as a function of cardiac cycle. Obstruction of the foramen magnum by the cerebellar tonsils during systole or reversal of CSF flow may be further evidence of a pathological condition.

Beyond observation, the sole treatment for a Chiari malformation is operative. The clear indications to operate include severe or disabling symptoms, symptomatic progression during observation, or radiographic evidence of an extensive or progressive syringomyelia. Many other patients may be candidates for surgery when factoring in the numerous variables elaborated earlier.

BASIC DECOMPRESSION

Given the central assumption that a symptomatic Chiari malformation and syringomyelia are a result of obstructed CSF flow and direct compression of neural structures at the level of the foramen magnum, the mainstay of surgical treatment is directed at decompression of the foramen magnum and reestablishment of CSF flow. Numerous variations of surgical techniques and options have been presented (21–29). The popularity of various surgical strategies has waxed and waned over time. Immediately following is the basic recommended approach for surgical decompression of the foramen magnum. Subsequently, other popular techniques and their indications are addressed.

The patient is operated under general endotracheal anesthesia. Consideration may be made of fiberoptic intubation. Regardless, the cervical spine should not be exposed to any large or excessive movements that may compromise an already attenuated brainstem and spinal cord. We do not routinely employ any form of intraoperative neurologic monitoring for this operation.

The patient is placed in a head-holding device and carefully turned to the prone position, whereupon the head and neck are fixed in neutral anatomic alignment. The scalp is shaved up to the level of the inion. The skin is initially cleaned with alcohol. This step serves several purposes. Hair from higher on the scalp may be combed back away from the operative site and will not require cutting. Oil buildup on the skin may be removed to allow skin markings to better adhere to the skin during surgical preparation and allow drapes to better adhere. The alcohol also serves as an additional bacteriocidal agent that potentially reduces infection.

The anesthesiologist is positioned at the head. The primary surgeon frequently stands to the patient's left side, depending on hand dominance and general surgeon preference. If an assistant surgeon is present, he or she stands across the table, and the scrub technician stands just caudal to the primary surgeon. Otherwise, the scrub technician may serve a secondary role as the assistant from across the table.

The midline incision extends from just below the inion to the level of the C2 spinous process. Lower incisions may be planned when the cerebellar tonsils extend more caudally into the cervical canal. The skin is prepared and draped in sterile fashion. Some surgeons give the patient an osmotic diuretic or steroid or both prior to incision. There are no solid scientific data to either support or refute this practice. The amount and subsequent frequency of dosing of steroid medication should be carefully weighed against the potentially increased risk of CSF leak and infection. Likewise, dehydration of the patient with diuretics should not be taken lightly. Antibiotics are generally given prior to incision. The antibiotic choice will be dependent on common pathogens within a given hospital and their drug resistance profile. We generally administer 2 grams of oxacillin.

The operating room setup includes equipment routinely used for other types of posterior cervical operations, including self-retaining retractors, a variety of rongeurs, suction and coagulation equipment, and a high-speed drill. The surgeon generally performs the operation with the aid of loupes and a headlight.

Prior to incision, the skin is infiltrated with 0.5% lidocaine with 1:200,000 epinephrine. The initial incision is made through the skin and subcutaneous fat. By placing the wound margins on a lateral stretch, a relatively avascular fascial plane may be developed between the bundles of paraspinal musculature. The prominent C2 spinous process can generally be readily identified during this dissection. With this as an initial land-mark, the base of the occiput and C1 lamina can be identified and safely dissected. Un-less necessary for the decompression, minimizing the removal of muscular attachments from C2 will help reduce postoperative pain. Care should be taken to avoid a vertebral artery injury when exposing the dorsal arch of C1.

The posterior fossa craniectomy and the cervical laminectomy are perhaps the most important and potentially the only definitive requirements in the operation. In-adequate bony removal may result in insufficient or no clinical improvement. Too much bony removal may predispose the patient to slumping of the cerebellum, a com-plication to be discussed later. The preoperative MRI will help to determine the caudal extent of the dural exposure, which generally only requires a C1 laminectomy. The en-tire width of the cervical canal should be exposed. In general, the posterior fossa cra-niectomy should be approximately 2.5 cm in width and should extend superiorly 2 cm (Fig. 17.2). It is important to remove bone laterally around the rim of the foramen magnum approaching the occipital condyles. As the surgeon moves more laterally, the orientation of the rim of the foramen magnum changes, and ultimately bone cannot be removed with rongeurs. At this junction, if lateral compression remains, further bony resection will have to be performed with a burr. In rare instances, there will be a very low-lying torcula. The position of the torcula, therefore, should be noted on the preoperative imaging studies, and the superior extent of the craniectomy adjusted accordingly.

Following the bony decompression, tight dural bands may prevent full expansion of cervicomedullary dura. Release of the bands, located most frequently beneath the C1 lamina, may produce a visible expansion of the dura. For highly selected patients, this limited operation may result in a good to excellent outcome.

If intraoperative ultrasound is available, evaluation of CSF flow may be performed. Sagittal ultrasound through the bony defect will allow visualization of the cervicomedullary

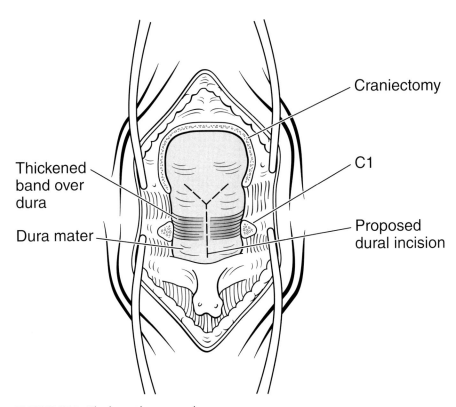

FIGURE 17.2. The bony decompression.

region and cerebellar tonsils. CSF in the retrocerebellar space and freely pistoning cerebellar tonsils should be observed; otherwise, additional decompression is necessary.

Should the surgeon determine that additional decompression is necessary, the authors have used a variety of techniques. The most common and widely recognized procedure is the duraplasty. Prior to dural opening, all bone edges are waxed. Oozing soft tissues are coagulated, and epidural spaces are lined with hemostatic agents. Both the surgeon and the patient may be rewarded by meticulous hemostasis at this juncture. Upon closure of dura, a relatively bloodless field will facilitate a rapid, watertight closure. In addition, because introduction of blood products intradurally may lead to symptomatic scarring and arachnoiditis, thorough hemostasis may reduce the likelihood of blood entering the spinal canal.

The dura is opened with a Y-shaped incision (Fig. 17.3). The long arm of the Y extends down the midline of the cervical canal, and the two short arms extend into the region of the posterior fossa craniectomy. The longitudinal dural incision can frequently be made by splitting the dura with a nerve hook. If possible, the arachnoid layer should not be violated. Although in some patients the circular sinus may be rudimentary, when crossing this sinus or dural venous lakes, the surgeon may confront rather brisk bleeding. Having bipolar electrocautery, suture, or surgical clips readily available is recommended.

A variety of materials may be used to patch and close the dura. The use of autologous pericranium, ligamentum nuchae, and fascia lata; synthetic dura; bovine pericardium; and cadaveric fascia lata and dura has all been reported, but few comparative

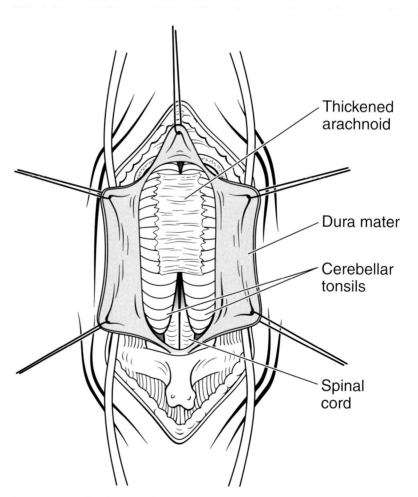

FIGURE 17.3. The dural incision.

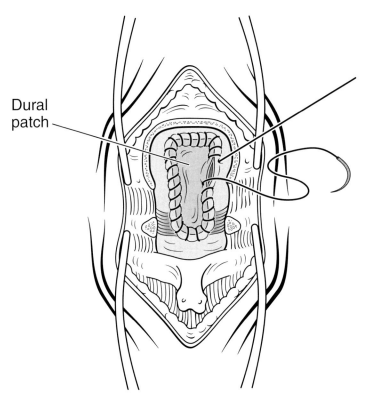

Dural patch

FIGURE 17.4. The dural graft.

studies have been performed (30). A triangular-shaped patch is created approximately the size of the dural opening (Fig. 17.4). A nonabsorbable suture should be utilized for closure. A fine monofilament suture with a small needle may reduce the likelihood of CSF leak through suture holes.

In 1993, Isu et al. (31) reported a technique of dural expansion by removal of the outer layer of dura.Gambardella et al. (32) reported on a variation of this technique by performing microincisions in the external layer of dura to allow for dural expansion. We have performed this technique on a limited number of patients with adequate results. Parasagittal or oblique transverse incisions are made in the outer dural layer, and stretching of the inner layer may be observed beneath the incision. In young children, where the dura may be more distensible, simple decompression with or without microincisions may be a preferred technique (33).

Because overcrowding of the foramen magnum and CSF flow obstruction may be the etiology of all symptoms associated with a Chiari malformation as well as serve as the pathophysiologic source for development of syringomyelia, simple decompression of the foramen magnum may independently lead to excellent results (33,34). Munshi et al. (35), in a small series of patients, suggested that combining this technique with duraplasty in patients with syringomyelia might lead to a more reliable symptomatic or radiographic improvement.

Following decompression with or without duraplasty, closure is performed. A Valsalva maneuver should be performed to evaluate the tightness of the duraplasty. The goal is to obtain a watertight primary closure. In almost all cases, this can be accomplished because a graft is used. If the patient's dura is exceptionally attenuated, fibrin glue may be of some assistance, although the efficacy of this substance when used to seal dura has never been clinically proven. Particular attention should be paid to closure of the fascial layer, which may prevent a developing pseudomeningocele from becoming a CSF fistula.

ADDITIONAL TECHNIQUES

Simple foramen magnum decompression with or without duraplasty frequently results in clinical or radiographic improvement of the patient. Numerous procedures and variations of this technique have been reported, and clearly defining the best therapeutic approach is difficult. The following is a brief discussion of other techniques and procedures that may be employed in the treatment of the Chiari malformation and syrinx.

Cerebrospinal Fluid Diversion

Although surgical decompression of the foramen magnum does not directly treat syringomyelia, because of the pathophysiologic relationship, one frequently observes clinical improvement in spinal cord symptoms or a radiologic improvement in the size of the syrinx. Although we do not consider shunting a primary treatment, in the past shunting has been the mainstay of treatment for a Chiari patient with a particularly large syrinx and few hindbrain symptoms (26,36,37). Other reports suggest that primary shunting results in poor outcome (38).

We prefer to address the primary pathophysiologic entity with decompression. Persistent syrinxes that are accompanied by unimproved spinal cord symptoms and not improved with CSF decompression may be good candidates for treatment with direct shunting. Prior to surgery, the patient should undergo repeat MRI of all portions of the neuraxis involved. Any site of significant CSF flow obstruction should be addressed before shunting the syrinx. Particular attention should be paid to the former surgical site to assess for adequacy of decompression, scarring, pseudomeningocele formation, or other entity that may invite revision surgery (39). Cardiac gated cine MRI may provide valuable information on whether normal CSF flow patterns have been established.

Once the need for shunting has been determined, the surgeon may select among syringopleural, syringoperitoneal, and syringosubarachnoid shunts. None of these procedures demonstrates clearly superior results. The syringosubarachnoid shunt offers the advantage of relative technical simplicity from a single incision. On the other hand, manipulation of a second catheter tip around the spinal cord invites an additional opportunity for injury. Furthermore, these shunts may function poorly if inserted in a region of arachnoid scarring or inadvertently in the subdural space. Iwasaki et al. (37) reported on their experience with syringosubarachnoid shunts and concluded that a dorsal root entry zone myelotomy combined with ventrolateral subarachnoid placement of the distal catheter resulted in the fewest cord injuries and shunt malfunctions.

The major advantage offered by pleural or peritoneal placements of the distal catheter is drainage into an environment of slightly negative pressure. Both insertion sites will require a separate incision and may require long and awkward tunneling and patient positioning requirements.

In any patient, direct shunting of a syrinx exposes the spinal cord to the potential for injury. If possible, selection of an entry site into the cord below the cervicothoracic junction may reduce the magnitude of an injury. At times, syrinxes may be discontinuous or separated. Endoscopic fenestration of septa may be a viable option to ensure communication of the entire syrinx with the shunt system. Alternatively, multiple shunt systems may need to be employed.

Lysis of Arachnoidal Adhesions and Resection of the Cerebellar Tonsils

Although many surgeons believe that equivalent clinical outcomes may be obtained with a less involved procedure to decompress the foramen magnum, others report that manipulation or resection (or both) of the cerebellar tonsils may enhance the surgical result for the Chiari I patient with syringomyelia (38). The rationale is that removal of the cerebellar tonsils and lysis of adhesions improves the ability of CSF to flow from the foramen of

Magendie into the cervical subarachnoid space. In addition, removal of the cerebellar tonsils provides direct relief of a compressive mass upon the brainstem and high cervical cord.

The procedure involves pial coagulation and incision. Subsequently, surgical suction or an ultrasonic aspirator is employed to perform a subpial dissection. This should be performed with minimal blood loss to minimize the development of postoperative arachnoidal adhesions. Removal is performed until access into the fourth ventricle can be directly visualized. A modification of the procedure may be to perform shrinkage of the tonsils with bipolar electrocautery until they have recoiled to the level of the posterior fossa (40).

The decision to perform this portion of the procedure must be carefully weighed against the risks of a surgical procedure that involves dissection around the brainstem. No particular neurologic function is directly attributable to the cerebellar tonsils; therefore, no clinical deficit should be observed from their removal. On the other hand, surgical dissection can lead to dense arachnoid adhesions that may present additional therapeutic challenges in the future.

If the surgeon chooses to either shrink the pia arachnoid surrounding the tonsils or remove them, the foramen of Magendie should always be inspected. There may be arachnoid adhesions or a thin membrane obstructing outflow from this foramen. If such entities are present, a fourth-ventricle-to-cervical-subarachnoid shunt should be placed. This shunt can be anchored to the pia arachnoid with a fine suture.

Obex Plugging

Early theories of syringomyelia suggested that the development of a syrinx was a result of direct CSF flow into the obex (41–43). As a result, plugging of the obex with muscle tissue has been advocated (5,44). Because this maneuver does not address the currently presumed pathophysiologic mechanism for syrinx development and because of the potential morbidity, plugging of the obex has fallen out of favor.

POSTOPERATIVE CARE

The patient is generally maintained in a monitored setting overnight following surgery. This will allow for close observation of the patient for early complications, which may include cardiac abnormalities or respiratory depression. Prophylactic antibiotics are discontinued within this 24-hour period. In addition, any steroid use is usually discontinued because prolonged use may lead to impaired wound healing. The head of the bed should be maintained in a semi-upright position to reduce the effects of intracranial pressure on any dural repair. Barring any complications, the patient may be observed for the remainder of the hospitalization in a ward setting.

An MRI should be obtained 8 to 12 weeks following surgery to evaluate the adequacy of cervicomedullary decompression. In addition, any syrinx present preoperatively may be assessed for radiographic resolution. This study also serves as a baseline for comparison should the patient present with any new clinical complaints that may warrant further intervention.

COMPLICATIONS

Posterior fossa operations, in general, can be associated with complications resulting in high morbidity and mortality. The scope and invasiveness of the operation performed will partly influence the incidence of specific complications. The most serious complications include respiratory depression, cardiac abnormalities, and profound neurologic deficits. The etiologies of these clinical changes are varied but include wound hematoma, vasospasm, edema, direct central nervous system injury, and vascular injury. Minimizing manipulation of neural tissues and their associated vascular structures and maintaining meticulous hemostasis will help reduce the incidence of these complications.

Infections may be a complication of any operation. Infection usually presents within days to weeks of the operation. Clearly identified superficial wound infections may be treated on an outpatient basis with oral antibiotics. If the patient shows signs of any meningeal irritation, a CSF sample will need to be obtained to differentiate between aseptic and bacterial meningitis. While laboratory results are pending, the patient should be started on broad-spectrum IV antibiotics and IV steroids. Treatment may be refined as the definitive diagnosis is obtained. Consideration should be given to the removal of certain implants. Prophylactic antibiotics, meticulous surgical prep, and careful control of the operating environment will aid in the prevention of a bacterial infection. Minimizing the exposure of the intradural contents to blood products and degradation products from soft tissues will also help reduce inflammation.

Wound healing is also of concern in any operation. Poor wound healing following Chiari decompressions may manifest as wound dehiscence, pseudomeningocele, and CSF fistula. One must always consider infection and nutritional status when encountering a poorly healing wound. Intraoperatively, one should obtain a watertight closure of the dura. To deter a pseudomeningocele from developing into a CSF fistula, tight closure of the fascial layer should be performed. Whenever a pseudomeningocele or CSF leak occurs, one should consider the possibility of concurrent hydrocephalus. If this complication is encountered early, an externalized drain may be sufficient to treat this complication. Although a small asymptomatic pseudomeningocele may not require intervention, any delayed symptomatic presentation of a pseudomeningocele will likely require open direct repair.

A delayed complication that may be seen following decompression of the foramen magnum is cerebellar slumping or ptosis. This results when the cerebellum sags through a decompressive craniectomy that is too large. The patient may present with new intractable headaches that are different from those associated with the Chiari malformation. The patient may have persisting or worsening spinal cord symptoms associated with syringomyelia. Because sagging of the cerebellum may cause traction on cranial nerves, new cranial neuropathies may develop. Suboccipital cranioplasty has been described to manage cerebellar ptosis (45).

Of course, with any surgical procedure a patient may fail to improve. Occasionally the surgeon may confront neurologic deterioration from arachnoid adhesions and scarring. Minimizing manipulation of intradural structures and avoiding blood product entrance into the spinal canal may avoid this complication. One report described the development of syringobulbia that was successfully managed with reexploration, lysis of adhesions, and shunting (46).

The previous paragraphs delineated the most commonly occurring complications. Acute hydrocephalus associated with hygromas has been reported and managed with a short course of ventricular drainage (47). Others have reported complications that include postlaminectomy kyphosis, spinal accessory mononeuropathy, intranuclear ophthalmoplegia, diplopia, and macroglossia (7,48–50).

REFERENCES

1. Chiari H. Concerning alterations in the cerebellum resulting from cerebral hydrocephalus. *Pediatr Neurosci* 1987;13:3–8. [Originally published in *Dtsch Med Wochenschr* 1891;17:1172–1175.]
2. Mesiwala AH, Shaffrey CI, Gruss JS, et al. Atypical hemifacial microsomia associated with Chiari I malformation and syrinx: further evidence indicating that Chiari I malformation is a disorder of the paraxial mesoderm. Case report and review of the literature. *J Neurosurg* 2001;95:1034–1039.
3. Milhorat T, Chou M, Trinidad E, et al. Chiari I malformation redefined: clinical and radiographic findings for 364 symptomatic patients. *Neurosurgery* 1999;44:1005–1017.
4. Nishikawa M, Sakamoto H, Hakuba A, et al. Pathogenesis of Chiari malformation: a morphometric study of the posterior cranial fossa. *J Neurosurg* 1997;86:40–47.

5. Batzdorf U. Syringomyelia, Chiari malformation and hydromyelia. In: Youmans JR, ed. *Neurological surgery,* 4th ed. Philadelphia: WB Saunders, 1996:1090–1109.

6. Dyste G, Menezes A, VanGilder J. Symptomatic Chiari malformations: an analysis of presentation, management, and long-term outcome. *J Neurosurg* 1989;71:159–168.

7. Menezes A. Chiari I malformations and hydromyelia—complications. *Pediatr Neurosurg* 1991;92: 146–154.

8. Oldfield EH, Muraszko K, Shawker TH, et al. Pathophysiology of syringomyelia associated with Chiari I malformation of the cerebellar tonsils: implications for diagnosis and treatment. *J Neurosurg* 1994;80:3–15.

9. Aboulker J. La syringomyelia et les liquardes intra-rachidiens. *Neurochirurgie* 1979;25(suppl 1):1–144.

10. Ball M, Dayan A. Pathogenesis of syringomyelia. *Lancet* 1972;2(7781):799–801.

11. Heiss JD, Patronas N, DeVroom HL, et al. Elucidating the pathophysiology of syringomyelia. *J Neurosurg* 1999;91:553–562.

12. Bejjani GK. Definition of the adult Chiari malformation: a brief historical overview. *Neurosurg Focus* 2001;11:Article 1.

13. Oakes WJ. Chiari malformations, hydromyelia, syringomyelia. In: Wilkins RH, Rengachary SS, eds. *Neurosurgery,* 2nd ed. St. Louis: McGraw-Hill, 1996:3593–3616.

14. Haroun RI, Guarnieri M, Meadow JJ, et al. Current opinions for the treatment of syringomyelia and Chiari malformations: survey of the Pediatric Section of the American Association of Neurological Surgeons. *Pediatr Neurosurg* 2000;33:311–317.

15. Nishizawa S, Yokoyama T, Yokota N, et al. Incidentally identified syringomyelia associated with Chiari I malformations: is early interventional surgery necessary? *Neurosurgery* 2001;49:637–641.

16. Klekamp J, Iaconetta G, Samii M. Spontaneous resolution of Chiari I malformation and syringomyelia: case report and review of the literature. *Neurosurgery* 2001;48:664–667.

17. Sun JC, Steinbok P, Cochrane DD. Spontaneous resolution and recurrence of a Chiari I malformation and associated syringomyelia. Case report. *J Neurosurg (Spine 2)* 2000;92:207–210.

18. Moriwaka F, Tashiro K, Tachibana S, et al. Epidemiology of syringomyelia in Japan: the nationwide survey. *Rinsho Shinkeigaku* 1995;35:1395–1397.

19. Mikulis DJ, Diaz O, Egglin TK, et al. Variance of the position of the cerebellar tonsils with age: preliminary report. *Radiology* 1992;183:725.

20. Armonda RA, Citrin CM, Foley KT, et al. Quantitative cine-mode magnetic resonance imaging of Chiari I malformations: an analysis of cerebrospinal fluid dynamics. *Neurosurgery* 1994;35: 214–223.

21. Alden TD, Ojemann JG, Park TS. Surgical treatment of Chiari I malformation: indication and approaches. *Neurosurg Focus* 2001;11:Article 2.

22. Decq P, Guerinel CL, Sol JC, et al. Chiari I malformation: a rare cause of noncommunicating hydrocephalus treated by third ventriculostomy. *J Neurosurg* 2001;95:783–790.

23. Dickman CA, Locantro J, Fessler RG. The influence of transoral odontoid resection on stability of the craniovertebral junction. *J Neurosurg* 1992;77:525–530.

24. Eule JM, Erickson MA, O'Brien MF, et al. Chiari I malformation associated with syringomyelia and scoliosis. A twenty-year review of surgical and nonsurgical treatment in a pediatric population. *Spine* 2002;27:1451–1455.

25. Goel A, Desai K. Surgery for syringomyelia: an analysis based on 163 surgical cases. *Acta Neurochir* 2000;142:293–302.

26. Hida K, Iwasaki Y. Syringosubarachnoid shunt for syringomyelia associated with Chiari I malformation. *Neurosurg Focus* 2001;11:Article 7.

27. Iskandar BJ, Hedlund GL, Grabb PA, et al. The resolution of syringomyelia without hindbrain herniation after posterior fossa decompression. *J Neurosurg* 1998;89:212–216.

28. Krieger MD, McComb JG, Levy ML. Toward a simpler surgical management of Chiari I malformation in a pediatric population. *Pediatr Neurosurg* 1999;30:113–121.

29. Sakamoto H, Nishikawa M, Hakuba T, et al. Expansive suboccipital cranioplasty for the treatment of syringomyelia associated with Chiari malformation. *Acta Neurochir* 1999;141:949–961.

30. Vanaclocha V, Saiz-Sapena N. Duraplasty with freeze-dried cadaveric dura versus occipital pericranium for Chiari type I malformation: comparative study. *Acta Neurochir* 1997;139:112–119.

31. Isu T, Sasaki H, Takamura H, et al. Foramen magnum decompression with removal of the outer layer of the dura as treatment for syringomyelia occurring with Chiari malformation. *Neurosurgery* 1993;33:845–850.

32. Gambardella G, Caruso G, Caffo M, et al. Transverse microincisions of the outer layer of the dura mater combined with foramen magnum decompression as treatment for syringomyelia with Chiari I malformation. *Acta Neurochir* 1998;140:134–139.

33. Yundt KD, Park TS, Tantuwaya VS, et al. Posterior fossa decompression without duraplasty in infants and young children for treatment of Chiari malformation and achondroplasia. *Pediatr Neurosurg* 1996;25:221–226.

34. Feldstein NA, Choudhri TF. Management of Chiari I malformations with holocord syringohydromyelia. *Pediatr Neurosurg* 1999;31:143–149.

35. Munshi I, Frim D, Stine-Reyes R, et al. Effects of posterior fossa decompression with and without duraplasty on Chiari malformation-associated hydromyelia. *Neurosurgery* 2000;46:1384–1390.

36. Alzate JC, Kothbauer KF, Jallo GI, et al. Treatment of Chiari type I malformation in patients with and without syringomyelia: a consecutive series of 66 cases. *Neurosurg Focus* 2001;11:Article 3.

37. Iwasaki Y, Hida K, Koyanagi I, et al. Reevaluation of syringosubarachnoid shunt for syringomyelia with Chiari malformation. *Neurosurgery* 2000;46:407–413.

38. Guyotat J, Bret P, Jouanneau E, et al. Syringomyelia associated with type I Chiari malformation. A 21-year retrospective study on 75 cases treated by foramen magnum decompression with a special emphasis on the value of tonsils resection. *Acta Neurochir* 1998;140:745–754.

39. Pare LS, Batzdorf U. Syringomyelia persistence after Chiari decompression as a result of pseudo-meningocele formation: implications for syrinx pathogenesis. Report of three cases. *Neurosurgery* 1998;43:945–948.

40. Won DJ, Nambiar U, Muszynski CA. Coagulation of herniated cerebellar tonsils for cerebrospinal fluid pathway restoration. *Pediatr Neurosurg* 1997;27:272–275.

41. Gardner WJ. Hydrodynamic mechanism of syringomyelia: its relationship to myelocele. *J Neurol Neurosurg Psychiatry* 1965;28:247–256.

42. Gardner WJ, Angel J. The mechanism of syringomyelia and its surgical correction. *Clin Neurosurg* 1959;6:131–140.

43. Williams B. The distending force in the production of "communicating" syringomyelia. *Lancet* 1969;2:604–609.

44. Levy WJ, Mason L, Hahn JF. Chiari malformation presenting in adults: a surgical experience in 127 cases. *Neurosurgery* 1983;12:377–390.

45. Holly LT, Batzdorf U. Management of cerebellar ptosis following craniovertebral decompression for Chiari I malformation. *J Neurosurg* 2001;94:21–26.

46. Takahashi Y, Tajima Y, Ueno S, et al. Syringobulbia caused by delayed postoperative tethering of the cervical spinal cord—delayed complication of foramen magnum decompression for Chiari malformation. *Acta Neurochir* 1999;141:969–973.

47. Elton S, Tubbs RS, Wellons JC, et al. Acute hydrocephalus following a Chiari I decompression. *Pediatr Neurosurg* 2002;36:101–104.

48. McLaughlin MR, Wahlig JB, Pollack IF. Incidence of postlaminectomy kyphosis after Chiari decompression. *Spine* 1997;22:613–617.

49. Pivalizza EG, Katz J, Singh S, et al. Massive macroglossia after posterior fossa surgery in the prone position. *J Neurosurg Anesthesiol* 1998;10:34–36.

50. Rescigno JA, Felice KJ. Spinal accessory mononeuropathy following posterior fossa decompression surgery. *Acta Neurol Scand* 2002;105:326–329.

18

CERVICAL SPINE TUMORS

ALAN M. LEVINE

Considerable advances have been made in the treatment of tumors of the cervical spine over the last decade. These include progress in diagnostic techniques as well as in the surgical treatment of tumors. Tumors of the cervical spine can be divided into three groups. The first group comprises benign cervical tumors, which occur most commonly in the posterior elements of children. They frequently present with pain; in the past, they were easily overlooked and diagnosis was delayed. The current use of both magnetic resonance imaging (MRI) and computed tomography (CT) scans has made the diagnosis of tumors such as osteoid osteoma considerably easier.

The second group comprises metastatic tumors of the cervical spine, which are less common than those in the thoracic and lumbar spine and constitute between 10% and 30% of all spinal metastases. Ninety percent of patients with cervical metastases have other spinal metastases; the mean survival with all tumor types is 15 months from the time of occurrence. The incidence of cervical spine metastases varies with the histologic type, with breast and myeloma being the most common.

For the third group, primary tumors of the spine, treatment has changed dramatically in the last decade. The concept of oncologic resection of primary malignant tumors has caused an evolution from mere palliation of patients with primary malignant spinal tumors to the potential for long-term survival and even cure. The concepts have evolved to closely resemble those applied to malignant tumors of the extremities. Piecemeal corpectomy is appropriate for patients with trauma or metastatic tumors but is inappropriate in most circumstances for treatment of the patient with a primary spinal tumor. En bloc resection combined with appropriate neoadjuvant modalities such as chemotherapy or radiation therapy has changed the overall intent of the treatment program as well as the prognosis. Because both the evaluation and the treatment vary so widely among these three major groups of tumors, the techniques involved in their treatment are subdivided in this chapter according to the type of tumor to be considered.

PRIMARY BENIGN TUMORS

Primary benign tumors of the cervical spine are seen primarily in children. In the thoracic and lumbar regions of the spine, benign tumors are more frequent than malignant tumors (1), but in the cervical spine, benign tumors are less frequent than malignant tumors. Within this group of patients with benign tumors, there is a wide variation in the radiographic appearance of the tumors. Some are minimally destructive, such as osteoid osteoma, whereas others such as osteoblastoma or aneurysmal bone cysts are highly destructive and easily visible on radiographs.

The primary clinical onset of benign tumors of the cervical spine is nonspecific and usually consists of diffuse or localized neck pain in a younger individual. Delays in diagnosis are now less common. Although some tumors are felt to have specific symptom complexes, such as osteoid osteoma, none has one that is truly diagnostic. Radicular symptoms may be present in benign tumors if a small lesion encroaches on a neuro-foramen, but it is unusual for these patients to have myelopathy. Radicular pain occurs in 20% to 50% of all patients, but radicular findings are present in less than 20% of all patients. The most common histologic diagnoses are osteoid osteoma, osteoblastoma, giant cell tumor, osteochondroma, Langerhans cell histiocytosis, and aneurysmal bone cysts. Tumors are generally well distributed equally throughout the seven levels of the cervical spine.

Radiographic Evaluation

In all cases, radiographic evaluation of the child or teenager with neck pain should begin with two-view plain radiographs. The majority of benign lesions in the cervical spine are commonly visible with plain radiographs; the only lesion that may not be at least partially visible is an osteoid osteoma. Occasionally, oblique views of the cervical spine will be used, especially in the patient with a small lesion within the pedicle. Although previously technetium 99 isotope labeling was thought to be of great value in detecting tumors not visible on standard radiographs, this technique has been superseded by the use of MRI. Some lesions that do have activity on bone scan are not clearly seen on MRI, and single-photon emission computed tomography (SPECT) may be helpful in detecting these. However, if the patient has definitive symptomatology involving the cervical spine, an MRI will generally be more effective than bone scan as a screening tool. Most benign tumors of the cervical spine will demonstrate decreased intensity on T1-weighted images compared with normal bone marrow, especially if they have any calcification, and will have variable to increased signal on T2-weighted images. Fat-suppressed T2-weighted images, a fast spin echo, or stir images can accentuate the amount of edema seen in the adjacent vertebral bodies and soft tissue (2). MRI is most helpful in those tumors that have marrow placement or soft tissue mass. It may be difficult to demonstrate the nidus of a very small osteoid osteoma with this technique. Therefore, CT scan remains effective in the assessment and planning of surgical intervention for benign tumors of the cervical spine. Generally, 2-mm cuts are necessary through the area of interest to obtain satisfactory definition to define small lesions.

Biopsy of benign lesions is rarely indicated prior to surgery. Most have such typical appearance on radiograph as to be definitive, although some highly destructive lesions, such as giant cell tumors, may be confused with metastatic disease. Those involving an interior body are best biopsied using needle biopsy techniques.

Surgical extirpation of benign tumors of the cervical spine rarely requires techniques other than those that are standard for other cervical procedures. Some tumors, such as a stage III osteoblastoma or large aneurysmal bone cysts, may not be amenable to surgical resection and may require adjuvant techniques such as megavoltage radiation therapy (3). The remainder of the tumors can generally be treated utilizing standard approaches. Because the majority of tumors in the cervical spine are posterior, laminectomy at one or more levels in a piecemeal fashion generally will provide long-term cure of the tumor. In children, it is necessary to add fusion across those levels; otherwise, postlaminectomy kyphosis may occur (1,4).

The only benign tumors that may require a specialized technique are giant cell tumors of the cervical spine. These usually occur within the vertebral bodies and can be quite destructive. The approach that is used for these tumors is a partial or complete corpectomy (depending on tumor size), which is similar to that for patients with metastatic tumors. Therefore, a patient with a giant cell tumor occurring between C3 and C7 can have a standard anterior approach to the cervical spine. Those with involvement at C2 or at C2 and C3 may require an extended anterior retropharyngeal approach to the upper portion of the cervical spine (5).

Cervical giant cell tumors, especially when recurrent, may require adjuvant treatment. The most commonly used adjuvant treatments for giant cell tumors within the spine are phenol, liquid nitrogen, and methylmethacrylate. Figure 18.1 shows a patient

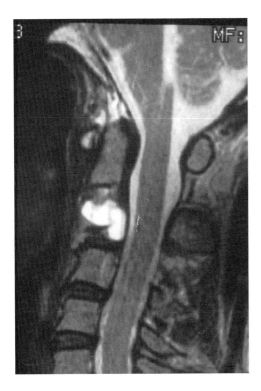

FIGURE 18.1. This patient presented with neck pain, and on the T2-weighted sagittal magnetic resonance image was noted to have an expansile lesion within the C3 vertebral body. The patient underwent an anterior approach to the cervical spine with curettage and bone grafting.

with a primary giant cell tumor involving C3 with little deformity. The initial procedure consisted of curettage and bone grafting, but shortly thereafter the patient had a recurrence with increased destruction, kyphosis (Fig. 18.2A), and extension into C2 (Fig. 18.2B,C).

Surgical Techniques

When using an anterior approach for upper cervical spine tumors, the patient is placed in the supine position on a radiolucent table, with Gardner-Wells tongs applied with 10 pounds of traction. A roll is placed between the shoulder blades, and the head is positioned in a ring and then taped to the table in the appropriate position. Evoked potential monitoring is generally utilized. Either the right or left side can be approached, depending on previous surgery and the surgeon's preference. A T-shaped incision is used, with a transverse submandibular branch and a vertical limb perpendicular to the submandibular limb (Fig. 18.3).

After the skin incision is made, the section is taken through the platysma and then mobilized in the subplatysmal plane. Care must be taken not to damage the mandibular branch of the fascial nerve when ligating the retromandibular vein. Direct damage or damage by traction will produce a droop of the ipsilateral side of the mouth secondary to denervation to the obiculare oris. After ligating the retromandibular vein, the section is taken deep to the retromandibular and anterior fascial veins while protecting the superficial branches of the fascial nerve. The submandibular gland is dissected out, ligated, and removed, and the digastric muscle is then divided. The fascial lingual and superior thyroidal vessels are individually ligated and then clipped before being divided (Fig. 18.4). The superficial layer of the deep cervical fascia is then opened along the anterior border of the sternocleidomastoid. At this point, the superior thyroidal artery and vein are ligated (Fig. 18.5). The remaining branches off the carotid artery and internal jugular vein are then ligated to allow retraction of the carotid sheath laterally. The posterior belly of the digastric muscle, which is confluent with the external hyoid muscle, is divided and

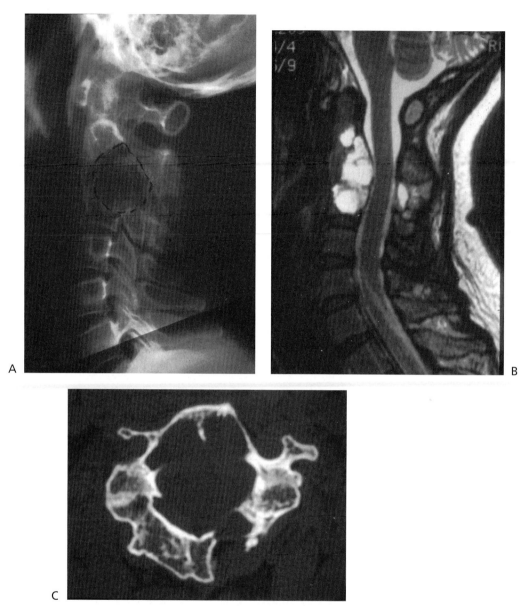

FIGURE 18.2. The patient returned 1 year after initial surgery complaining of increased pain and some deformity, with the head somewhat forward, and decreased range of extension-flexion motion. The patient was neurologically intact. **A:** The radiograph demonstrated kyphosis, with a larger lytic lesion that involved all of C3 and part of C4, with extension into C2. **B:** Magnetic resonance imaging was performed; the T2-weighted sagittal image demonstrated a much expanded area of bright signal involving the base of the dens, the C2 body, all of the C3 body, and most of the C4 body, with posterior bulging of the tumor and slight compression of the dural sac. **C:** On the axial cut, the computed tomography scan demonstrated a very thin rim of anterior bone with destruction of most of the anterior vertebral body. A small lytic area was also noted posteriorly.

then tagged for later repair. This allows mobilization of the hyoid bone and oral pharynx. The alar and prevertebral fascia are then split longitudinally, exposing the longus colli. At this level, the longus colli muscles converge toward the midline as they attach to the anterior tubercle of the atlas. The midline can be located by this tubercle.

At this point, image intensification can be used to ascertain exact localization, especially if there is destruction of both the C2 and C3 bodies (Fig. 18.6). The first intact disc below the area of tumor is generally opened first. In the case shown in Figure 18.6, the C3–4 disc was intact and the endplate of C3 was intact; thus, the dissection was

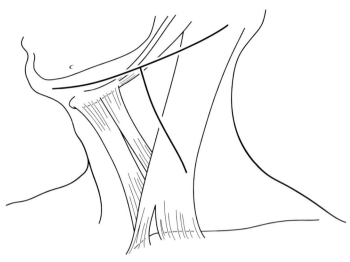

FIGURE 18.3. The approach to the upper cervical spine when reconstructing tumors generally requires a transverse incision paralleling the inferior edge of the mandible; for more distal extension, one can use a vertical limb that begins in the midportion of the transverse incision and is carried as far distally as necessary. It usually does not directly parallel the anterior portion of the sternocleidomastoid, but traverses it in order to maintain appropriate angles with the transverse incision.

begun in the C3 body (Fig. 18.7). The lesion for giant cell tumors can be removed intralesionally. Care must be taken, however, not to implant tumor in the surgical bed, because this tumor can seed into the incision line. A curette is used to carefully loosen the tumor within the body, and the pituitary rongeur is used to remove small pieces of the specimen.

Once all of the tumor within the cavity of the C2 and C3 bodies is removed and the disc between C2 and C3 is removed, the cavity is thoroughly inspected and copiously irrigated. Generally, the vertebral body will demonstrate small interstices where residual tumor remains. A high-speed, round, diamond-tipped burr can be used to thoroughly clean each cortical surface of the tumor cavity until there are no punctate areas left. In

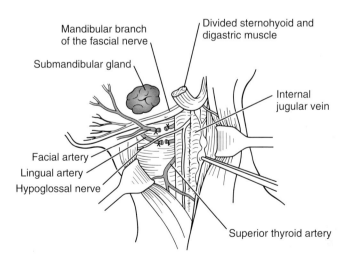

FIGURE 18.4. After the skin incision is made, the platysma is divided. Care must be taken not to damage the mandibular branch of the fascial nerve. The fascial, lingual, and superior thyroidal vessels are individually ligated and clipped before being divided.

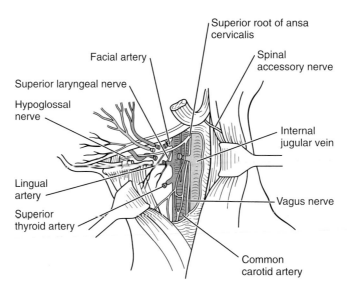

FIGURE 18.5. The superficial layer of the deep cervical fascia is opened along the anterior border of the sternocleidomastoid. The superior thyroidal vein and artery are also ligated. The digastric muscle is divided, allowing mobilization of the hyoid bone and the oral pharynx. This then allows the alar and prevertebral fascia to be split longitudinally, exposing the longus colli.

the upper cervical spine, there will be some portion of the dens process or one of the lateral masses of C2. Effort is made to burr into normal bone at both the proximal and distal extents of the resection. If there is no normal bone at the inferior aspect of C3, then the C3–4 disc should be removed until the superior endplate of C4 can be visualized. If an anchoring cavity in the inferior portion of C3 cannot be made, then a metallic anchor needs to be placed in the superior endplate of C4. However, in the case illustrated, there was remaining bone, and a cavity could be hollowed into the dens process, thus making a defined cavity within C2–3 in spite of this being a recurrent tumor.

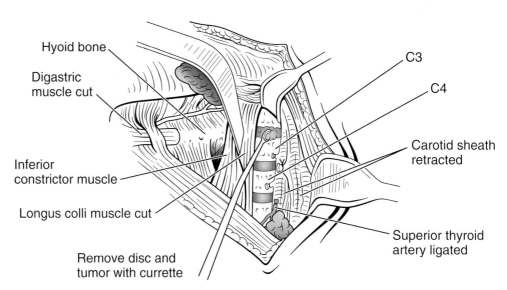

FIGURE 18.6. Generally, resection for any tumor is begun at the disc space just below the tumor. This allows establishment of appropriate anatomy. It also establishes the distal margin for the resection of the tumor. Cautery can be utilized to open the annulus. The disc is then removed using a pituitary rongeur. A ring curette is used, but only on the superior endplate of the distal body. Care is taken not to enter the tumor at this point, especially if it is vascular in nature.

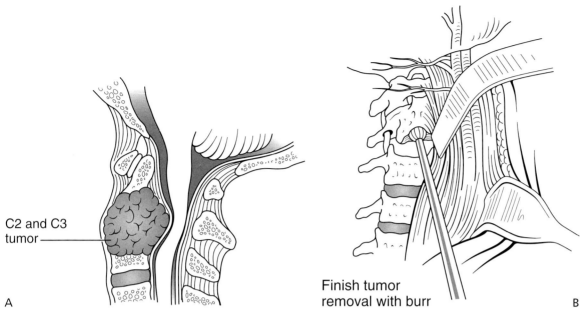

C2 and C3
tumor

A

Finish tumor
removal with burr

B

FIGURE 18.7. A: Once the borders of the resection are established, the tumor can be entered (assuming that this is a benign lesion that is to be removed using the technique of a piecemeal corpectomy). For tumors such as giant cell tumors, the tumor can be carefully separated from the remaining bone of the vertebral body. Special care should be taken not to allow pieces of the tumor to fall within the surgical bed because giant cell tumors have been reported to implant in distant sites or in the incision line. Only small amounts of tumors should be moved at any time. **B:** Once all of the gross tumor has been removed from the cavity of the vertebral bodies, the cavity is inspected. Any areas where there is residual bone along the edge of the cavity should then be burred, using a diamond-tipped high-speed air burr. This allows removal of small bits of tumor that are stuck in the interstices of the bone. At the surgeon's discretion, other adjuvant modalities also can be utilized.

Once the cavity is well defined and there is no further interstitial disease as indicated by punctate areas of tumor, the cavity can be filled with methylmethacrylate both as an adjuvant modality and as a method for stabilization. If the posterior wall of the body has been removed and either the dural sac or the posterior longitudinal ligament is visible, an alternative technique needs to be used. If a large mass of methylmethacrylate is packed in, compression of the dural sac can occur as the methylmethacrylate expands. In that case, one batch of methylmethacrylate is mixed and a very thin layer is placed along the posterior longitudinal ligament or directly on top of the dura and out toward the vertebral arteries on both sides (Fig. 18.8A,B). The layers should be kept extremely thin so that pulsation of either the vertebral arteries or the dural sac can change the position of the methylmethacrylate. The thin layer is allowed to harden, and then the cavity created by the hardening of the methylmethacrylate can be filled completely with more methylmethacrylate without concern for compression of the dural sac. If the posterior walls of the vertebral bodies are intact, the methylmethacrylate can be placed directly. This should form a tight seal, with no evidence of soft tissue or space between the methylmethacrylate and the surrounding bone (Fig. 18.8C,D).

Once this procedure is completed, there should be excellent hemostasis, and the closure is done in a routine fashion. Bone graft should not be used in this circumstance because recurrence becomes difficult to discern. In circumstances with circumferential involvement or extensive anterior disease, a posterior stabilization with autologous graft or fusion can then be performed (Fig. 18.9). This can either be accomplished as a one-sitting, two-stage procedure or in two separate sittings, depending on the patient's condition or the length of the procedure. Stabilization should be accomplished over the same levels. The occiput does not need to be included, since fixation can either be achieved

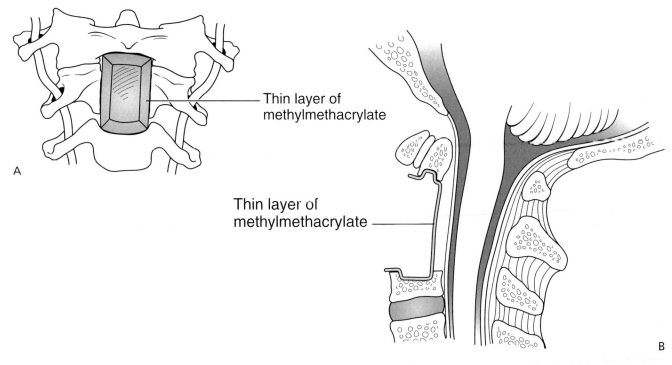

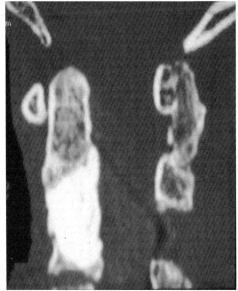

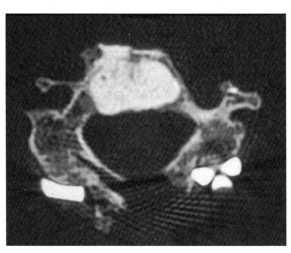

FIGURE 18.8. A: Placement of methylmethacrylate into vertebral bodies from an anterior approach can be done in several different fashions. If there is residual bone remaining proximally and distally, or if the areas can be undercut to provide a tab for stabilization of the tumor, no instrumentation is necessary in the vertebral bodies. If the anterior longitudinal ligament is left so that the dura is not exposed, the procedure becomes somewhat easier. However, even if the anterior longitudinal ligament has been removed, methylmethacrylate can be placed essentially directly on the dural sac, usually with a thin layer of Surgicel interposed. To prevent the methylmethacrylate from compressing the dural sac as it polymerizes and expands, the procedure is generally done in two phases. In the first phase a small amount of methylmethacrylate is mixed and a thin coating of methylmethacrylate is placed over the dura on the endplates proximally and distally and on the lateral borders of the corpectomy defect. If the methylmethacrylate is doughy, it will stay in that form; if it is thin enough, the pulsations of the dural sac will maintain a straight posterior wall, preventing any compression of the dural sac **(B). C:** This clinical example demonstrates the close proximity of the methylmethacrylate to the remaining bone, and the straight posterior contour that can be achieved using this method. Once the thin box of methylmethacrylate is polymerized, then the center of the box is filled with additional methylmethacrylate, which, as it polymerizes, can only expand anteriorly and not posteriorly toward the dural sac. **D:** This axial computed tomography scan at 2 years from the time of surgery demonstrates the complete filling of the defect and the sharp demarcation of the posterior wall.

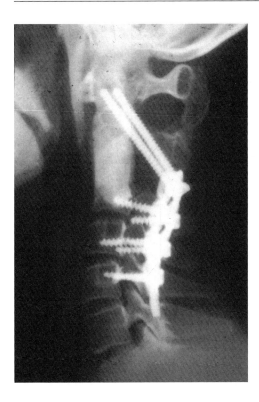

FIGURE 18.9. This lateral radiograph demonstrates a 4-year follow-up of the patient shown in Figures 18.1 and 18.2. There is no recurrence of disease. The patient has a stable construct in anatomic alignment with the fusion achieved posteriorly with autologous bone.

with transarticular screws incorporated into the plate or with screws placed in the C1 lateral masses if transarticular screws cannot be used with the plate.

METASTATIC DISEASE

In patients with osseous metastases from solid tumors, the spinal column is the most common site of involvement, though the exact incidence is quite difficult to quantitate. Based on a number of autopsy series, somewhere between 40% and 70% of all patients who develop solid tumors will have vertebral metastases. Neural compression, however, occurs in only 5% to 10% of all patients, with the annual number of patients with neural compression resulting from metastasis estimated to be about 20,000. The incidence of spinal metastases at autopsy varies with the primary tumor pathology. In patients with prostate cancer, up to 90% of patients may have vertebral metastases; about 75% of patients with breast cancer, 45% with lung cancer, and 30% with renal cell carcinoma have spinal metastases (6). The incidence of clinically significant or symptomatic spinal cord compression also varies with the tumor, being highest in patients with breast cancer and renal cell carcinoma and lowest in those with metastases from prostate carcinoma.

Although the locale of spinal metastases varies somewhat with tumor type, only about 10% of all spinal metastases occur in the cervical spine; the majority occur in the thoracic spine. When neural compression occurs, approximately 75% of the time it occurs from tumor that is in the body anteriorly, whereas only 15% of the time is the tumor mass posterior, and 10% of the time lateral. As mentioned previously, cervical metastases are often a later stage in bony metastases, with 90% of patients already having other spinal metastases by the time they have cervical involvement. Mean life expectancy for a patient having a cervical metastasis is 15 months, but varies widely with the tumor type.

Patients with bony metastases present either asymptomatically on routine screening follow-up such as bone scan, with pain, or finally with neurologic deficit. Pain, which is the most common presentation, can be based on neural compression, tumor replacement of the body, pathologic fracture, or instability. Duration of symptoms is a critical parameter in evaluation, and the rapidity of onset of neurologic deficit is a prognostic factor.

Radiographic Evaluation

Evaluation of the cervical spine in patients with metastatic disease always begins with biplanar plain radiographs. Although bone scan is frequently used to assess the presence of metastases, it is less effective than either CT scan or MRI in finding the presence of cervical metastases (7). Radiologically, the differentiation between vertebral compression fractions secondary to osteopenia and compression fractures secondary to tumor can be very difficult. Enhancement and signal intensity are not always predictive, but MRI is an excellent screening tool and will define well the degree of neural compression. CT scan better defines the extent of bony and especially cortical disruption, whereas MRI better describes the degree of marrow replacement.

Patients for whom surgery is contemplated for metastatic disease of the cervical spine should have an MRI of the entire spine. In a study done of multiple sites of epidural compression, 9% of all patients who presented with dural compression had a second level involved, and the mean separation between levels was 12 (8). Thus, to prevent complications as well as to assess the patient prognostically, midsagittal screening of the entire spine from the cervical spine through the lumbar spine is necessary prior to contemplating surgery. In patients presenting with simultaneous areas of cord compression (not simply spinal involvement), the mean survival irrespective of histologic type was generally only about 3 months. Patients should also undergo a routine screening workup for other metastases. Prognosis in terms of visceral metastases and anesthetic risk is based on the involvement of liver and lung. Thus, a patient undergoing surgery should have appropriate bone scans as well as CT scans of the chest and abdomen.

To plan surgery more appropriately, attempts have been made to assess potential survival for patients with metastatic disease. Tokuhashi et al. (9) developed a 12-point scale in 1994 based on six general parameters: general condition, number of extra spinal bone metastases, number of metastases in vertebral bodies, major internal organ involvement, primary site, and severity of spinal cord paresis. The authors found that those with fewer than 6 points lived less than 6 months, whereas three-quarters of those with more than 8 points lived more than 12 months. This factor of survival bears critically on the technical aspects of reconstruction of patients undergoing surgery for metastases to the cervical spine. The mean survival in most series that reviewed surgical treatment of spinal metastases has ranged from 8 to 14 months. Survival in all series, however, varied with histologic diagnosis when that factor was analyzed separately.

Although radiation or chemotherapy (or both) may be appropriate treatment alternatives for some patients with metastatic disease, the two major surgical alternatives are kyphroplasty/vertebroplasty and surgical decompression and stabilization. To date, kyphroplasty and vertebroplasty have not been used in the cervical spine. Thus, the remaining surgical alternative is decompression and stabilization.

Surgical Technique

Depending on the location of the metastasis in the cervical spine, various techniques may apply. However, prior to dealing with those, some general concepts regarding reconstruction of the cervical spine for metastatic disease should be addressed. Basically, three questions need to be answered:

1. Should the surgeon use titanium or stainless steel instrumentation?
2. What methodology should be used to fill in gaps in achieving stabilization?
3. Does the surgery need to be done anteriorly or posteriorly or both?

The overriding principle in treatment of all metastatic disease is that the reconstruction should be stable enough so that the patient can be mobilized immediately without requiring healing to achieve sufficient stability. This is critical for two reasons. First, the patient with metastatic disease to the cervical spine has a limited life expectancy. As previously noted, in most series the life expectancy is between 8 and 14 months. If patients need to be immobilized in a halo or some other orthosis for 3 months or more after surgery to achieve stability, they may not survive long enough beyond that to acquire a quality-of-life benefit from the procedure. Second, most patients with cervical metastases have either had radiation to the area or will be receiving radiation or chemotherapy or both postoperatively. Both modalities diminish the ability of the local tissues to heal and the ability of the spine to achieve a solid arthrodesis. Thus, the need for bone healing as a prerequisite for achieving stability after reconstruction due to cervical metastases has little merit. The ultimate goal is to achieve a pain-free stable spine as soon after surgery as technically possible.

When metallic implants are necessary, the use of titanium is clearly superior to the use of stainless steel in patients who have metastatic disease of the spine. This is not an issue of relative strength or modulus of elasticity, but simply one of enhancing future imaging. If the patient has neural deficit preoperatively or develops neural deficit postoperatively, it is often necessary to take MRIs at given intervals. The use of titanium implants allows much more effective imaging. The patient with a stainless steel implant in the anterior column of the spine will effectively have obliteration of imaging capabilities throughout that region, whereas the patient with titanium in the anterior column of the spine will have perfectly adequate re-imaging capabilities for the spinal canal.

The next consideration is the choice of materials for reconstruction of corpectomy defects, which can be done with bone graft (allograft or autograft), prosthetics or cages, methylmethacrylate, or combinations of these materials. In general, the advantage of using bone graft to fill in a defect after a corpectomy is that the construct is extremely durable after the fusion has occurred. However, in patients with metastatic disease, bone grafts have several major disadvantages. First, there is a need for fusion to occur in order to produce long-term stability, and thus a potential need for the use of an external orthosis while healing is occurring. Second, any bone graft may be invaded by recurrent tumor, and thus its integrity may be compromised. Finally, pseudoarthrosis with bone grafts is extremely common in the face of a previously radiated spinal bed.

The data concerning the effectiveness of the use of bone graft in patients with metastatic disease are very limited. In a series by Singh et al. (10), seven patients were treated with long structural allografts in the anterior portion of the cervical spine. All were immobilized postoperatively, and only one of the seven patients lived long enough to determine whether the allograft had actually incorporated (12-month follow-up). In a review article by Wetzel and Phillips (11) in 2000, it was suggested that "in cases in which bone quality is of concern, additional stability may be afforded by the use of polymethylmethacrylate (PMMA). This material should not be used in lieu of grafting, however, in cases in which survivorship is expected to exceed 6 months because of the high likelihood of cement loosening and migration." However, in the more than 60 references listed, not a single one was given for either the durability or the complication rates associated with the use of any reconstructive material, although it was suggested that rib grafts, iliac crest grafts, or allografts were optimum reconstruction methods.

Because the majority of patients undergoing surgery for symptomatic metastatic disease of the cervical spine have a life expectancy of 12 months or less, routine use of bone graft alone has little advantage. It is unlikely to heal because of the use of radiation and chemotherapy, and may provide limited initial stability. Even for those with longer life expectancy, bone grafting combined with either a cage or methylmethacrylate is a better choice. The initial reports on the use of PMMA occurred in the 1970s, with Scoville et al. (12) and then subsequently Dunn (13) reporting on its use for corpectomy replacement in metastatic disease. Methylmethacrylate has several advantages for spinal reconstruction, especially for corpectomy defects. It gives early initial stability, is impervious to tumor, and does not require external immobilization, although either plate or rod fixation across the affected levels is advocated. Methylmethacrylate is strongest in axial compression and weakest in tension. It has poor resistance to distraction or rotation, and therefore any constructs need to be augmented with instrumentation to counteract those forces. It does not bond to any adjacent bone, requires a method to augment stability and prevent dislodgment, and may be associated with a slightly higher rate of infection, although this is not well documented in the literature.

The use of PMMA for cervical corpectomies for neoplasms has evolved. Dunn (13) initially reported on 10 cases, and 20% of the patients experienced failure of the construct. Other series throughout the 1980s used various types of stabilization, but finally, in the mid-1990s, plate fixation became routinely used in concert with methylmethacrylate for vertebral body placement in the cervical spine. In 1995, Timlin et al. (14) reported 26 cases with plate fixation with a 0% failure rate, and in 2000, Miller et al. (15) reported 29 cases augmented with placement fixation with a 7% failure rate. Thus, when used properly, the combination of methylmethacrylate and an anterior plate can give adequate long-term stability.

Most of the unfavorable clinical and biomechanical data regarding the use of methylmethacrylate actually concern its use in a posterior position, where it is subjected to tension and rotation (16,17). The use of methylmethacrylate in the posterior portion of the cervical spine has been largely abandoned because of the wound problems and the fact that the material is being used in a suboptimal mechanical fashion. Thus, optimal use of methylmethacrylate as a vertebral body replacement for metastatic tumors seems to be most appropriate.

The final issue is the necessity of anterior or posterior surgery (or both) for achievement of stability. This choice is predominantly based on the lesion's location within the cervical spine and the degree of vertebral disruption. The occipital cervical junction and the cervicothoracic junction generally require at least posterior fixation, and when anterior stabilization is done, it may need to be augmented in the majority of cases with posterior stabilization. However, between C3 and C7, where most metastases occur, anterior corpectomy with methylmethacrylate body replacement and plate stabilization is generally effective as long as there is retention of the posterior elements. If there is destruction of the pedicles and facets, then it may be necessary to augment the anterior construct with posterior screw and plate fixation. Posterior constructs alone can be used in patients who have disruption of the posterior elements or have some instability without loss of anterior column stability.

In the upper cervical spine, pathologic fractures and the necessity for reconstruction of lesions are even more unusual than in the remainder of the cervical spine. In a number of reported series, anterior decompression was rarely necessary because of the spacious anatomic configuration of the neural canal in the upper cervical spine. Severe neurologic involvement is infrequent and quite late in most series (18). Deformity and instability are much more common reasons for the need for operative intervention (18–22). In the majority of these series, essentially all of the patients with upper cervical spine lesions or fractures presented with pain. Half of all the reported patients had surgery, and all had a posterior approach.

For patients with involvement of C1 or C2 or both, most commonly an occipitocervical stabilization is required. These patients generally have gross instability as the reason for their pain. The patient should undergo an awake nasotracheal intubation with positioning in a three-prong headrest, and should be turned into the prone position and positioned for surgery while awake so that neurologic reexamination can be performed. Once the position is found to be satisfactory and the patient's neurologic status is carefully reassessed, the patient can then be anesthetized fully. Procedures are generally done through a midline posterior approach with exposure of the occiput, C1, C2, and generally at least to C3 if not to C4 to gain adequate stability (Fig. 18.10). Segmental fixation

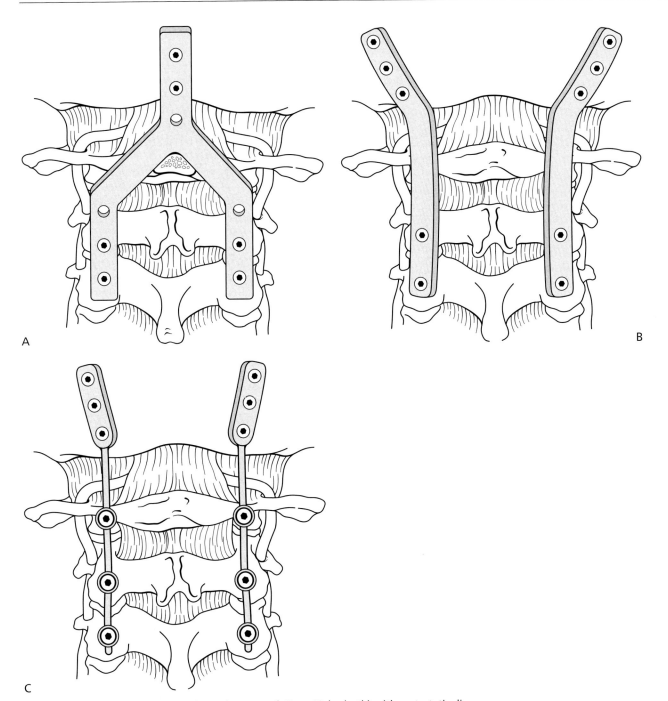

A

B

C

FIGURE 18.10. A: For patients with involvement of C1 or C2 (or both) with metastatic disease, the most common procedure required is occipital cervical stabilization. Because of the large diameter of the canal, generally neural compression is a less common reason for requiring surgery than instability. Most procedures are done through a posterior approach, and a variety of different plates are available for reestablishing stability. The critical feature of the plates is the ability to achieve adequate fixation in the occiput as well as either in C1 or C2 and potentially in C3 so that immediate stability is obtained by the patient without the necessity for a bony fusion to occur to achieve the required stability. **B:** Bilateral plates are often effective techniques. A minimum of six screw holes in the skull with screw lengths ranging from 6 to 10 mm can generally suffice. Fixation in the cervical spine can be achieved with pedicle screws in C2 and/or transarticular screws from C2 into C1; if additional length is needed, a lateral mass screw at C3 can be used. **C:** Alternatively, a rod-plate combination with multiaxial screws allows fixation at optimal position in C1, C2, and C3. The plate portion is then attached to the skull, and the multiaxial screws can be attached to the rod portion of the construct.

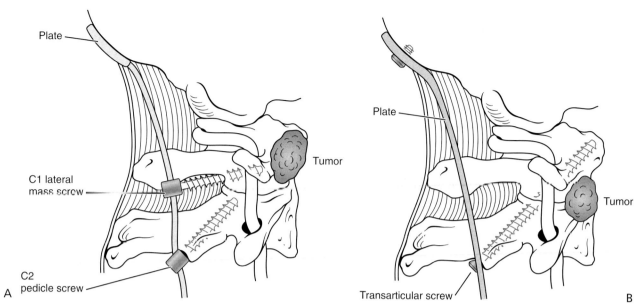

Plate

C1 lateral
mass screw

C2
pedicle screw

A

Plate

Tumor

Tumor

Transarticular screw

B

FIGURE 18.11. The stabilization of the C1–2 articulation in combination with the fixation to the skull can be achieved in either of two fashions. **A:** A multiaxial head screw can be placed in the lateral mass of C1 and a pedicle screw placed in the pedicle of C2. Connecting this to a rod stabilizes the C1–2 articulation. **B:** Alternatively, a transarticular screw can be placed from the lateral aspect of the lamina of C2 across the C1–2 joint into C1 in a standard fashion. This can either be done through a plate or connected to a rod-plate construct to the skull.

is optimal, and a combination of screws into the C2 pedicle or transarticular screws from C2 into C1 incorporated into the plate allows reasonable fixation to the upper cervical spine. It is generally optimal to place at least six screws in the occiput (Fig. 18.11).

For metastatic lesions of the lower cervical spine, between C3 and C7, the most effective route for exposure is the anteromedial approach. This can be done either through a transverse incision if disease is limited to one level or through a more vertical incision paralleling the anterior portion of the sternocleidomastoid if the approach needs to be extended to several levels. Generally, patients without kyphosis are positioned in light traction (10 pounds) applied by Gardner-Wells tongs in the supine position at the time of surgery. If the patient has kyphosis secondary to collapse of the involved vertebra (as in the patient shown in Figure 18.12, with a first recurrence of breast cancer with C4 collapse and kyphosis 10 years postmastectomy), the deformity can usually be improved prior to surgery. Traction is applied 24 hours in advance of surgery, beginning at 10 pounds and gradually increasing to 20 or 25 pounds, sufficient to gradually correct the kyphosis. Because kyphosis generally will increase the amount of pressure on the dural sac, there is usually little danger in applying gentle extension and longitudinal traction to reduce the deformity prior to beginning surgery. In this patient after correction of kyphosis, CT scan and MRI (Fig. 18.13) still showed marked dural compression. However, preoperative reduction makes the approach easier and obviates the need for correction of the deformity during the course of the surgery.

A rolled towel is placed between the shoulders, and an awake nasotracheal intubation is done so that the patient's neurologic status can be checked after final positioning. For most tumors of the lower cervical spine, a left-sided approach is utilized. Appropriate landmarks for a single-level transverse incision, such as a carotid tubercle at C2 to C6, can be palpated. The incision is taken from the midline just over the anterior portion of the belly of the sternocleidomastoid on the lateral side. If a transverse incision is used (Fig. 18.14A), the platysma is divided in the same direction as the skin incision; similarly, if a vertical incision is used (Fig. 18.14B), the platysma is split in the same direction as the incision.

The superficial layer of the deep fascia is then divided over the anterior border of the sternocleidomastoid, with the strap muscles taken medially and the sternocleidomastoid

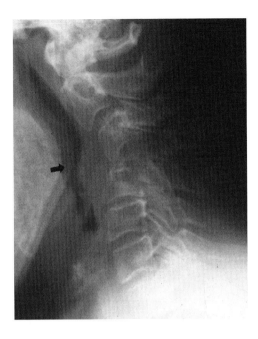

FIGURE 18.12. This patient had a known history of carcinoma of the breast; however, she was without recurrence for 10 years. She then began to have neck pain, and a radiograph demonstrated collapse of the C4 body with kyphosis. This was her first evidence of metastatic disease.

laterally. As with all anterior approaches, the plane of dissection is taken medial to the carotid sheath down through the intermediate layers of the deep cervical fascia. The carotid sheath can be retracted laterally with either a thyroid or appendiceal retractor, and then the dissection proceeds through the fascia down between the alar and visceral fascia behind the esophagus. A second appendiceal retractor can be placed behind the esophagus,

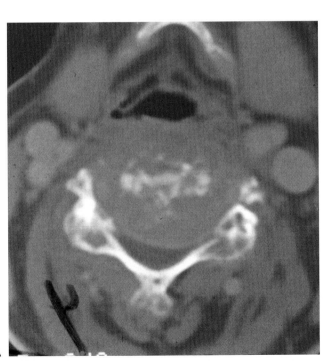

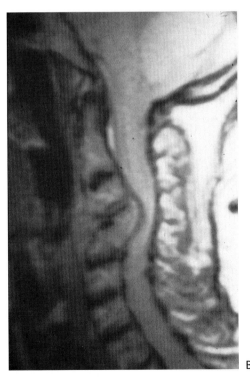

FIGURE 18.13. A: Computed tomography scan demonstrated complete destruction of the C4 body with compression of the dural sac as a result of the kyphosis. **B:** The midsagittal magnetic resonance image demonstrated the kyphosis, loss of sagittal alignment, and marked compression of the dural sac even after realignment using 20 pounds of skeletal traction.

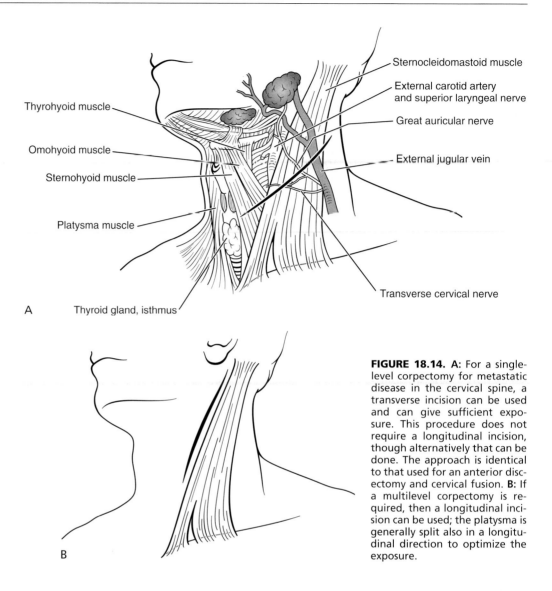

Thyrohyoid muscle

Omohyoid muscle

Sternohyoid muscle

Platysma muscle

Sternocleidomastoid muscle

External carotid artery
and superior laryngeal nerve

Great auricular nerve

External jugular vein

Transverse cervical nerve

A   Thyroid gland, isthmus

B

FIGURE 18.14. A: For a single-level corpectomy for metastatic disease in the cervical spine, a transverse incision can be used and can give sufficient exposure. This procedure does not require a longitudinal incision, though alternatively that can be done. The approach is identical to that used for an anterior discectomy and cervical fusion. **B:** If a multilevel corpectomy is required, then a longitudinal incision can be used; the platysma is generally split also in a longitudinal direction to optimize the exposure.

retracting it across the midline. Blunt dissection with a Kitner dissector is used to clear along the fascial sheath. At this point, the only structure remaining is the prevertebral fascia. It is critical, especially in cases of metastatic disease to the cervical spine, to locate the right and left longus colli muscles. The anatomy can be quite distorted, and ascertaining the midline can be difficult. Dissection above and below the area of tumor is necessary to clearly identify the midline. An attempt should be made when opening the prevertebral fascia to do it exactly in the midline. If the tumor is not readily evident because of the bulging of the prevertebral fascia, then a needle marker should be placed and the location clearly identified using image intensification. Dissection in essentially all cases will require a full vertebral body above and below the area of tumor.

Generally, cautery will be necessary to dissect the longus colli muscle back. It should be done beginning at an area of normal bone either above or below the tumor so that a decision can be made whether the longus colli is involved and whether it needs to be resected or can be easily dissected back off the surface of the tumor mass. This should be done both on the right and on the left (Fig. 18.15). Unless the tumor mass is bulging out over the surface of the discs above and below, it should not be removed first. The initial dissection should be into the discs above and below the tumor—in the case shown in Figure 8.15, at C4–5 and C5–6. After dissecting the longissimus colli back, the cautery should be used to remove the anterior portion of the annulus as extensively from side to

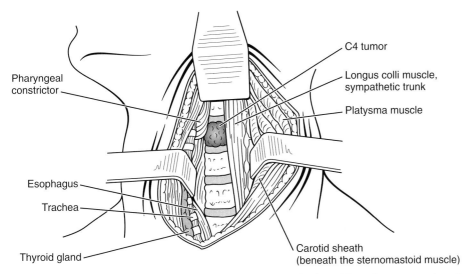

C4 tumor

Longus colli muscle, sympathetic trunk

Platysma muscle

Pharyngeal constrictor

Esophagus

Trachea

Thyroid gland

Carotid sheath (beneath the sternomastoid muscle)

FIGURE 18.15. The approach to the anterior cervical spine in the mid portion, as mentioned previously, is similar to that for a single-level anterior cervical discectomy and fusion, the only difference being that exposure needs to be somewhat broader than normally utilized. The longissimus colli is dissected back off the surface of the vertebral body almost completely so that the lateral aspects of the vertebral bodies can be well visualized. To do this effectively at the index level, often the longissimus colli needs to be dissected both at the level superior to and the level inferior to the vertebral body.

side as possible (Fig. 18.16). Then, using a ring or an angled curette, the disc material should be loosened up and removed with a pituitary rongeur (Fig. 18.17). Fully dissecting the disc spaces first will allow more optimal localization for the surgeon of his or her position within the vertebral body.

After the tumor is fully exposed, excision of the tumor is the next step. Tumor can be excised using a variety of instruments. Assuming that bleeding is minimal, a pituitary rongeur is usually optimal for removing the initial two-thirds of the tumor (Fig. 18.18). Once both disc spaces are emptied and the anterior two-thirds of the tumor are removed,

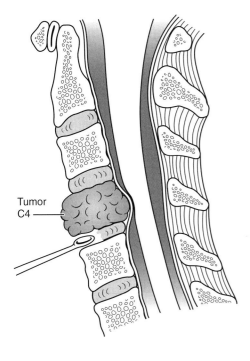

Tumor C4

FIGURE 18.16. Unless the tumor within the vertebral body bulges out significantly over the discs above and below, removal of the tumor should be reserved until after the discs above and below it and the involved vertebral body have been removed completely. The technique is similar to other discectomies with the exception of a much broader dissection being necessary using a cautery. The annulus is removed in toto, beginning from the lateral aspect of the body, continuing across the anterior aspect, and coming to the near-side lateral aspect, removing as much as possible of the annulus. The nucleus can then be removed using a ring curette, with care being taken not to penetrate the tumor but to clean the superior aspect of the body below and inferior aspect of the body above prior to manipulating the tumor.

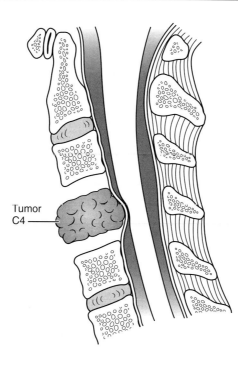

FIGURE 18.17. Once the procedures described in the legend to Figure 18.16 are complete, the endplates of the involved body are generally respected and the tumor can now be removed using those endplates as a guide. A pituitary rongeur is used to remove all of the tumor.

any residual bony endplate of the affected vertebral body is also removed. From this point on, a curette can be used to carefully remove the tumor down to the posterior longitudinal ligament. Either an angled or straight small curette is used to carefully loosen bits of tumor, which can then be removed using a pituitary rongeur (Fig. 18.19A).

The decision whether to open the posterior longitudinal ligament if it appears to be intact is a difficult one. Some tumors will penetrate through the posterior longitudinal ligament and thus will compress the dural sac. Other tumors will essentially stop, and most of the compression will have been the result of loss of height and kyphosis; once the pressure of the tumor is removed, that compression of the dural sac is removed. In part,

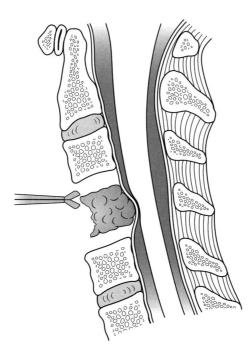

FIGURE 18.18. The tumor is removed approximately two-thirds of the way back using a pituitary rongeur. Generally, the tumor can be loosened with a curette and then picked up with the pituitary rongeur.

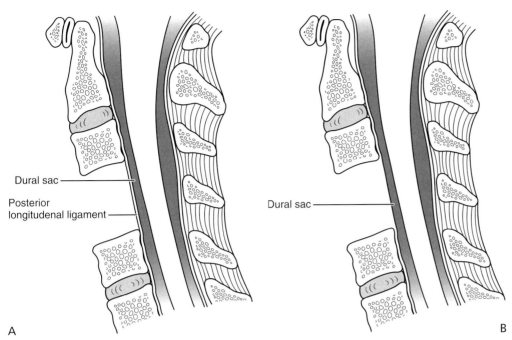

FIGURE 18.19. A: The posterior extent of resection varies with both the type of tumor and the appearance of the preoperative magnetic resonance image. In many tumors, the posterior longitudinal ligament is not involved. Leaving it intact makes reconstruction somewhat easier, but failing to remove it when there is tumor behind it compressing the dural sac will leave residual neural compression. However, for tumors such as breast cancer, most frequently the ligament is respected as a barrier, and the tumor can be gently peeled off the ligament by using a curette, leaving the ligament in place. **B:** In tumors such as lung carcinomas, it is not unusual to find that the tumor has penetrated through the posterior longitudinal ligament, and when it is opened, there is still tumor compressing the dural sac that needs to be removed.

this decision depends on whether the posterior longitudinal ligament can be visualized on the MRI preoperatively. If it is clearly visualized and the degree of compression is not great, then the posterior longitudinal ligament can in some cases be retained. If it is questionable or the degree of compression is significant without a tremendous amount of kyphosis, then generally the posterior longitudinal ligament should be opened (Fig. 18.19B). A small angled curette can be used to dissect between the posterior aspect of either the superior or inferior vertebral body and the posterior longitudinal ligament; once freed, the posterior longitudinal ligament can be opened longitudinally with a Penfield elevator and then removed carefully using a 2-mm Kerrison punch. If the patient has had preoperative radiation, the dura will appear white and thickened, and the posterior longitudinal ligament may in fact be scarred to it. In patients who have not received preoperative radiation, the plane is freer and the dural sac has a bluer tint.

Dissection is also carried laterally using an angled curette until all of the soft tumor is removed. Because the vertebral artery may be involved, this artery should be carefully assessed on the MRI prior to beginning the procedure. It is frequently quite evident whether the vertebral artery is contiguous with the tumor mass or whether it remains surrounded by bone within its foramen and will not be encountered during the decompression. Very often, small branches directly from the vertebral artery feed the tumor. These can usually be controlled with a small clip. Bipolar cautery is also an effective technique for small vessels. The use of Surgicel for gentle packing is also effective. If there is a question about the extent of decompression, the cavity can be filled with radiopaque contrast material, and a cross-table lateral and anteroposterior radiograph can be taken to ascertain the extent of decompression when visualizing anatomy is difficult.

Once the decompression has been completed, reconstruction must be addressed. As discussed previously, bone graft is rarely indicated in patients with metastatic disease of

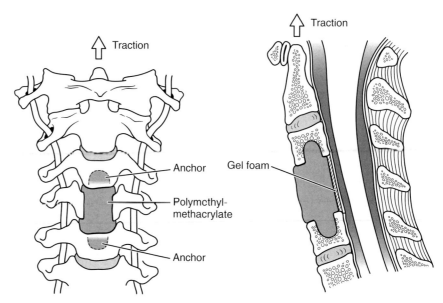

FIGURE 18.20. Once the decompression has been completed, reconstruction must be addressed. Polymethylmethacrylate anteriorly in the spine is an excellent reconstructive material. It gives immediate stability in compression, allowing the patient to be mobilized with minimal or no external immobilization if plate fixation is also utilized. The methylmethacrylate can be anchored to the levels above and below, using a variety of different techniques. Some authors advocate simply excavating holes through the endplate of the body above and below and into the cancellous bone, then allowing the methylmethacrylate that is placed in the cavity to form a small bud, which then prevents it from dislodging.

the spine. Polymethylmethacrylate gives immediate stability and is durable over the long term. Although PMMA alone can be utilized simply by excavating holes within the vertebral body above and below (Fig. 18.20), in most cases it is stabilized by fixation into the bodies above and below. This can be done either with screws or with a small rod (Fig. 18.21). Although Steinmann pins have been used in the past, they have been known to migrate, making them somewhat less desirable. Additionally, they are sharp on the ends and may more easily damage the esophagus when being placed. The screws can be placed using a right-angle drill and then a right-angle screwdriver. They can be placed at approximately a 45-degree angle (Fig. 18.21A) and screwed in sufficiently so that the heads are below the anterior edge of the vertebral body. Generally, a screw between 10 and 15 mm in length is sufficient. Alternatively, rods can be placed by making a perforation in the endplate of the vertebral body above. This can be done with either a right-angle drill or a right-angle clamp. A rod is cut to twice the length of the vertebral body. The rod is slid superiorly into the level above until the inferior end of the rod clears the bottom of the open space. A second hole is perforated into the inferior endplate. The rod can then be pushed down into the space to enter that hole and then pulled down approximately half a length of a vertebral body until it is centered across the corpectomy defect (Fig. 18.21B). Another alternative is to place a cage (Fig. 18.22).

If PMMA is to be used to fill the space, at this point a decision needs to be made about the way in which it will be placed. Because methylmethacrylate expands during its polymerization, care must be taken that it does not recompress the dural sac. A thin layer of either gel foam or Surgicel can be placed directly over the dural sac. If there is no posterior longitudinal ligament, the methylmethacrylate should be placed in two steps. The first step is to take a very thin layer of slightly doughy methylmethacrylate and place it directly over the Surgical and up along the endplates and lateral sides of the body. It is important that this layer be continuous but quite thin (Fig. 18.23A). Thus, the pulsations of the dural sac will keep it from compressing the dural sac if the overall volume is

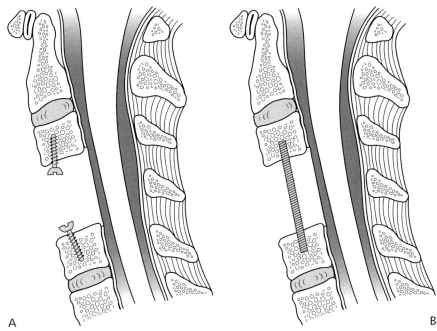

A   B

FIGURE 18.21. It is critical to give stability to the methylmethacrylate in some fashion, especially if an anterior plate is not being utilized. **A:** A very easy technique that creates less bleeding than excavating a cavity through an endplate is to simply place a 20-mm cancellous screw obliquely from the disc space through the endplate approximately half-way into the vertebral body. The heads should be left protruding into the disc space but should not be left anterior to the anterior edge of the vertebral body. **B:** Alternatively, a small rod can be placed into the space as well. This can be done in one of two fashions. Using a small right-angle clamp, the endplate can be penetrated superiorly and inferiorly and along the entire length of the bodies above and below until the opposite endplate is reached. The rod is then cut to be long enough to span both the defect as well as the length of one additional vertebral body. The rod is then placed in the inferior hole and moved down through the entire inferior vertebral body until the endplate is encountered; the superior end can then be placed into the corpectomy defect. The rod is then advanced superiorly, with half of the excess rod in the inferior vertebral body and half in the superior one, giving excellent fixation. Alternatively, a slot can be made in the anterior surface of the superior vertebral body and a perforation in the superior endplate of the inferior vertebral body. The rod is slid into the inferior vertebral body and dropped into the slot anteriorly. That slot is later filled with methylmethacrylate.

small. This will leave a cavity in the center that can then be filled at will with PMMA once the peripheral methylmethacrylate is set completely (Fig. 18.23B). Care must be taken not to have the methylmethacrylate come out anterior to the anterior edge of the vertebral bodies, especially if a plate is to be used.

If the posterior longitudinal ligament is intact and has not been opened, then the methylmethacrylate can be placed directly into the space without significant risk of compression of the dural sac as long as excessive amounts of PMMA are not used. The posterior longitudinal ligament will act as a barrier. Care should be taken, however, not to overly compress the methylmethacrylate into the space. Again, it is important that as the PMMA expands, it does not extend beyond the anterior surface of the adjacent vertebral bodies.

Once the methylmethacrylate is hardened, if only an anterior procedure is to be done, it is usually advisable to place a plate over the three levels. The plate is contoured and care is taken that the methylmethacrylate in the corpectomy spaces does not interfere with the plate; screw holes are then placed in the proximal and distal bodies (Fig. 18.24). It is not necessary to place screws into the methylmethacrylate. This construct is usually sufficient so that patient mobilization can occur immediately. Once this step has

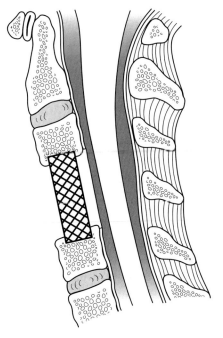

FIGURE 18.22. Alternatively, a cage can be placed into the defect. This is either filled with methylmethacrylate or, less optimally, with bone graft prior to placing a plate across the defect and anchoring it to the body above and below. Bone graft is less effective for metastatic disease than methylmethacrylate in that its ultimate stability is achieved by fusion. This is less likely to occur in patients with metastatic disease because the area will undergo radiation, thus delaying potential healing, and the patient's overall metabolic status is such that the achievement of fusion is less predictable.

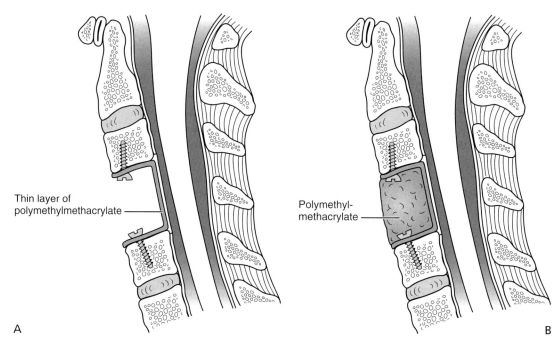

Thin layer of polymethylmethacrylate

Polymethylmethacrylate

A   B

FIGURE 18.23. A: A similar technique to that described for lesions in the upper cervical spine can be utilized for filling corpectomy defects in the lower cervical spine. If screws are placed as anchors, again a thin layer of doughy methylmethacrylate is used to coat the superior and inferior endplates of the corpectomy defect as well as the posterior aspect either along the posterior longitudinal ligament or along the dural sac and the lateral aspects, creating a very thin box, which is then allowed to harden. Once hardened, the methylmethacrylate box is filled with additional methylmethacrylate, creating a solid block of methacrylate. Care must be taken to be certain that the methacrylate does not bulge anteriorly or have any sharp edges that could potentially be detrimental to the esophagus **(B).**

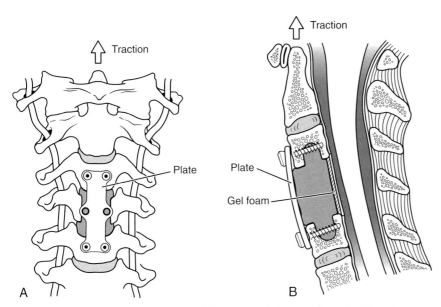

FIGURE 18.24. In most circumstances, this construct is then reinforced with a plate. The plate will enhance the stability of the construct because it provides rotational stability, which is less optimally obtained using a methylmethacrylate block alone or in concert with a rod or screw fixation. The axial stability is maintained by the methacrylate block. It is critical when applying the plate that all traction be off the cervical spine. Even with screws placed in the vertebral bodies above and below or with a rod, rarely it is difficult to place the four screws anchoring the plates superiorly and inferiorly.

been completed, a lateral roentgenogram is taken to ascertain that the methylmethacrylate has not bulged posterior to the wall of the vertebral bodies. If it looks satisfactory, then the wound is closed in a routine fashion.

The patient can be mobilized the next day in a soft collar for approximately 7 to 10 days until the musculature is healed, and then can be released from all external immobilization. With this construct, no bone graft is necessary; its durability is sufficient to exceed the life expectancy of the majority of patients. If there is a long life expectancy, such as a long duration of disease-free interval in a patient with breast cancer as illustrated in this example, then this construct can be augmented with a posterior procedure done during the same procedure with internal fixation and autologous bone graft. In long-term follow-up of 10 years postsurgery and 20 years following the original breast cancer, this example demonstrated the durability of the construct (Fig. 18.25).

Only occasionally is it necessary to do an isolated posterior procedure in the mid-cervical spine for metastatic disease. If there is tumor compressing the dural sac in the area of the lamina or pedicles, a standard laminectomy or partial pediculectomy can be done for direct decompression (Fig. 18.26A). In that case, posterior stabilization is necessary. Standard plate-and-screw or screw-and-rod stabilization can be done on both sides, with at least one solid level above the defect in the posterior elements (Fig. 18.26B). If this is at C6 or C7, extension into the thoracic spine is necessary. Fixation to C7, unless the pedicles are used, is suboptimal, and extension to T1 is generally necessary. Posterior bone graft can be placed on the contralateral side from the area of the tumor; however, because postoperative radiation is generally used, the probability of achieving a solid fusion is small. The use of methylmethacrylate posteriorly as a tension band, which was done in the past, is now contraindicated. The rate of posterior wound complications from the use of methylmethacrylate was excessive (17). Additionally, methylmethacrylate is relatively poor in tension. An anterior fusion is preferable if it is felt that the ability to achieve stability posteriorly is limited by the amount of resection or the quality of the bone.

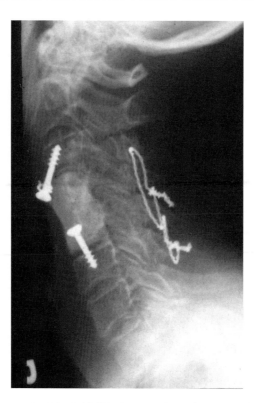

FIGURE 18.25. A lateral roentgenogram taken 10 years after the surgery for the patient shown in Figure 18.12. The screw technique was utilized. Because this was a solitary metastasis and the patient was to receive radiation therapy, the patient was turned prone after completion of the anterior procedure, and a wiring was also done with autologous bone graft placed along the lateral masses, achieving a solid arthrodesis. Note that there are no lucencies or other changes in position 10 years postsurgery and 20 years after the original occurrence of the breast cancer, demonstrating the durability of this construct.

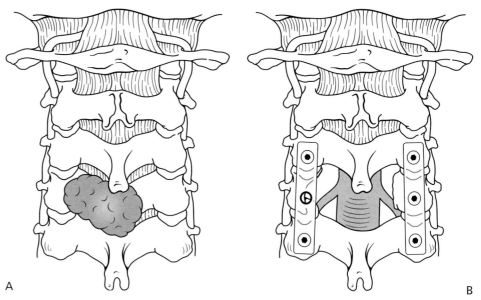

A

B

FIGURE 18.26. A: Occasionally, metastatic disease can occur as a tumor in the posterior elements of the cervical spine. It frequently involves the pedicle and/or lateral mass and lamina. This can cause either root compression or dural compression with myelopathy. If the tumor is limited to the posterior elements and pedicle, decompression can be achieved adequately using a piecemeal laminectomy and pediculectomy **(B).** The patient can be stabilized using a plate construct or, alternatively, multiaxial screws connected with rods. The constructs should be rigid enough that the patient is able to be mobilized without needing to achieve solid arthrodesis. If there is also anterior disease, an anterior corpectomy may be necessary. Bone graft or bone graft substitutes in these patients can be added, but the probability of achieving a solid arthrodesis in tumors that are more aggressive, such as lung or renal carcinomas, is low.

MALIGNANT TUMORS

The technical problem with resection of primary tumors of the cervical spine is that of anatomy. By the time of diagnosis, tumors of the cervical spine frequently encase either one or both of the vertebral arteries (Fig. 18.27). Although it is possible to bypass the vertebral arteries once the tumor is of sufficient size, involvement of the dura is also part of the anatomic problem. Most certainly, the key principle in terms of resection of malignant tumors of the cervical spine is proper oncologic care of the patient. A primary intralesional resection of an osteosarcoma of the spine is not a satisfactory oncologic solution to the clinical problem. Appropriate neoadjuvant chemotherapy prior to resection of the tumor is a key component of success even before considering the technical elements of the surgery. Although there has been a recent report of a "total cervical spondylectomy" for osteosarcoma of the cervical spine, this was not in fact an en bloc resection as described by the authors, but was a piecemeal procedure with contaminated margins (23). However, when the tumor is confined to the vertebral body and either does not involve a vertebral artery or involves only one vertebral artery, a true en bloc resection is feasible, especially for chordomas (24).

Radiologic Evaluation

The assessment of the patient with a potentially malignant tumor always begins with biplanar radiographs. The clinical presentation of patients with malignant tumors can range from pain to difficulty swallowing to either radiculopathy or myelopathy in a wide age range of patients, dependent on the histology. Either the anterior or posterior elements can be involved; however, the vertebral body is more commonly the primary site. After plane radiographs localize the lesion, MRI can be used to define soft tissue, vascular, and neural element involvement. CT scan is almost always also necessary to precisely define the extent of bony destruction and anatomy.

Histologic diagnosis should be made whenever possible using core needle biopsy (not fine needle aspiration). Open biopsy should be avoided because the extent of tissue contamination from an open procedure may compromise the surgeon's ability to do the definitive resection. Complete systemic workup should be done prior to treatment planning and varies slightly with the histology of the tumor. Essentially all patients with malignant tumors of the cervical spine should have a chest CT scan and bone scan, with positron emission tomography scan and CT scan of the abdomen used when indicated. Multidisciplinary planning and sequencing of treatment modalities is critical for malignant tumors and should never be circumvented. Chemotherapy or radiation or both can play an indispensable role in the treatment of malignant tumors, and a poorly conceived "emergent" spinal procedure may compromise the patient's ultimate survival and function.

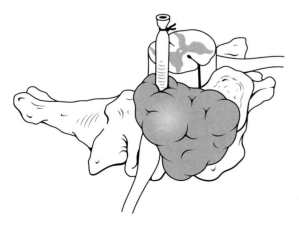

FIGURE 18.27. For patients with malignant tumors of the lower cervical spine, en bloc resections are indeed possible. This is especially true of chordomas. The position and involvement of the vertebral artery is probably the most critical feature. If only one vertebral artery is involved, it can be embolized with coils prior to surgery if it is the nondominant vertebral artery or if both vertebral arteries are comparable in diameter. This allows subsequent ligation and resection of the vertebral artery at the time of surgery. Involvement of both vertebral arteries is problematic.

Surgical Technique

For this procedure, the patient can be placed in the supine position, as done for other tumors of the cervical spine. Either a longitudinal or transverse incision can be used to resect the carotid sheath on the side of the involved vertebral artery. To control bleeding and decrease complications, the vertebral artery can be occluded preoperatively using interventional radiologic techniques. This allows the cerebral circulation to be examined prior to the surgery; in fact, a balloon can be inserted into the vertebral artery and inflated to ascertain the dominance of the involved vertebral artery as well as the effect on the patient's cerebral circulation. If it is not the dominant vertebral artery, it can be occluded using coils to minimize risk during the operative procedure. Through the anterior approach, the tumor mass can be identified anteriorly, and as long as the tumor remains confined by the anterior longitudinal ligament, it can be resected after retracting the carotid sheath and sternocleidomastoid laterally, exposing the transverse processes of the appropriate vertebral bodies. If necessary, a portion of the longus colli muscle can be resected as part of the specimen in order to obtain an adequate margin. The vertebral artery can then be ligated above and below the level of resection, and if it has been previously occluded using coils, blood loss will be minimal.

Using a diamond burr, a trough can be made on the contralateral side of the vertebral body beyond the level of the tumor margin lateral to the tumor margin. Troughs can then be made above and below the involved disc space, with transverse troughs at the body above and below (Fig. 18.28). If using the Tomita procedure (24), the t-saw can then be slid through the troughs across to the involved pedicle and cut sharply through the pedicle with sacrifice of the root at that level. The entire mass can then be removed. If the vertebral artery is not involved, a trough can be made just medial to the vertebral arteries on each side with a diamond-tipped burr. For small tumors with the discs uninvolved, the discs can be excised and the vertebral body removed as a block.

Because of the position of the spinal cord, a circumferential en bloc resection is not possible if there is involvement of the pedicles bilaterally. If there is no involvement of the pedicles bilaterally, the procedure can be made somewhat easier by beginning with a posterior approach. The posterior elements can be taken off piecemeal, and the vertebral arteries exposed from the posterior approach and mobilized. The spine can then be restabilized from the posterior approach with screw-and-rod or plate-and-screw fixation.

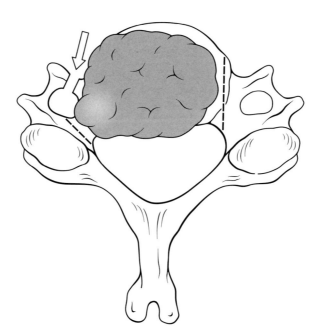

FIGURE 18.28. En bloc resection of a lesion involving the vertebral body and/or one vertebral artery can be achieved by establishing the limits of the tumor above and below. This is done by removing the discs above and below, making sure not to enter the tumor. The osteotomy can be made through the foramen for the vertebral artery. Once the vertebral artery has been ligated and resected, the pedicle can then be divided. If there is sufficient space on the contralateral side, the osteotomy can come just medial to the opposite vertebral artery, preserving it while allowing the tumor to be taken out as a single block of bone with negative margins.

Thus, when the body is to be removed anteriorly, the resection with either a single vertebral artery or through the pedicles will have been facilitated by the previous posterior approach. With more extensive initial tumor involvement, the only realistic option may be to consider appropriate preoperative treatment with chemotherapy to try to minimize the cell viability and thus the potential for spread, subsequently followed by aggressive intralesional or marginal debulking when an en bloc resection is not feasible (23). However, to date there is no long-term evidence concerning the success of that approach. For tumors such as chordomas with more extensive involvement, the only other surgical option is to resect all of the visible tumor (as directed by the preoperative MRI) in a piecemeal fashion. This procedure should be reassessed postoperatively with a gadolinium-enhanced MRI and then followed up with appropriate radiation therapy, such as the use of a proton beam in the immediate postoperative period (25).

Reconstruction depends on the need for adjuvant treatment. Those patients subjected to either chemotherapy or radiation may have delayed healing or lack of healing of bone graft in the radiated bed. Thus, planning for the reconstruction needs to include consideration of the postoperative modalities. Further success in the treatment of malignant tumors may be dependent on the development of adjuvant modalities because the anatomic constraints to a true en bloc resection with negative margins are significant in the cervical spine.

REFERENCES

1. Levine AM, Boriani S, Donati D, et al. Benign tumors of the cervical spine. *Spine* 1992;17: S399–S406.
2. Kahnna AJ, Carbone JJ, Kebaish KM, et al. Magnetic resonance imaging of the cervical spine. *J Bone Joint Surg Am* 2002;84(suppl 2):70–80.
3. Feigenberg SJ, Marcus RB, Zlotecki RA, et al. Megavoltage radiotherapy for aneurysmal bone cysts. *Int J Radiat Oncol Biol Phys* 2001;49:1243–1247.
4. Boriani S, Capanna R, Donati D, et al. Osteoblastoma of the spine. *Clin Orthop* 1992;278:37–45.
5. McAfee PC, Bohlman HH, Riley LH, et al. The anterior retropharyngeal approach to the upper part of the cervical spine. *J Bone Joint Surg Am* 1987;69:1371–1383.
6. Gerszten PC, Welch WC. Current surgical management of metastatic spinal disease. *Oncology (Huntingt)* 2000;14(7):1013–1024.
7. Petren-Mallmin M, Andreasson I, Nyman R, et al. Detection of breast cancer metastases in the cervical spine. *Acta Radiol* 1993;34(6):543–548.
8. Bernat JL, Greenberg ER, Barrett J. Suspected epidural compression of the spinal cord and cauda equina by metastatic carcinoma. Clinical diagnosis and survival. *Cancer* 1983;51:1953–1957.
9. Tokuhashi Y, Matsuzaki H, Kawano H, et al. The indication of operative procedure for a metastatic spine tumor: a scoring system for the preoperative evaluation of the prognosis. *Nippon Seikeigeka Gakkai Zasshi* 1994;68(5):379–389.
10. Singh K, DeWald CJ, Hammerberg KW, et al. Long structural allografts in the treatment of anterior spinal column defects. *Clin Orthop* 2002;394:121–129.
11. Wetzel FT, Phillips FM. Management of metastatic disease of the spine. *Orthop Clin North Am* 2000;31(4):611–621.
12. Scoville WB, Palmer AH, Samrak, et al. The use of acrylic plastic for vertebral replacement or fixation in metastatic disease of the spine: technical note. *J Neurol* 1967;27(30):274–279.
13. Dunn EJ. The role of methylmethacrylate in the stabilization or replacement of tumors in the cervical spine: a project of the CSRS. *Spine* 1997;2:25.
14. Timlin M, Thalgott J, Ameriks J, et al. Management of metastatic tumors to the spine using simple plate fixation. *Am Surg* 1995;61(8):704–708.
15. Miller DS, Lang FF, et al. Coaxial double-lumen methylmethacrylate reconstruction of the anterior cervical and upper thoracic spine. *J Neurosurg* 2000;92:181–190.
16. Panjabi MM, Guel VK, Clark CR, et al. Biomechanical study of cervical spine stabilization with methylmethacrylate. *Spine* 1985;10(3):198–203.
17. McAfee PC, Bohlman HH, Ducker T, et al. Failure of stabilization of the spine with methylmethacrylate: a retrospective analysis of 24 cases. *J Bone Joint Surg* 1986;68(8):1145–1157.
18. Phillips E, Levine AM. Metastatic lesions of the upper cervical spine. *Spine* 1989;14(10):1071–1077.
19. Hastings DE, Macnab I, Lawson V. Neoplasms of the atlas and axis. *Can J Surg* 1968;11:290–296.

20. Sundaresan N, Galicich JH, Lane JM, et al. Treatment of odontoid fractures. *J Neurosurg* 1981;54: 187–192.
21. Atanasiu JP, Badatcheff F, Pidhorz L. Metastatic lesions of the cervical spine: a retrospective analysis of 20 cases. *Spine* 1993;18(10):1279–1284.
22. Nakamura K, Tayama Y, Suzuki N, et al. Metastasis to the upper cervical spine. *J Spinal Disord* 1995;9:195–201.
23. Cohen ZR, Fourne DR, et al. Total spondylectomy for primary osteosarcoma: case report and description of operative technique. *J Neurosurg* 2002;97:386–392.
24. Fujita T, Kawhara N, Matsumoto T, et al. Chordoma in the cervical spine managed with an en block excision. *Spine* 1999;24:1848–1854.
25. Noel G, Habrand JL, Mammar H, et al. Combination of photon and proton radiation therapy for chordomas and chondrosarcomas of the skull base: the Centre de Protontherapie D'Orsay experience. *Int J Radiat Oncol Biol Phys* 2001;51(2):392–398.

SURGICAL MANAGEMENT OF INTRADURAL PATHOLOGY: VASCULAR MALFORMATION

ERIC M. MASSICOTTE
MICHAEL G. FEHLINGS

The topic of decompression of vascular lesions is broad and includes many different lesions. Table 19.1 provides a primary classification of the vascular lesions of both spine and spinal cord (1). Different classifications have been put forward for spinal cord vascular malformations based on angioarchitecture and the relationship to the parenchyma of the spinal cord (2–5). These classification systems provide some assistance in management. For the purpose of this chapter, attention will be focused on spinal dural arteriovenous fistulas (SDAVFs) and spinal cord arteriovenous malformations (SCAVMs) because these represent the majority of the lesions encountered. Table 19.2 represents an adaptation of the Anson and Spetzler classification published in 1992 (6).

TABLE 19.1. SPINAL CORD VASCULAR LESIONS

Spinal vascular lesions
Spinal dural arteriovenous fistulas
  Isolated
  Multiple
Spinal extradural and paraspinal arteriovenous lesions
  Fistula
  Isolated (vesicovaginal fistula and other locations)
  Associated (systematized dysplasia, e.g., von Recklinghausen disease)

Spinal cord vascular lesions
Spinal cord vascular malformation
  Isolated
    Arteriovenous malformations
    Arteriovenous fistulas
  Multiple
    Metameric (Cobb and other syndromes and associations)
    Nonmetameric (Rendu-Osler-Weber and Klippel-Trenaunay syndromes and others)
Spinal cord telangiectasias
Cavernous vascular malformations (cavernoma)

Adapted from Berenstein A, Lasjaunias P. *Surgical neuroangiography.* Heidelberg: Springer-Verlag, 1992, p. 2, with permission.

TABLE 19.2. CLASSIFICATION OF SPINAL CORD ARTERIOVENOUS MALFORMATIONS

Type I: An arteriovenous fistula located between a dural branch of the spinal ramus of a radicular artery and an intradural medullary vein

Type II: An intramedullary glomus malformation with a compact nidus within the substance on the spinal cord

Type III: An extensive arteriovenous malformation, often extending into the vertebral body and paraspinal tissues

Type IV: An intradural perimedullary arteriovenous fistula

     A: Single perimedullary fistula fed by a single arterial branch

     B: Intermediate-sized perimedullary fistula with multiple dilated arterial feeders

     C: Large perimedullary fistula with multiple giant perimedullary arterial feeders

Adapted from Anson JA, Spetzler RF. Classification of spinal arteriovenous malformations and implications for treatment. *Barrow Neurological Institute Quarterly* 1992;8:2–8, with permission. Further subdivisions of type IV malformations are from Gueguen B, Merland JJ, Riche MC, et al. Vascular malformations of the spinal cord: intrathecal perimedullary arteriovenous fistulas fed by medullary arteries. *Neurology* 1987;37:969–979.

INDICATIONS AND CONTRAINDICATIONS; BENEFITS AND LIMITATIONS

The role of resection or disconnection of spinal cord arteriovenous malformations (AVMs) and arteriovenous fistulas (AVFs) has been justified based on the natural history of these entities. Limited studies are available on the natural history, and in light of the more recent evolution in our collective understanding of these malformations, critical appraisal of available information is needed. Aminoff and Logue (7) presented a group of 60 patients in 1974. The profile of this group suggested a heterogenous population of SCAVMs and SDAVFs. Older men represented the majority of this group and presented with progressive myelopathy and claudication symptoms, whereas a smaller number of younger patients presented with acute exacerbations. Table 19.3 details the clinical findings for each category of AVM. The conclusions reached by Aminoff and Logue were based on combined pathologies and demonstrated that 19% of patients deteriorated within 6 months; this number increased to 50% by 3 years. More recent studies also support the poor prognosis observed if left untreated (8,9).

Absolute contraindications are few, but the risk of resection or embolization for some of these lesions needs to be weighed against the potential benefits. The elderly patient with complete paraplegia who is incontinent and not in significant or uncontrollable pain may not benefit from surgical intervention. Even partial embolization targeting obliteration of anatomic weaknesses, such as aneurysm, can decrease the risk of hemorrhage (10,11). Certain lesions, such as juvenile or type III AVM, may prove to be

TABLE 19.3. CLINICAL CHARACTERISTICS ASSOCIATED WITH SPINAL CORD ARTERIOVENOUS MALFORMATIONS

Classification	Frequency (%)	Predominant pathophysiology	Presentation	Age (yr) and sex
Type I	60–80	Venous hypertension	Progressive myelopathy, claudication	40–70, male > female
Types II and III	20	Hemorrhage, compression, steal phenomena	Subarachnoid hemorrhage (one-third)	Childhood and early adulthood
Type IV	20	Hemorrhage, venous hypertension, compression	Progressive sensory/motor deficits	20–40

too formidable for resection (6). Even by combining modalities, the risk involved with resection of some lesions involving multiple compartments (i.e., intradural, extradural, and spinal column) may not be to the patient's benefit. The limitations of our technologies need to be respected.

Intervention for most lesions, however, can be managed using embolization, surgery, or both. Several groups have demonstrated improvement in neurologic status following treatment (12–16). Micturition disability was observed by Song et al. (15) to be improved if treatment was performed within 13 months of onset of symptoms. They also noted improvement with gait in their patients. However, not all interventions are met with permanent improvements. Tacconi et al. (17) found decline in functionality when looking at the long-term outcome of their 25 patients taken from a larger group of 78. The length of follow-up was between 18 months and 24 years. These authors speculated that "irreversible deterioration of spinal cord function occurred as a consequence of the hemodynamic changes of its blood supply." The acute progression of neurologic deterioration, as seen with type IV lesions, compels the treating physician to act urgently.

RECOMMENDED APPROACHES

Approaches are based on the location of the specific pathology. The majority of lesions will be exposed using a posterior approach by laminectomy. The amount of bony removal is dictated by the size and location of the lesion. For example, an SDAVF with a single arterial feeder coming from the left L1 can be disconnected using a hemilaminectomy or a standard laminectomy at the L1 level (Fig. 19.1). Multilevel laminectomy becomes necessary only when multiple arterial feeders are involved, requiring exposure for their resection. Previously, the dissection of the dilated tortuous venous plexus on the dorsal aspect of the spinal cord was deemed necessary. This incurred significant morbidity by either direct trauma or compromise of the venous outflow segmentally. Based on improved knowledge of the angioarchitecture and pathophysiology of SDAVFs, it is now recognized that these lesions can be treated effectively by disconnection of the abnormal communication between the arterial and venous compartment, thus addressing the venous overflow and hypertension.

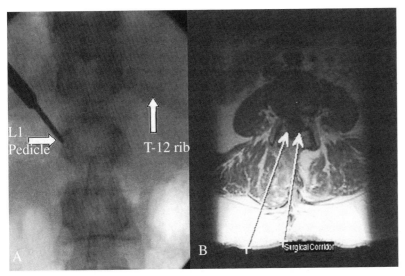

FIGURE 19.1. A: Intraoperative x-ray demonstrating the localization of the L1 pedicle used to identify the spinal dural arteriovenous fistula. **B:** Postoperative axial magnetic resonance imaging scan showing the surgical corridor used to gain exposure to the dura and disconnect the vascular lesion.

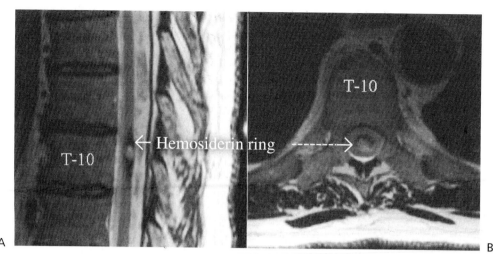

A   B

FIGURE 19.2. Sagittal **(A)** and axial **(B)** magnetic resonance imaging scans with T2 sequences showing a cavernous malformation at the T10 level. A typical hemosiderin ring is demonstrated.

Anterior approaches may be required when dealing with SCAVMs predominantly fed by the anterior spinal artery. Lesions with extension into the extradural compartments such as the vertebral body and paraspinal muscles may also be easier to manage by surgical means using anterior or combined approaches.

PREOPERATIVE CONSIDERATIONS

Preoperative investigations will require the use of standard imaging techniques such as x-ray, computed tomographic (CT) scan, and magnetic resonance imaging (MRI) (Fig. 19.2). Myelography is seldom used except when MRI is contraindicated. Certain pathologies such as cavernous malformations do not require more invasive investigation such as angiography. The use of new magnetic resonance sequences has provided better illustrations of certain vascular lesions (Fig. 19.3). Magnetic resonance angiography can assist the angiographer by not only making the diagnosis but also localizing the vascular lesion. High-resolution selec-

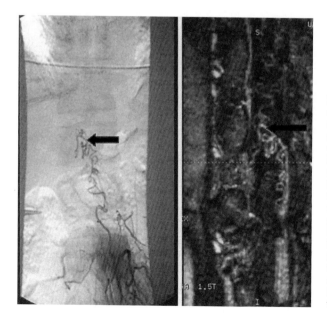

FIGURE 19.3. Conventional digital subtraction angiography on the left is compared with autotriggered elliptic centric ordered three-dimensional gadolinium-enhanced magnetic resonance (MR) angiography on the right for the same lesion. Use of the MR angiographic technique to make the diagnosis and localize the specific level involved provides assistance to the angiographer, who can subsequently focus on fewer levels and possible treatment with embolization. The green arrows in both panels correspond to the same loop.

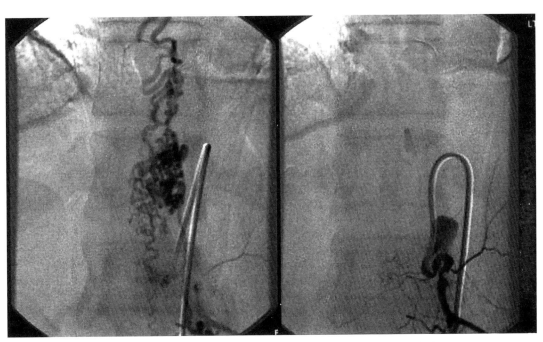

FIGURE 19.4. A T12 arterial feeder **(left)**, and a postembolization injection of the same feeder **(right)**.

tive digital angiography still represents the gold standard. Confirmation of the sensitivity and specificity of these new magnetic resonance techniques is still required.

Interventions such as embolizations can play a role in the management of certain lesions, either by assisting with subsequent surgery or as the sole treatment (Fig. 19.4). In the event of eventual surgery, the interventional neuroradiologist in our institution places a skin marker at the level of the pedicle to assist in localization.

OPERATING ROOM SETUP

Anesthetic considerations consist of tight regulation of blood pressure and good intravenous access. Rapid blood loss can be encountered with high-flow lesions such as the type III juvenile AVM or the type IVC. Steroid administration prior to intramedullary resection or manipulation has been part of our routine to reduce intramedullary edema.

Operative setup requires the use of a radiolucent table for the possibility of intraoperative fluoroscopy or x-ray. Intraoperative angiography or temporary balloon occlusion of large lesions such as type IVC may be indicated to gain control of bleeding during the resection. In some cases intraoperative angiography has been used to confirm complete resection. Alternatively, intraoperative Doppler ultrasound monitoring to confirm complete obliteration has been described (18). We prefer to use the Jackson table when the posterior approach is used. This allows the radiolucent frame to rotate and therefore facilitate visualization of intradural lesions. Patient comfort can also be maximized in order to reduce the chances of pressure palsy during long procedures.

The role of surgical navigation is growing, and merging images from different modalities is certainly becoming more popular (19). Combining angiograms and CT scans would be useful in these cases; however, this has yet to be introduced in clinical applications.

Intraoperative monitoring with somatosensory and motor evoked potentials is considered routine in our institution for intramedullary lesions. The use of both sensory and motor evoked potentials provides a more complete and continuous assessment of the spinal cord, and case studies have been reported on their usefulness (20,21).

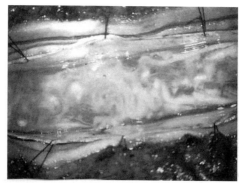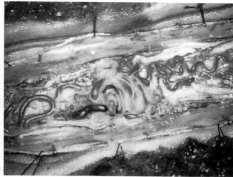

FIGURE 19.5. Intraoperative pictures showing the arachnoid layer intact **(left)** and the opened layer **(right)**. Sharp microsurgical dissection is essential to identify and isolate the vessels involved and the exact point of resection. The embolization and thrombosis of the coronal venous plexus are seen (*arrow*).

INTRAOPERATIVE CONSIDERATIONS

The need for adequate exposure and microsurgical principles cannot be overstated. A clear field will allow the surgeon to identify the vascular anatomy of the spinal cord and precisely locate the pathology. Compromise of the arterial supply or venous outflow of the native spinal cord can be disastrous. Figures 19.5 and 19.6 give the reader a perspective as seen by the surgeon under the operative microscope. Minimal manipulation of the spinal cord is observed and can be performed safely if the dentate ligaments at several continuous levels are released. Meticulous microsurgical principles need to be applied under the microscope in order to minimize the surgical trauma to the spinal cord and surrounding vascular anatomy. An intraoperative microscope with two binocular eyepieces provides the surgeon and the assistant the necessary magnification and illumination to work simultaneously.

Intradural identification of the angioarchitecture is critical for disconnection of SDAVFs, perimedullary AVFs, and dissecting SCAVMs. Removal of the dilated venous plexus from the pial surface is no longer deemed necessary and is actually detrimental. By removing or interfering with venous outflow, venous hypertension may be aggravated and therefore contribute to postoperative neurologic worsening. Correlation with the preoperative angiogram will assist the experienced surgeon in achieving complete resection or disconnection. The use of intraoperative micro-Doppler monitoring for confirmation of obliteration of the SDAVF is safe and useful according to Kataoka et al. (18). Other techniques include the use of intraoperative angiography (Fig. 19.7). This more

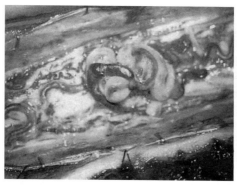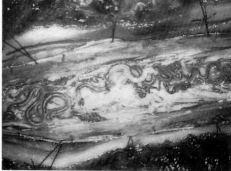

FIGURE 19.6. Intraoperative photograph illustrating partial **(left)** and complete **(right)** resection of the embolized and thrombosed vessels. Resection of the dilated coronal venous plexus is not recommended based on the added morbidity and possible compromise of the venous outflow, but this situation required resection for visualization of the arterial feeders coming from the anterior spinal artery.

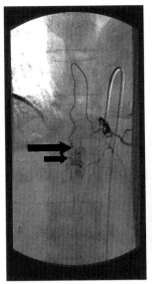
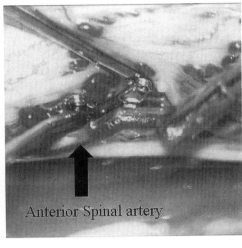

FIGURE 19.7. Angiogram **(left)** demonstrating two small feeders to a nidus (*green arrows*), and corresponding intraoperative pictures with two small aneurysm clips on the same arterial feeders coming off the anterior spinal artery.

A   B   C

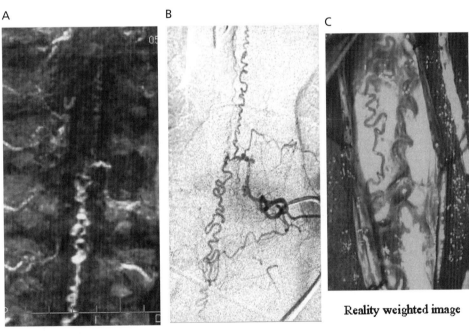

Gd-MRA   IADSA   Reality weighted image

FIGURE 19.8. The three images **(A, B, C)** represent the same spinal dural arteriovenous fistula. **A:** Represents an MR angiographic technique after multiplanar volume reformatting. The enlarged dural feeding artery arising from the left T6 intercostal artery can by identified. The high signal, seen in this coronal view, allows delineation of the course of the abnormal vessels from below the rib, through the neural foramen and into the dural compartment. Dilated medullary veins can be easily visualized extending caudally. **B:** Oblique view of intraarterial digital subtraction angiographic image (IADSA) shows the injection of contrast into the left T6 intercostal artery. **C:** Intraoperative picture or Reality weighted image of the same spinal dural AVF. (Adapted from Farb RI, et al. Spinal dural arteriovenous fistula localization with a technique of first-pass gadolinium-enhanced MR angiography: initial experience. *Radiology* 2002;222:843–850, with permission.)

invasive procedure can present some technical challenges because the patient is often prone, leaving access to the groin difficult.

Intraoperative complications range from catastrophic blood loss and death to inaccurate localization of the level and the need for extension of the bony exposure. Neurologic deterioration can result from compromised arterial supply or venous hypertension from outflow obstruction and surgical trauma. A detailed vascular anatomy, identified during angiography, allows the surgical team to navigate and correlate the angiogram pictures with specific live anatomy. The precise locus of the abnormal arteriovenous connection or the location of all the feeders of the AVM needs to be clearly identified before disconnection or resection (Figs. 19.8–19.10).

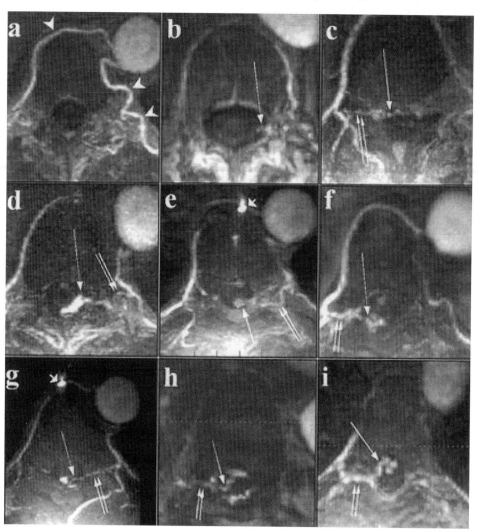

FIGURE 19.9. Transverse multiplanar volume reformatted images of the spine obtained with autotriggered elliptic centric ordered three-dimensional gadolinium-enhanced magnetic resonance angiography. **A:** A normal intercostal level that shows both intercostal arteries (*arrowheads*) as they arise from the aorta and course over the neural foramen. **B to I:** A spinal dural arteriovenous fistula is depicted in patients 1, 2, 3, 4, 5, 7, 8, and 9, respectively. Note the abnormal enlarged dural branch (*double arrow*), which courses through the neural foramen toward the thecal sac, and the abnormal early-draining intradural medullary vein (*single arrow*) that arises from the dural fistula within the subarachnoid space. The short arrow in E and G indicates a magnetic resonance system artefact. (Adapted from Farb RI, Kim JK, Willinsky RA, et al. Spinal dural arteriovenous fistula localization with a technique of first-pass gadolinium-enhanced MR angiography: initial experience. *Radiology* 2002;222:843–850, with permission.)

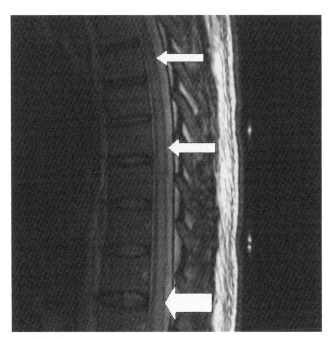

FIGURE 19.10. Sagittal magnetic resonance image with T2 sequence showing the signal changes in the entire thoracic spinal cord. Radiographic changes on T2 magnetic resonance images have been correlated with successful treatment of spinal dural arteriovenous fistulas, but do not always correspond to a clinical improvement (22).

POSTOPERATIVE CONSIDERATIONS

Close monitoring by clinical neurologic assessment provides the most accurate evaluation of the spinal cord. Avoidance of hypotension in the postoperative period is essential (23). Principles learned from the trauma literature regarding control of blood pressure can be used in this setting. Keeping the patient euvolemic can often present a challenge if large amounts of fluids were lost intraoperatively or if there were long anesthetic times. Primary use of volume resuscitation to avoid hypotension can sometimes fail and require the use of dopamine to maintain blood pressure. Alpha-agonist vasopressors have been demonstrated to cause a reduction in spinal cord perfusion (24). Any related transfusion coagulopathy needs to be corrected aggressively.

Temporary cerebrospinal fluid (CSF) diversion may also be required. If the primary dural repair is unsatisfactory, CSF may need to be diverted to allow closure of the wound. Another such circumstance may arise when significant spinal cord swelling occurs. The technique of CSF diversion in this scenario has been used in the setting of thoracoabdominal aortic aneurysm repair. By draining CSF, the intradural pressure is reduced, thus decreasing the effect on venous outflow and spinal cord perfusion (25).

Steroids can also be used to reduce the surgical trauma to the surrounding spinal cord. We routinely continue a short course of steroids for patients who develop some new neurologic deficits.

The need for delayed postoperative spinal angiography may require consideration. SDAVFs are believed to be acquired lesions arising from thrombosis of the dural spinal veins (8,26–29). The disconnection of one such lesion may not be enough. In a dynamic pathological process, it may be wise to repeat the spinal angiogram in a delayed fashion. The dynamic nature of these lesions is emphasized by Rodesch et al. (5) in a review of experience at the Bicêtre. A new classification for these spinal cord arteriovenous shunts would include genetic and hereditary factors (5). The authors emphasize clinical and radiographic follow-up. By recording serial images for these patients, the need for noninvasive techniques is greater.

In summary, considerable advances in diagnostic imaging, interventional neuroradiology, and microsurgery have greatly improved the diagnosis and treatment of spinal vascular malformations. Further work on the natural history of these lesions will provide for a greater depth of understanding.

REFERENCES

1. Niimi Y, Berenstein A. Endovascular treatment of spinal vascular malformations. *Neurosurg Clin N Am* 1999;10:47–71.
2. Bao YH, Ling F. Classification and therapeutic modalities of spinal vascular malformations in 80 patients. *Neurosurgery* 1997;40:75–81.
3. Heros RC, Debrun GM, Ojemann RG, et al. Direct spinal arteriovenous fistula: a new type of spinal AVM. Case report. *J Neurosurg* 1986;64:134–139.
4. Marsh WR. Vascular lesions of the spinal cord: history and classification. *Neurosurg Clin N Am* 1999;10:1–8.
5. Rodesch GMD. Classification of spinal cord arteriovenous shunts: proposal for a reappraisal—the Bicêtre experience with 155 consecutive patients treated between 1981 and 1999. *Neurosurgery* 2002;51:374–380.
6. Anson JA, Spetzler RF. Classification of spinal arteriovenous malformations and implications for treatment. *Barrow Neurological Institute Quarterly* 1992;8:2–8.
7. Aminoff MJ, Logue V. Clinical features of spinal vascular malformations. *Brain* 1974;97:197–210.
8. Detweiler PW, Porter RW, Spetzler RF. Spinal arteriovenous malformations. *Neurosurg Clin N Am* 1999;10:89–100.
9. Grote EH, Voigt K. Clinical syndromes, natural history, and pathophysiology of vascular lesions of the spinal cord. *Neurosurg Clin N Am* 1999;10:17–45.
10. Lasjaunias LP, Berenstein A. *Surgical neuroangiography: endovascular treatment of spine and spinal cord lesions.* New York: Springer-Verlag, 1992:5–24.
11. Rodesch G, Lasjaunias P. Multiple arteriovenous fistulae in the Klippel-Trenaunay-Weber syndrome (KTW). *Neuroradiology* 1993;35:561–562.
12. Behrens S, Thron A. Long-term follow-up and outcome in patients treated for spinal dural arteriovenous fistula. *J Neurol* 1999;246:181–185.
13. Huffmann BC, Gilsbach JM, Thron A. Spinal dural arteriovenous fistulas: a plea for neurosurgical treatment. *Acta Neurochir (Wien)* 1995;135:44–51.
14. Lee TT, Gromelski EB, Bowen BC, et al. Diagnostic and surgical management of spinal dural arteriovenous fistulas. *Neurosurgery* 1998;43:242–246.
15. Song JK, Vinuela F, Gobin YP, et al. Surgical and endovascular treatment of spinal dural arteriovenous fistulas: long-term disability assessment and prognostic factors. *J Neurosurg* 2001;94:199–204.
16. Ushikoshi S, Hida K, Kikuchi Y, et al. Functional prognosis after treatment of spinal dural arteriovenous fistulas. *Neurol Med Chir (Tokyo)* 1999;39:206–212.
17. Tacconi L, Lopez Izquierdo BC, Symon L. Outcome and prognostic factors in the surgical treatment of spinal dural arteriovenous fistulas. A long-term study. *Br J Neurosurg* 1997;11:298–305.
18. Kataoka H, Miyamoto S, Nagata I, et al. Intraoperative microdoppler monitoring for spinal dural arteriovenous fistulae. *Surg Neurol* 1999;52:466–472.
19. Weber DA, Ivanovic M. Correlative image registration. *Semin Nucl Med* 1994;24:311–323.
20. Katayama Y, Tsubokawa T, Hirayama T, et al. Embolization of intramedullary spinal arteriovenous malformation fed by the anterior spinal artery with monitoring of the corticospinal motor evoked potential—case report. *Neurol Med Chir (Tokyo)* 1991;31:401–405.
21. Sala F, Niimi Y, Krzan MJ, et al. Embolization of a spinal arteriovenous malformation: correlation between motor evoked potentials and angiographic findings: technical case report. *Neurosurgery* 1999;45:932–937.
22. Horikoshi T, Hida K, Iwasaki Y, et al. Chronological changes in MRI findings of spinal dural arteriovenous fistula. *Surg Neurol* 2000;53:243–249.
23. Sumann G, Kampfl A, Wenzel V, et al. Early intensive care unit intervention for trauma care: what alters the outcome? *Curr Opin Crit Care* 2002;8:587–592.
24. Tator CH, Fehlings MG. Review of the secondary injury theory of acute spinal cord trauma with emphasis on vascular mechanisms. *J Neurosurg* 1991;75:15–26.
25. Bethel SA. Use of lumbar cerebrospinal fluid drainage in thoracoabdominal aortic aneurysm repairs. *J Vasc Nurs* 1999;17:53–58.

26. Aminoff MJ, Barnard RO, Logue V. The pathophysiology of spinal vascular malformations. *J Neurol Sci* 1974;23:255–263.
27. Borden JA, Wu JK, Shucart WA. A proposed classification for spinal and cranial dural arteriovenous fistulous malformations and implications for treatment. *J Neurosurg* 1995;82:166–179.
28. Hassler W, Thron A, Grote EH. Hemodynamics of spinal dural arteriovenous fistulas. An intraoperative study. *J Neurosurg* 1989;70:360–370.
29. Niimi Y, Berenstein A, Setton A, et al. Embolization of spinal dural arteriovenous fistulae: results and follow-up. *Neurosurgery* 1997;40:675–682.

SURGICAL APPROACHES FOR THE RESECTION OF INTRADURAL TUMORS

L. FERNANDO GONZALEZ
CURTIS A. DICKMAN

Decompression of intradural pathology includes the surgical treatment of intramedullary spinal cord lesions as well as lesions inside the dural envelope but outside the spinal cord. Spinal intradural tumors constitute 2% to 4% of all tumors that involve the central nervous system (CNS) (1). Spinal intramedullary tumors constitute about 10% of all spine tumors. Several types of tumors can affect the cervical spinal cord. Intrinsic lesions include astrocytomas, ependymomas, hemangioblastomas, metastases, and other tumors. Intradural extramedullary lesions primarily include schwannomas, neurofibromas, and meningiomas; they arise outside the spinal cord but eventually compress the spinal cord as they grow.

The goal of surgery in patients with a neoplasm is to maximize surgical resection of the lesion without damaging or worsening preexisting neurologic deficits. This chapter reviews the surgical approach and technical nuances of this type of surgery as performed at the Barrow Neurological Institute. The chapter reviews general technical aspects of resecting spinal cord tumors and focuses on particular considerations involved with common intramedullary or extramedullary intradural lesions involving the cervical spine. Cavernous malformations, arteriovenous malformations (AVMs), and dural arteriovenous fistulas constitute a special group of vascular entities that are beyond the scope of this chapter.

DIAGNOSIS

It is important to differentiate intradural lesions that arise from within the spinal cord from those that arise outside the spinal cord but within the dura. Although a patient's clinical history is important, it does not always predict the precise location of a lesion.

Clinical Examination

Some of the signs and symptoms caused by these lesions are pain, motor and sensory disturbances, sphincter abnormalities, and autonomic disturbances. Pain usually appears before motor signs in a radicular distribution. Pain is often associated with extramedullary intradural lesions (e.g., schwannomas). Intramedullary lesions also often become symptomatic with pain (2), which may be ill-defined, diffuse, and funicular (3,4). Such pain has little value in localizing a lesion and may correspond to irritation of long sensory pathways such as the spinothalamic tracts or posterior columns. Pain develops over several weeks or months when neoplastic diseases are present (5). In contrast, with nontumoral entities such as inflammation (e.g., myelitis), pain develops acutely over days or weeks. This time frame can be used as a diagnostic aid.

In patients with intramedullary lesions, motor disturbances can manifest with upper motor neuron deficits such as spasticity, hyperreflexia, and weakness. Intradural extramedullary lesions may be associated with early focal segmental motor deficits and lower motor neuron compromise such as weakness, atrophy, and areflexia if specific nerve roots are compromised. After some growth, intradural extramedullary lesions may compress the corticospinal tract.

Segmental sensory deficits in a dermatomal distribution may indicate the presence of either an intradural extramedullary or an extradural lesion. Sensory changes are the second most common finding in patients with intradural lesions after pain. Intrinsic spinal cord lesions are often associated with sacral sparing. In this phenomenon, sensibility in the sacral area is preserved consistent with the somatotopic distribution of the spinothalamic fibers inside the spinal cord. Sacral fibers are located in the periphery of the tract, whereas fibers from the arms are located more medially (6). The lower cranial nerves (i.e., IX, X, XI, and XII) should be examined carefully when a lesion extends proximally into the craniovertebral junction.

Children often exhibit spinal deformity, kyphoscoliosis, or torticollis caused by compromise of the paraspinal nucleus. This same mechanism has been proposed to underlie deformity associated with syringomyelia.

Hydrocephalus and increased intracranial pressure can occur and may reflect intracranial neoplastic seeding that obstructs cerebrospinal fluid (CSF) circulation or an exaggerated protein content in the CSF, which mostly is associated with ependymomas (4).

A number of nontumoral entities can mimic neoplastic lesions. No definitive guidelines are available. As a general rule, however, nontumoral inflammatory lesions have a more acute course (days to weeks) than tumors, which have a longer evolution (months) and tend to compromise neurologic functions significantly.

Systemic diseases should be ruled out with complementary CSF studies: cell counts for infection, oligoclonal bands and brain magnetic resonance imaging (MRI) for multiple sclerosis, angiotensin converting enzyme for sarcoidosis, and serology for human immunodeficiency virus (7).

Diagnostic Imaging

MRI is the most useful modality for identifying and characterizing spinal cord tumors. Although there are exceptions, tumors typically enlarge the spinal cord whereas inflammatory lesions do not affect its diameter. T1- and T2-weighted MRIs provide important anatomic details that help identify the position of certain lesions (intramedullary or intradural extramedullary) with great accuracy. Gadolinium-enhanced T1-weighted images are extremely helpful in differentiating tumor from normal tissue. Nontumoral lesions can enhance with gadolinium (i.e., acute multiple sclerosis plaques or inflammatory processes). Gadolinium-enhanced images also help to identify tumoral nodules within cysts. Cysts are associated with 50% of intraspinal tumors and are easily identified on sagittal sequences. Axial views help determine whether a lesion is intra- or extramedullary (8). Special sequences such as fat-suppression images are invaluable in distinguishing fat from normal tissue when lipomas are present (9).

If MRI is precluded because a patient has a cardiac stent, pacemaker, or other contraindication, computed tomography (CT) with intrathecal contrast (myelographic CT) can be very useful in determining the exact location of these lesions.

Plain radiography may show bony erosion or remodeling if chronic expansive lesions are present. Radiographs also may show abnormalities in the curvature of the cervical spine. In syringomyelic curvature the scoliotic apex often points toward the left, whereas in idiopathic scoliosis the vertex points to the right (2).

SURGICAL TECHNIQUE

The surgical approach for resecting intradural tumors in the cervical spine should be tailored according to the location of the lesion. The standard posterior approach is the

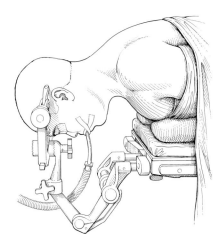

FIGURE 20.1. The patient is placed in the prone position and the head is fixed in a Mayfield (three-pin fixation system) head holder. Slight flexion of the head improves visualization of the entire cervical region. (Reproduced with permission from Barrow Neurological Institute.)

main route used for tumor removal through a laminoplasty or laminectomy. The patient is placed in the prone position, and the head is fixed with a three-point fixation head holder (Mayfield headrest, Ohio Medical, Inc., Cincinnati, OH; Fig. 20.1). We prefer to use the prone position instead of the sitting or semi-sitting position to reduce the risk of air embolism and hypotension. All pressure points are padded with gel rolls. The abdomen and the thorax must be free of pressure to avoid venous hypertension and limitations to chest expansion, respectively. Prophylactic antibiotics are routinely administered (10). For intramedullary tumors, surgeons may elect to administer high doses of methylprednisolone (2) based on the steroid dosages used in the spinal cord injury protocol (10,11). Monitoring motor evoked potentials (MEPs) has been described as very useful in identifying when to stop surgical resection, although the technique requires special anesthetic techniques and may be associated with artifacts related to exemic coagulation. A 50% drop in MEPs is the recommended criterion for terminating resection (12–14).

The appropriate level for the skin incision is determined with the aid of fluoroscopy (C-arm) and skin palpation, remembering that C7 has the longest spinous process. These findings are correlated with preoperative MRI. The skin incision should be long enough to grant access beyond the caudal and rostral edges of the lesion. The skin is opened on the midline with a scalpel. Subcutaneous dissection is performed with monopolar cauterization. The dissection must remain in the midline to prevent excessive muscular bleeding and to facilitate closure once the procedure is completed. Subperiosteal dissection of the paraspinal muscles over the cervical laminae is performed with a periosteal dissector. If facet resection is required to expose the lesion or if fixation of the cervical spine is required, the facets are exposed bilaterally. The bony exposure should include one level below and one level above the intradural lesion. We routinely use a cerebellar retractor to retract the cervical paraspinal muscles laterally. Once the cervical laminae are exposed, we often retract the soft tissue laterally and anteriorly with fishhooks attached to Leyla bars. This retraction diminishes the working depth of the incision.

Laminoplasty

The laminae are exposed on both sides, and the ligamentum flavum underneath the caudal and rostral laminae is dissected free with a curved curette. We use a pneumatic craniotome (Fig. 20.2) with a pediatric B1 or B5 footplate (Medtronic, Midas Rex, Forth Worth, TX) to cut the laminae. The dissection begins on the caudal edge of the laminae so that the laminar flap can be elevated smoothly and easily. A unilateral osteotomy is created by advancing the drill bit rostrally, with the footplate of the drill hugging the undersurface of the laminae, avoiding compression of the tumor or spinal cord. Multiple laminae can be osteotomized rapidly in sequence with this technique (15). After the

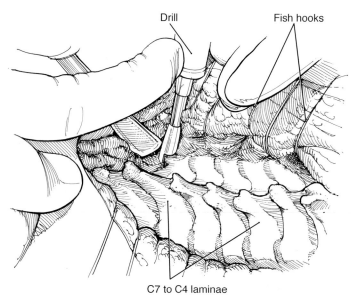

Drill   Fish hooks

C7 to C4 laminae

FIGURE 20.2. Once the soft tissues are opened through the midline and retracted laterally with fishhooks, the posterior elements become evident. The pneumatic drill with a footplate attachment is inserted beneath the most caudal lamina to be removed. The osteotomy is made in a caudal-to-rostral direction through several laminae, carefully hugging the undersurface of the laminae with the footplate of the drill. (Reproduced with permission from Barrow Neurological Institute.)

laminotomy is performed on one side, the contralateral osteotomy is performed. The interspinous ligament is cut caudally and rostrally to the involved segment, and the laminar flap is elevated (Fig. 20.3).

In children, a laminoplasty is used rather than a laminectomy to diminish scar tissue over the dura and to prevent postlaminectomy kyphosis from developing. Reimer and Onofrio (4) reported the incidence of postlaminectomy spinal deformity in children to

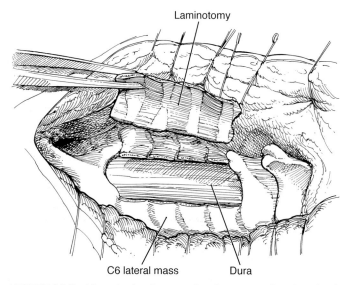

Laminotomy

C6 lateral mass   Dura

FIGURE 20.3. After the laminotomy has been completed on both sides, the flap is lifted off the dura. The lateral masses are exposed so the laminae can be reattached with miniplates after the tumor has been removed and the dura is closed. (Reproduced with permission from Barrow Neurological Institute.)

be as high as 50%. They also reported that 33% of patients who underwent a laminectomy required posterior fixation.

Laminectomy

Laminectomy or laminoplasty can be performed in adults to approach intradural tumors. Laminectomy is performed with a relatively simple technique. The laminae are removed using sharp dissection with Leksell rongeurs and Kerrison rongeurs to expose the pathology and a margin of normal dura rostral and caudal to the tumor.

As the laminectomy is performed, the bone is removed without impinging on the spinal canal with any of the tools. Small Kerrison rongeurs (2-mm footplate) and the tips of the Leksell rongeurs are used to carefully remove the bone. The laminae can also be removed efficiently with a fine, footplated drill bit in a manner identical to the technique used for laminoplasty.

Dural Preparation and Opening

Epidural hemostasis is obtained with bipolar coagulation and Surgicel strips. The bony edges are waxed with bone wax and covered with 1-inch by 3-inch cottonoid patties. The dura is raised with jeweler forceps, and a small dural incision is performed carefully with a no. 11 blade. The dural incisions are extended to expose the pathology using sharp dissection or traction and countertraction with dural forceps. Dural edges are tacked up and sutured to the wound margins with 4–0 Nurolon sutures to retract the dural edges upward and laterally to prevent epidural blood from entering the subarachnoid space (Fig. 20.4). A midline, linear dural incision is used for intramedullary tumors and for most extramedullary intradural tumors. If needed, a **T** incision can be used to obtain lateral exposure. Alternatively, a curved dural incision can be used to obtain lateral access to the spinal canal.

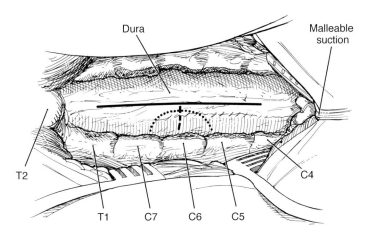

FIGURE 20.4. The posterior dural surface is widely exposed. Epidural bleeding is controlled with bipolar cauterization and thin strips of Surgicel, and the surgical field is ready for the dural opening. Malleable suction helps keep the surgical field clean from cerebrospinal fluid and blood. The dura can be opened in three ways: a midline incision (*solid lines*) for intramedullary tumors; a midline incision with a perpendicular extension (**T** incision, *dashed line*) when one side of the spinal cord must be accessed; and an arcuate incision (*dotted line*) with a lateral base when intradural and extramedullary lesions are treated. (From Spetzler RF, Koos WT, Richling B, et al. *Color Atlas of Microneurosurgery,* 2nd ed. Vol. III, *Intra- and extracranial revascularization and intraspinal pathology.* New York: George Thieme Verlag, 1999, with permission.)

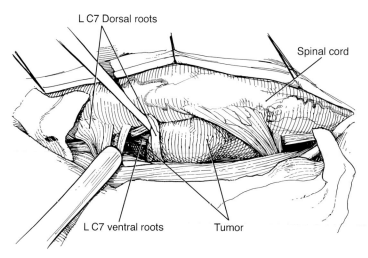

L C7 Dorsal roots

Spinal cord

L C7 ventral roots

Tumor

FIGURE 20.5. Intradural extramedullary tumors are resected after the arachnoid plane between the spinal cord, nerve roots, and lesion is defined. The dentate ligament can be sectioned to mobilize the spinal cord. This technique minimizes retraction and improves visibility. Dural edges are lifted with 4–0 Nurolon to prevent bleeding in the surgical field. (From Spetzler RF, Koos WT, Richling B, et al. *Color Atlas of Microneurosurgery*, 2nd ed. Vol. III, *Intra- and extracranial revascularization and intraspinal pathology.* New York: George Thieme Verlag, 1999, with permission.)

Once the dura is opened, the microscope is brought into the surgical field. Microscopic illumination and magnification are invaluable for resecting these intradural tumors. It is helpful to insert a fixed, medium, malleable stainless steel suction device (PMT Corp., Chanhassen, MN) near the edge of the dura in the wound to remove CSF and blood to facilitate the microsurgical dissection.

Microsurgical Tumor Removal

If a lesion is intradural extramedullary (e.g., meningiomas or schwannomas), the plane between the tumor and the pia is identified and preserved. The lesion is removed carefully with microscissors and microsurgical dissection instruments by progressively isolating the tumor from the spinal cord. Bipolar coagulation is used to devascularize the feeding vessels to the tumor. In meningiomas, the dural-based feeding vessels are cauterized during the early phases of tumor dissection to minimize bleeding. Bipolar cauterization is used sparingly with intramedullary tumors to minimize tissue damage to the spinal cord. During the resection of ventral intradural extramedullary lesions, the dentate ligament is cut to mobilize the spinal cord to facilitate exposure of the tumor (16).

A posterior approach can be extended laterally by resecting the ipsilateral lamina, facet, and pedicle and then opening the dura around the dorsal root and posterior section of the dentate ligament (17). This modification exposes the ventral aspect of the spinal canal through a posterolateral corridor (Fig. 20.5). Anterior approaches to intradural lesions in the cervical region are of limited value because of restricted access laterally and difficulty with dural closure.

INTRAMEDULLARY SPINAL CORD TUMORS

For lesions inside the spinal cord, the surgical plane between the lesion and the spinal cord is identified and followed until the lesion is removed completely. Some infiltrating lesions show no external signs on the surface of the spinal cord, and it becomes necessary to find the best route to minimize spinal cord injury. There are two possible routes for exposing these lesions: a posterior midline myelotomy through the sulcus between the dorsal columns, or a posterolateral myelotomy through the dorsal root entry zone. A posterior midline approach is usually used for centrally located intramedullary tumors. A lateral approach is used for eccentric or exophytic lesions. Deficits of proprioception and vibration sensation are expected after a dorsal myelotomy. Dermatomal sensory deficits are produced by myelotomy through the dorsal root entry zone. A myelotomy is performed with a no. 59 Beaver blade (Fig. 20.6) (13) or a no. 11 blade. Some centers prefer carbon dioxide laser or neodymium:yttrium-aluminum-garnet (Nd-YAG) contact laser for dissecting the tumor; however, we prefer sharp dissection to create the myelotomy for removing the tumor (13).

Sometimes swelling and enlargement make it difficult to identify the midline on the posterior surface of the cord. Vessels are usually displaced from the midline and do not constitute a reliable marker. A midpoint between both dorsal root entry zones can be used to determine the starting site for a midline myelotomy (7).

During a posterolateral approach, the spinal cord is opened though the dorsal root entry zone. The point at which the posterior roots enter the spinal cord offers an avenue for resecting intramedullary lesions. A posterolateral approach is seldom used for myelotomy because most intramedullary tumors are within the center of the spinal cord. A decision about the myelotomy site should be based on a patient's symptoms and MRI findings.

Traction stitches (6–0) are often used (Fig. 20.7) (2,5) to retract the pia to hold the spinal cord open while the intramedullary tumor is being exposed and removed. Others, however, have questioned their efficacy (13).

We start the resection of intramedullary astrocytomas within the tumor and dissect toward the periphery (centrifugal resection) toward normal tissue (Fig. 20.8). Ependymomas, however, are resected by establishing the tumor margins peripherally before debulking the central portion of the tumor. A clear surrounding normal tissue plane can be established and the tumor can be isolated from the normal spinal cord, allowing a gross total resection to be achieved. Ultrasonic aspiration is useful for internally debulking large ependymomas (18). If the tumor is small, it can be resected as a single specimen.

Cysts often form in the normal spinal cord tissue adjacent to ependymomas or hemangioblastomas and help demarcate the margins of the tumor. The cysts can be drained

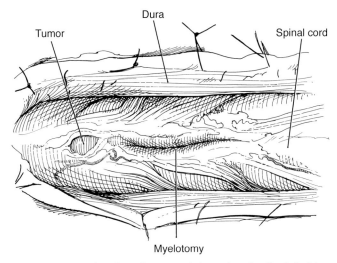

FIGURE 20.6. The dura is opened in a longitudinal fashion through the midline and its edges are retracted up and laterally with sutures to prevent blood from entering the intradural surgical field. The myelotomy is usually performed in the midline within the posterior median sulcus to expose the intramedullary tumor. (From Spetzler RF, Koos WT, Richling B, et al. *Color Atlas of Microneurosurgery,* 2nd ed. Vol. III, *Intra- and extracranial revascularization and intraspinal pathology.* New York: George Thieme Verlag, 1999, with permission.)

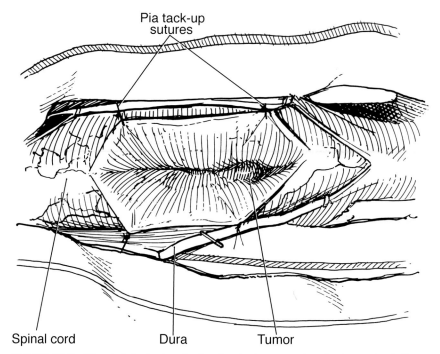

Pia tack-up
sutures

Spinal cord   Dura   Tumor

FIGURE 20.7. The pia is tacked up to the dural edge, exposing the tumor bed. (From Spetzler RF, Koos WT, Richling B, et al. *Color Atlas of Microneurosurgery,* 2nd ed. Vol. III, *Intra- and extracranial revascularization and intraspinal pathology.* New York: George Thieme Verlag, 1999, with permission.)

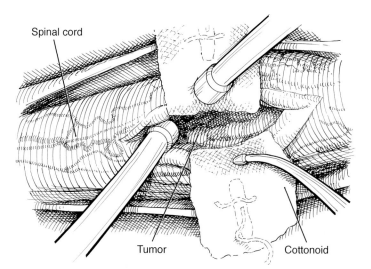

Spinal cord

Tumor   Cottonoid

FIGURE 20.8. The tumor is exposed through a linear, longitudinal myelotomy. The tissue planes separating the normal spinal cord from the tumor are followed carefully to define the tumor boundaries. The tumor is microsurgically detached from the adjacent normal spinal cord. (From Spetzler RF, Koos WT, Richling B, et al. *Color Atlas of Microneurosurgery,* 2nd ed. Vol. III, *Intra- and extracranial revascularization and intraspinal pathology.* New York: George Thieme Verlag, 1999, with permission.)

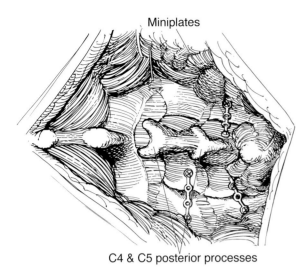

Miniplates

C4 & C5 posterior processes

FIGURE 20.9. Once the tumor resection is complete and hemostasis is obtained, the dura is closed with running stitches of Nurolon 4–0. The laminae are replaced and reapproximated from the respective lateral mass to the lamina with titanium miniplates. (From Spetzler RF, Koos WT, Richling B, et al. *Color Atlas of Microneurosurgery,* 2nd ed. Vol. III, *Intra- and extracranial revascularization and intraspinal pathology.* New York: George Thieme Verlag, 1999, with permission.)

early during the procedure to alleviate pressure within the spinal cord and to facilitate resection of the tumor (11). The surgical removal of the walls of tumor cysts is not advocated because the walls of the cysts are composed of normal tissue (19).

Once the tumor has been resected and hemostasis has been obtained, the tumor bed is irrigated with saline solution. Bipolar coagulation is used sparingly, as needed. The pia can be reapproximated with interrupted stitches of 8–0 nylon (20); we prefer not to close the pia. The dura is closed with a running suture of 4–0 Nurolon or 6–0 Prolene in a watertight fashion. The dura can be patched if part of it was resected with the tumor base (e.g., meningiomas). Dural patching has been used to prevent the formation of postoperative scar tissue and to reduce the risk of spinal cord tethering (7). Once the dura is closed and hemostasis is obtained, the laminar flap can be reattached with titanium microplates and screws (Fig. 20.9).

After an intramedullary tumor has been resected, patients usually experience variable deficits of dorsal column function. These symptoms reflect microvascular damage to the posterior columns during the myelotomy (5). Other sensory deficits or motor deficits occur less frequently and are often transient.

INTRADURAL EXTRAMEDULLARY SPINAL CORD TUMORS

Schwannomas and Neurofibromas

Neurilemomas, also called neurinomas or schwannomas, are the most common intradural extramedullary tumors of the spine. The cervical spine is the most common location for these tumors. Seventy percent are intradural, 15% are purely extradural, and 15% are dumbbell shaped and follow the nerve root along its trajectory (21). Rare cases of intramedullary schwannomas have been described. The genesis of intramedullary schwannomas has been attributed to the invasion of a nerve tumor into the spinal cord following vascular structures (22) and to schwannosis, a hyperplastic nerve reaction to a previous injury (8).

Central myelin is produced by oligodendrocytes, whereas peripheral myelin is produced by Schwann cells. Schwannomas arise from the nerve sheath that invests the peripheral nerve, specifically at the transition area where central myelin joins peripheral myelin (1). Both schwannomas and neurofibromas arise from the sensory root (23). In the posterior entry zone the nerve becomes displaced by the tumor, growing eccentrically and forming a globoid mass with a discrete attachment to the nerve. The tumor can be dissected from the nerve and its function preserved intact. Nerve sheath tumors are usually isointense on T1-weighted MRI and enhance dramatically after the administration of gadolinium (Fig. 20.10).

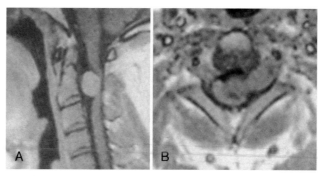

FIGURE 20.10. Sagittal **(A)** and axial **(B)** T1-weighted magnetic resonance images with gadolinium show a contrast-enhanced anterolateral intradural tumor compressing the spinal cord at C2-C3. On the axial plane the extension of this lesion to the neural foramen creates a dumbbell shape, characteristic of schwannomas. (From Spetzler RF, Koos WT, Richling B, et al. *Color Atlas of Microneurosurgery*, 2nd ed. Vol. III, *Intra- and extracranial revascularization and intraspinal pathology.* New York: George Thieme Verlag, 1999, with permission.)

Intradural schwannomas are often ball shaped and located dorsally or dorsolaterally. They are clearly demarcated, which permits their safe microdissection. The pial surfaces of the spinal cord are preserved. Small tumors can be removed as a single piece after detaching the tumor from the sensory rootlets of origin using sharp dissection with microscissors. Large tumors need to be debulked internally with a Cavitron ultrasonic surgical aspirator (CUSA) (Cooper Medical, Stanford, CT) to relieve the mass effect on the spinal cord. The edges of the tumor are then folded inward to separate the surfaces of the tumor from the spinal cord. Dumbbell tumors occasionally require sacrifice of the facet and preservation of the vertebral artery.

Staged anterior or posterior approaches may be needed if a dumbbell schwannoma extends into the brachial plexus. The first stage is posterior and limited to decompressing the spinal cord. The second stage is surgical exploration of the brachial plexus through an anterior incision. This two-stage approach is recommended to prevent CSF leaks after spinal cord decompression (24).

Neurofibromas are tumors that arise from the nerve itself, specifically from fibroblasts around the nerve. They manifest with abundant fibrous tissue and cause diffuse enlargement of the nerve (23). Neurofibromas compromise the entire fascicle, making it difficult to remove the tumor without sacrificing the nerve (23,25,26).

Neurofibromas are commonly associated with neurofibromatosis type I or von Recklinghausen's disease, a genetic disorder transmitted in an autosomal dominant fashion and characterized by a mutation on chromosome 17q. Neurofibromas can be either intradural or extradural but never intramedullary (26). Neurologic symptoms, usually pain, are caused by compression of nervous structures.

Plexiform neurofibromas constitute a special group of tumors characterized by multiple slow-growing lesions that can reach significant proportions without causing major symptoms or signs. Unlike common neurofibromas, plexiform tumors compromise large extensions of a single nerve or an entire neural plexus, involving vascular structures during their course. Surgery is indicated when the spinal cord is markedly compressed. Root compression at the foramen can be managed conservatively and followed with MRI. Surgery is considered only when multiple radiculopathies are present (27).

Meningiomas

Meningiomas are the second most common intradural tumor after schwannomas. Like intracranial meningiomas, they are most common in middle-aged women (28). Although extremely rare, extradural meningiomas have been reported (16). Meningiomas are benign tumors that arise from the arachnoid layer, specifically from cap cells around the spinal nerve roots (23,29).

Meningiomas affect the thoracic spine more often than the cervical spine (29,30), with a 4:1 ratio (28). In about two-thirds of patients, meningiomas are located lateral to the spinal cord, compressing it from the side. One-third are located anterior and posterior to the spinal cord (28). Cervical lesions often have a component anterior to the spinal cord (29). Technically, anteriorly located meningiomas are the most difficult to remove (29,31) because some degree of spinal cord mobilization is required by cutting the dentate ligaments and working from a posterolateral approach. Also, the dura of origin cannot be excised with anteriorly based meningiomas.

Pain is the most common symptom, followed by sensory loss and weakness (29,31). En plaque meningiomas may appear as calcified lesions around the spinal cord that can be confused with ossification of the posterior longitudinal ligament (32,33).

Meningiomas are isointense on T1- and T2-weighted MRI and enhance significantly after the administration of gadolinium (Fig. 20.11) (16,31).

Macroscopically, there are two types of meningiomas: the common globoid, encapsulated tumors and the rare diffuse, fusiform, enlarged meningiomas (en plaque). The latter is associated with a high incidence of scarring (arachnoiditis) (34) and recurrence after resection (33).

The meningothelial (syncytial) type is the most common meningioma, followed by psammomatous tumors (29,30). Only a few cases of transitional meningiomas have been described. In other series, however, psammomatous tumors have been more prevalent (28,31).

Meningiomas are removed in an orderly sequence. The lesion is exposed and the tumor is detached from the surface of the dura by coagulating and cutting the dural-based blood vessels feeding the tumor. After the tumor is devascularized, the tumor can be debulked internally with a CUSA. Using microdissection, the tumor is separated from the pial surfaces of the spinal cord and nerve roots. If the tumor is fully accessible, it can be removed with sharp, en bloc dissection. If possible, the dural origin of the tumor should be resected.

Rather than blunt tissue dissection, sharp dissection with microscissors is recommended, especially to establish the normal pial tissue planes around the margins of the tumor and to remove arachnoid scarring around the tumor (34). The dura that gave rise to a posterior meningioma can be resected, but this maneuver is extremely difficult to accomplish with anterior lesions. No difference has been found in the rate of recurrence after the base of anterior lesions has been coagulated or resected (28). In both cases the rate of recurrence has been reported to be as low as 3% to 7% (28,29). Surgery is the definitive and most gratifying treatment for these lesions, and complete removal is often possible. Postoperative radiotherapy is rarely advocated because of the slow-growing and benign nature of meningiomas (31). Patients should be monitored on a long-term basis to detect tumor recurrence.

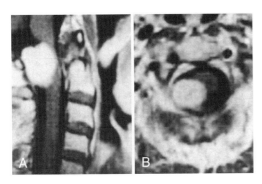

FIGURE 20.11. A: Sagittal T1-weighted magnetic resonance image (MRI) with gadolinium shows a hyperintense, rounded, intradural extramedullary lesion compressing the high cervical spinal cord. **B:** Axial T1-weighted MRI with gadolinium shows a hyperintense intradural meningioma compromising most of the spinal canal. (From Spetzler RF, Koos WT, Richling B, et al. *Color Atlas of Microneurosurgery,* 2nd ed. Vol. III, *Intra- and extracranial revascularization and intraspinal pathology.* New York: George Thieme Verlag, 1999, with permission.)

INTRADURAL INTRAMEDULLARY LESIONS

Astrocytomas

Spinal cord astrocytomas are more common in children than in adults (13,35). They have been reported early in life and are considered congenital astrocytomas (36). Spinal cord astrocytomas are predominantly low-grade lesions (Kernohan grades I and II) (37). Pilocytic and fibrillar astrocytomas constitute the majority. Of all intramedullary tumors, 95% are pilocytic astrocytomas (38). Fortunately, highly malignant tumors (Kernohan grades III and IV) constitute less than 7.5% of all intraspinal tumors (3,35).

The cervical region is more often affected (5,39,40) than the thoracic or lumbar spine. A special subset of cervical tumors represents an extension from brainstem lesions. Known as *cervicomedullary astrocytomas*, these tumors are more aggressive than pure spinal tumors but less aggressive than isolated brainstem tumors (18,41). Astrocytomas that compromise the entire spinal cord, *holocord astrocytomas*, have been described. Their exact incidence is unknown but has been reported to be as high as 75% in one series (42).

On MRI the spinal cord appears expanded, and this appearance can be confirmed during surgery. On MRI it is impossible to distinguish between low- and high-grade tumors. However, malignant tumors are most often associated with leptomeningeal enhancement and, in some cases, seeding to other sites within the CNS (39). In one series, enhancement was present in 83% of the patients with malignant lesions. Enhancing lesions were either low- or high-grade astrocytomas (41). They usually appear isointense on T1-weighted MRIs and hyperintense on T2-weighted MRIs (Fig. 20.12).

During surgical resection, the myelotomy is performed on the dorsal median sulcus or through the dorsal root entry zone, according to the position of the lesion on MRI and the patient's symptoms. A frozen biopsy should be obtained immediately to rule out inflammatory diseases or a high-grade malignancy. The extent of tumor resection is dictated by the presence or absence of borders demarcating the tumor. Well-demarcated tumors are resected aggressively. Poorly demarcated tumors are debulked internally. A less aggressive resection should be attempted for highly malignant tumors or poorly demarcated infiltrative lesions (3,25,43). The goal during surgical removal of malignant tumors is to maximize resection while preserving motor and sensory function. MEPs can be used to guide surgery.

Adjuvant chemotherapy has no clear role in the management of spinal cord astrocytomas (40). Radiotherapy after surgery remains controversial, especially the criteria for selecting candidates for this form of treatment. Low-grade tumors are not clearly

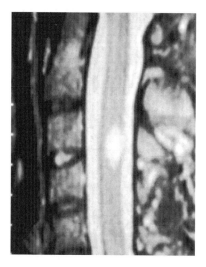

FIGURE 20.12. Sagittal T2-weighted magnetic resonance image with gadolinium shows an intramedullary astrocytoma at C3-C4. (From Spetzler RF, Koos WT, Richling B, et al. *Color Atlas of Microneurosurgery,* 2nd ed. Vol. III, *Intra- and extracranial revascularization and intraspinal pathology.* New York: George Thieme Verlag, 1999, with permission.)

radiosensitive. They occur in young patients, in whom radiation has deleterious effects on the development of tissues. Therefore, children constitute a poor group of patients for radiotherapy (42). High-grade, partially resected astrocytomas may be considered for postoperative radiotherapy in an effort to prevent further seeding and recurrence (43).

Functional outcome is related to the patient's preoperative status (5,42). Patients with higher levels of preoperative functional status do better after surgery than severely compromised patients (3). A 57% survival rate was reported 5 years after the resection of low-grade lesions (37), whereas 79% of patients with malignant astrocytomas (Kernohan grades III or IV) had a 6-month median survival (11). Patients with low-grade tumors have a longer history of symptoms than patients with high-grade tumors, who have a briefer symptomatic period before diagnosis (39).

Some authors argue that histologic pattern is the most important prognostic factor (44,45). In one series of pediatric astrocytomas, the survival period ranged from 12 to 18 years after complete resection of high-grade astrocytomas (46). A series of adults with partially resected astrocytomas followed by radiotherapy had poorer outcomes than patients who underwent more radical surgery without radiotherapy (3).

Ependymomas

Ependymomas are the most common intramedullary tumor in adults (3). Their incidence has been described as almost 60% of all intramedullary tumors (4). They are rare in children (35). Ependymomas are located inside the spinal cord, close to the central canal. They most commonly occur in the cervical and cervicothoracic junction (12), followed by the conus medullaris or filum terminale (4). An increase in the CSF content of protein (ranging between 58 mg% to 700 mg%) is a common finding (19) and may be responsible for some cases of hydrocephalus.

On MRI the spinal cord appears expanded (47). Ependymomas are isointense to hypointense on T1-weighted MRI. Signal intensity on T2-weighted MRI is high. In all cases homogeneous enhancement is present after gadolinium administration and usually reveals clearly defined caudal and rostral poles (Fig. 20.13) (48,49). Ring enhancement has been described in some patients. Some lesions are surrounded by hemosiderin, which has been considered characteristic for ependymomas (50). Subarachnoid hemorrhage may be the first symptom of intramedullary ependymomas (47).

The first surgical goal is to find a plane between normal spinal cord and the tumor (7). When it is impossible to delineate tumor boundaries intraoperatively, intraoperative ultrasonography can be very useful (51). Ependymomas are echogenic and their poles are easily identifiable with ultrasonography (48). Cystic lesions also can be identified easily.

Macroscopically, ependymomas are reddish gray, glistening, sausage-shaped lesions with well-circumscribed limits (7,23). A clear cleavage plane is often present and allows complete piecemeal removal in most patients. Consequently, complete macroscopic resection is more often obtained with ependymomas than with astrocytomas (70% vs.

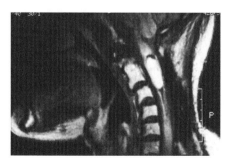

FIGURE 20.13. Sagittal nonenhanced T1-weighted magnetic resonance image shows an intramedullary tumor, evidence of acute intratumoral bleeding, and a characteristic sausage shape, typical of intramedullary ependymomas.

33%, respectively) (44). When tumor boundaries are difficult to define, the tumor can be decompressed from inside using ultrasonic aspiration and progressive resection of the periphery (48). There are three histologic types of ependymomas: cellular, myxopapillary, and anaplastic. The first cellular variety is the most common (7,52).

The vascular supply of ependymomas is anterior to the tumor and predominantly from perforating branches that arise from the anterior spinal artery. Sometimes the anterior spinal artery is engulfed in the tumoral mass (19,48). Devascularization must proceed carefully by isolating perforating vessels that irrigate the normal spinal cord from those that feed the tumor. The anterior spinal artery must be preserved to avoid spinal cord infarction.

The histologic type is not as important for predicting postoperative outcomes as it is in astrocytomas (43). Apparently, the extent of surgical removal is key to the survival of patients with ependymomas (total removal, 219 months; partial removal, 130 months) (44). Patients with ependymomas can be cured if the tumor is resected completely (48). One report showed a 100% survival rate during a 10-year follow-up of patients who underwent complete resection without radiotherapy (53). Preoperative neurologic status is the most important prognostic factor (19,54).

Patients who undergo gross total resection require no postoperative radiotherapy (12,20,53) and should be followed. Patients with a poorly differentiated lesion or a partially removed lesion should be considered for postoperative radiotherapy (19,52). Radiation dosages (43) are controversial, as is whether to irradiate adjacent levels to prevent further drop metastasis (52).

Hemangioblastomas

Hemangioblastomas represent the third most common intramedullary tumor after astrocytomas and ependymomas. They constitute 2% to 3% of intramedullary lesions. They can occur outside the spinal cord or dura (55). Two-thirds of all hemangioblastomas occur as isolated entities; one-third occur as part of von Hippel-Lindau disease. Von Hippel-Lindau disease is caused by a deletion in chromosome 3p (56). It has an autosomal dominant pattern of inheritance with low penetrance. Patients become symptomatic with CNS vascular tumors, visceral tumors, or retinal tumors. The most common location for intramedullary lesions is the cervical region, followed by the thoracic region (57). Retinal lesions are present in 33% of patients with spinal hemangioblastomas (55). Patients with spinal hemangioblastomas usually complain of pain and symptoms related to spinal cord compression, such as weakness or sensory deficits.

These highly vascular tumors are often associated with cysts and significant edema. Because of the exaggerated presence of blood vessels and draining veins (5), hemangioblastomas somewhat resemble AVMs. During surgical resection the arterial feeders should be coagulated first. Then the lesion is circumscribed but not opened. Finally, drainage veins are coagulated (55). These principles are the same as those used to remove AVMs. If the draining veins are cauterized before the feeding arteries are controlled, the tumor can bleed catastrophically.

Angiography shows a dense blush (tumor nodule) and sometimes feeding vessels that can be embolized. Venous drainage also can be assessed during the same procedure (56). These tumors may be solid or be associated with a cyst that contains blood.

The vascularity of these lesions can be assessed preoperatively with angiography. In some patients preoperative embolization should be considered. Angiography is not always necessary and should be reserved for when the diagnosis is doubtful or embolization is considered (58). Embolization should never be considered as the only therapeutic option (59).

T1-weighted MRIs reveal a homogenous lesion that enhances with gadolinium (Fig. 20.14). T2-weighted MRIs show the edematous and cystic components (57). Cysts may have different signal intensities on T1- and T2-weighted MRIs because of the different concentrations of protein inside the cyst (47). Syringomyelia is almost always present (57). MRI often shows tortuous, serpentine vessels around the lesion that appear as a sig-

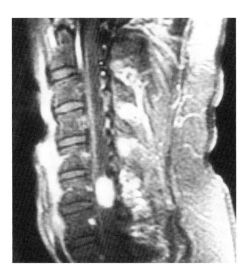

FIGURE 20.14. Sagittal T1-enhanced magnetic resonance image shows a large hemangioblastoma at C5-C6.

nal void inside the lesion (56). The solid areas enhance with gadolinium. Cystic walls are covered by glial tissue and not by tumor, explaining why cysts do not enhance.

Patients with hemangioblastomas should undergo a complete systemic evaluation to rule out von Hippel Lindau disease (57) and to provide adequate genetic counseling. Adjuvant radiotherapy has no role in the treatment of hemangioblastomas (57,58,60).

INTRAMEDULLARY METASTASIS

Once rare, intramedullary metastasis is becoming more common as cancer patients survive longer and detection techniques become more sensitive and widespread. Before MRI, spinal cord metastasis was rarely found. Metastases enhance significantly with gadolinium. The diagnosis should be made in the context of a known primary cancer (47). Lung and breast cancers are the most common primary tumors involved. On MRI, metastases expand the spinal cord. Edema is significant and enhancement is diffuse (21). Outcome depends on the grade of control achieved with the primary disease. Surgery follows the same technical principles.

REFERENCES

1. Miller DC. Surgical pathology of intramedullary spinal cord neoplasms. *J Neurooncol* 200;47: 189–194.
2. Houten JK, Cooper PR. Spinal cord astrocytomas: presentation, management and outcome. *J Neurooncol* 2000;47:219–224.
3. Epstein FJ, Farmer J-P, Freed D. Adult intramedullary astrocytomas of the spinal cord. *J Neurosurg* 1992;77:355–359.
4. Reimer R, Onofrio BM. Astrocytomas of the spinal cord in children and adolescents. *J Neurosurg* 1985;63:669–675.
5. McCormick PC, Stein BM. Intramedullary tumors in adults. *Neurosurg Clin N Am* 1990;1: 609–630.
6. Brazis PW, Masdeu JC, Biller J. The localization of lesions affecting the spinal cord. In: Brazis PW, Masdeu JC, Biller J, eds. *Localization in clinical neurology.* New York: Little, Brown and Company, 1996:79–108.
7. Schwartz TH, McCormick PC. Non-neoplastic intramedullary pathology. Diagnostic dilemma: to Bx or not to Bx. *J Neurooncol* 2000;47:283–292.
8. Riffaud L, Morandi X, Massengo S, et al. MRI of intramedullary spinal schwannomas: case report and review of the literature. *Neuroradiology* 2000;42:275–279.
9. Preul MC, Leblanc R, Tampieri D, et al. Spinal angiolipomas. Report of three cases. *J Neurosurg* 1993;78:280–286.

10. Pietilä TA, Stendel R, Schilling A, et al. Surgical treatment of spinal hemangioblastomas. *Acta Neurochir (Wien)* 2000;142:879–886.

11. Cohen AR, Wisoff JH, Allen JC, et al. Malignant astrocytomas of the spinal cord. *J Neurosurg* 1989;70:50–54.

12. Asazuma T, Toyama Y, Suzuki N, et al. Ependymomas of the spinal cord and cauda equina: an analysis of 26 cases and a review of the literature. *Spinal Cord* 1999;37:753–759.

13. Jallo GI, Kothbauer KF, Epstein FJ. Intrinsic spinal cord tumor resection. *Neurosurgery* 2001; 49:1124–1128.

14. Kothbauer KF, Deletis V, Epstein FJ. Comment on: Intraoperative monitoring. *Pediatr Neurosurg* 1998;29:54–55.

15. Raimondi AJ. Reflection of a laminar flap for exposure of the spinal canal in children. *Clin Neurosurg* 1978;25:504–511.

16. Souweidane MM, Benjamin V. Spinal cord meningiomas. *Neurosurg Clin N Am* 1994;5:283–291.

17. Martin NA, Khanna RK, Batzdorf U. Posterolateral cervical or thoracic approach with spinal cord rotation for vascular malformations or tumors of the ventrolateral spinal cord. *J Neurosurg* 1995; 83:254–261.

18. Robertson PL, Allen JC, Abbott IR, et al. Cervicomedullary tumors in children: a distinct subset of brainstem gliomas. *Neurology* 1994;44:1798–1803.

19. Fischer G, Mansuy L. Total removal of intramedullary ependymomas: follow-up study of 16 cases. *Surg Neurol* 1980;14:243–249.

20. Iwasaki Y, Hida K, Sawamura Y, et al. Spinal intramedullary ependymomas: surgical results and immunohistochemical analysis of tumour proliferation activity. *Br J Neurosurg* 2000;14:331–336.

21. Miller DC, McCutcheon IE. Hemangioblastomas and other uncommon intramedullary tumors. *J Neurooncol* 2000;47:253–270.

22. Lesoin F, Delandsheer E, Krivosic I, et al. Solitary intramedullary schwannomas. *Surg Neurol* 1983; 19:51–56.

23. McCormick PC, Post KD, Stein BM. Intradural extramedullary tumors in adults. *Neurosurg Clin N Am* 1990;1:591–608.

24. Long DM. Surgery for cervical spine tumors. In: Sherk HH, ed. *The cervical spine: an atlas of surgical procedures.* Philadelphia: Lippincott, 1994:289–306.

25. Guidetti B, Mercuri S, Vagnozzi R. Long-term results of the surgical treatment of 129 intramedullary spinal gliomas. *J Neurosurg* 1981;54:323–330.

26. Levy WJ Jr, Latchaw J, Hahn JF, et al. Spinal neurofibromas: a report of 66 cases and a comparison with meningiomas. *Neurosurgery* 1986;18:331–334.

27. Pollack IF, Colak A, Fitz C, et al. Surgical management of spinal cord compression from plexiform neurofibromas in patients with neurofibromatosis 1. *Neurosurgery* 1998;43:248–256.

28. Solero CL, Fornari M, Giombini S, et al. Spinal meningiomas: review of 174 operated cases. *Neurosurgery* 1989;125:153–160.

29. Levy WJ Jr, Bay J, Dohn D. Spinal cord meningioma. *J Neurosurg* 1982;57:804–812.

30. Roux F-X, Nataf F, Pinaudeau M, et al. Intraspinal meningiomas: review of 54 cases with discussion of poor prognosis factors and modern therapeutic management. *Surg Neurol* 1996;46: 458–464.

31. Gezen F, Kahraman S, Çanakci Z, et al. Review of 36 cases of spinal cord meningioma. *Spine* 2000;25:727–731.

32. Gamache FW Jr, Wang JC, Deck M, et al. Unusual appearance of an en plaque meningioma of the cervical spinal canal. A case report and literature review. *Spine* 2001;26:E87–E89.

33. Stechison MT, Tasker RR, Wortzman G. Spinal meningioma en plaque. Report of two cases. *J Neurosurg* 1987;67:452–455.

34. Klekamp J, Samii M. Surgical results of spinal meningiomas. *Acta Neurochir* 1996;65:77–81.

35. Houten JK, Weiner HL. Pediatric intramedullary spinal cord tumors: special considerations. *J Neurooncol* 2000;47:225–230.

36. Kaufman BA, Park TS. Congenital spinal cord astrocytomas. *Childs Nerv Syst* 1992;8:389–393.

37. Sandler HM, Papadopoulos SM, Thornton AF Jr, et al. Spinal cord astrocytomas: results of therapy. *Neurosurgery* 1992;30:490–493.

38. Rossitch E Jr, Zeidman SM, Burger PC, et al. Clinical and pathological analysis of spinal cord astrocytomas in children. *Neurosurgery* 1990;27:193–196.

39. Kulkarni AV, Armstrong DC, Drake JM. MR characteristics of malignant spinal cord astrocytomas in children. *Can J Neurol Sci* 1999;26:290–293.

40. Nishio S, Morioka T, Fujii K, et al. Spinal cord gliomas: management and outcome with reference to adjuvant therapy. *J Clin Neurosci* 2000;7:20–23.

41. Poussaint TY, Yousuf N, Barnes PD, et al. Cervicomedullary astrocytomas of childhood: clinical and imaging follow-up. *Pediatr Radiol* 1999;29:662–668.

42. Epstein F, Epstein N. Surgical treatment of spinal cord astrocytomas of childhood. A series of 19 patients. *J Neurosurg* 1982;57:685–689.

43. Isaacson SR. Radiation therapy and the management of intramedullary spinal cord tumors. *J Neurooncol* 2000;47:231–238.

44. Innocenzi G, Raco A, Cantore G, et al. Intramedullary astrocytomas and ependymomas in the pediatric age group: a retrospective study. *Childs Nerv Syst* 1996;12:776–780.
45. Innocenzi G, Salvati M, Cervoni L, et al. Prognostic factors in intramedullary astrocytomas. *Clin Neurol Neurosurg* 1997;99:1–5.
46. Przybylski GJ, Albright AL, Martinez AJ. Spinal cord astrocytomas: long-term results comparing treatments in children. *Childs Nerv Syst* 1997;13:375–382.
47. Lowe GM. Magnetic resonance imaging of intramedullary spinal cord tumors. *J Neurooncol* 2000; 47:195–210.
48. Epstein FJ, Farmer J-P, Freed D. Adult intramedullary spinal cord ependymomas: the result of surgery in 38 patients. *J Neurosurg* 1993;79:204–209.
49. Lonjon M, Goh KYC, Epstein FJ. Intramedullary spinal cord ependymomas in children: treatment, results and follow-up. *Pediatr Neurosurg* 1998;29:178–183.
50. Fine MJ, Kricheff II, Freed D, et al. Spinal cord ependymomas: MR imaging features. *Radiology* 1995;197:655–658.
51. Venes J. Spinal cord astrocytomas: results of therapy [Letter]. *Neurosurgery* 1992;31:1136.
52. Waldron JN, Laperriere NJ, Jaakkimainen L, et al. Spinal cord ependymomas: a retrospective analysis of 59 cases. *Int J Radiat Oncol Biol Phys* 1993;27:223–229.
53. Sgouros S, Malluci CL, Jackowski A. Spinal ependymomas—the value of postoperative radiotherapy for residual disease control. *Br J Neurosurg* 1996;10:559–566.
54. Hoshimaru M, Koyama T, Hashimoto N, et al. Results of microsurgical treatment for intramedullary spinal cord ependymomas: analysis of 36 cases. *Neurosurgery* 1999;44:264–269.
55. Yasargil MG, Antic J, Laciga R, et al. The microsurgical removal of intramedullary spinal hemangioblastomas. Report of twelve cases and a review of the literature. *Surg Neurol* 1976;6:141–148.
56. Hoff DJ, Tampieri D, Just N. Imaging of spinal cord hemangioblastomas. *Can Assoc Radiol J* 1993;44:377–383.
57. Roonprapunt C, Silvera VM, Setton A, et al. Surgical management of isolated hemangioblastomas of the spinal cord. *Neurosurgery* 2001;49:321–328.
58. Porter RW, Spetzler RF. Comments on: Roonprapunt C, Silvera VM, Setton A, et al. Surgical management of isolated hemangioblastomas of the spinal cord. *Neurosurgery* 2001;49:328.
59. Spetzger U, Bertalanffy H, Huffmann B, et al. Hemangioblastomas of the spinal cord and the brainstem: diagnostic and therapeutic features. *Neurosurg Rev* 1996;19:147–151.
60. Batson OV. The function of the vertebral veins and their role in the spread of metastases. *Ann Surg* 1940;112:138–149.

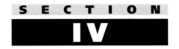

SECTION

IV

GRAFT TECHNIQUES

21

PRINCIPLES OF HARVESTING
ILIAC CREST

WILLIAM F. DONALDSON III
ERIC J. GRAHAM

When autogenous bone graft is mandated, the iliac crest remains the most reliable and popular graft material to date. The iliac crest is unique in its ability to provide either cancellous flakes or cortical struts or a combination. The surgeon only needs to modify the harvest technique to obtain a tricortical wedge for an anterior decompression and fusion or to obtain cancellous chunks for a posterior spinal instrumentation and fusion. The graft supplied by the crest is plentiful, nonimmunogenic, completely histocompatible, and devoid of blood-borne pathogens.

Additionally, the bone harvested from the iliac crest does not result in significant structural instability; however, there is obvious donor site morbidity and pain. The normal anatomy allows for four potential sites of harvesting the iliac bone. The left and right iliac crest both possess a large reservoir of bone that is easily accessed from either the anterior or posterior approach.

ANTERIOR APPROACH

As with all surgery, preoperative planning is essential. The right or left crest should be elevated with a stack of towels or a small sandbag. This places the crest at a more advantageous position by not only elevating the crest, but also by internally rotating the crest to facilitate the removal of graft. This site should be draped separately in most cases. Finally, prep with standard surgical scrub techniques and drape the entire crest to be harvested. The length of the incision should be based on the amount of desired exposure. The skin overlying the iliac crest is fortunately very pliable. A 5- to 8-cm incision should suffice in most instances.

Knowledge of the anatomy is essential prior to the incision. Palpate the iliac crest along its entirety. The incision should follow the arc of the crest. One must be cognizant of the anterior superior iliac spine (ASIS). Attached to the leading edge anteriorly is the origin of the inguinal ligament. Injury to this structure may compromise the integrity of the inguinal triangle, leading to an increased frequency of inguinal herniations and groin pain. This applies to males more than to females. Attached anteriorly to the female ASIS is the round ligament. Although this is not a vestigial structure, injury to the round ligament does not destabilize the inguinal triangle. We recommend leaving at least 2 to 3 cm of the iliac crest immediately adjacent to the ASIS. This provides an adequate zone of structural integrity to protect against fracture or avulsion (Fig. 21.1).

Also located adjacent to the ASIS is the lateral femoral cutaneous nerve. This supplies sensation to the anterolateral thigh in most people. Although injury to this sensory-only nerve seldom results in disability, the patient will gladly remind the surgeon of the numbness over the anterior thigh on each successive office visit. On rare occasions the nerve damage may result in persistent paresthesias and painful dysesthesias.

Therefore, mark the ASIS using a skin marker, and draw a 3- to 8-cm line along the curve of the crest starting approximately 3 cm lateral to the ASIS. The incision should be centered over the widest portion of the crest, which is the location of an abundance of cancellous bone. The incision should be superior to the top of the crest. This avoids another potential postoperative complication. If the incision is inferior to the crest, the scar tissues are constantly irritated by compression between the pelvic bone and the belt line.

Sharply incise the skin with a no. 20 blade scalpel. Utilize Bovie cauterization for skin bleeders. Place a Weitlaner retractor into the wound to help with exposure. Use the Bovie to dissect Scarpa and Camper's fascia in line with the incision and over the iliac crest. The dissection should reveal a deep fascial layer immediately overlying the crest. Carefully inspect the fascial thickness. This fascia condenses into a dense white band over the crest. Here the origins of the external oblique and internal oblique superiorly share the fascial anchor with the tensor fasciae latae inferiorly (Fig. 21.2). One must leave an adequate rim of fascia along either side of the incision to allow for successful closure. This is best accomplished with a Bovie incising the fascia midline between the respective muscle bellies. The cauterization should be full-thickness down to the iliac crest itself. This strip of fascia provides a true internervous plane. Once a leading edge of fascia is present, the dissection is more safely carried out utilizing a Cobb instrument for blunt dissection.

Gently strip the crest along the inner and outer walls of the ilium. As the dissection proceeds, the gluteus minimus and medius are stripped off the ilium (Fig. 21.3). Fortunately, the innervation of these muscles is distal to the operative field, minimizing the possibility of denervation. To minimize bleeding, avoid injury to the surrounding muscle by staying subperiosteally in the iliac wall dissection. If tricortical graft is desired, dissect the iliacus muscle subperiosteally to protect the contents of the pelvis and abdomen as well as to minimize bleeding. If cancellous graft alone is needed, window the iliac crest tubercle and remove the desired amount of bone via curettes. If both cortical and cancellous bone are needed, remove the outer table in strips using an AO gouge or osteotome. The cancellous bone is readily harvested with a Capner gouge or curette. If possible, do not violate the inner table of the pelvis.

Once the desired amount of bone has been obtained, irrigate the wound. Some form of fibrin polymer may be placed against the bleeding bone to encourage coagulation. If not, a drain may be indicated. This is based on surgeon preference. In our experience, a sheet of Gelfoam against the inner table followed by an interlocking running no. 1 Vicryl suture obviates the need for postoperative drainage. The deep fascia should be closed in either a running fashion or interrupted fashion with a no. 1 Vicryl suture on a cutting needle. The skin is closed in layers with a 2–0 Vicryl for the skin, followed by a 3–0 Vicryl running subcuticular. The skin is covered with sterile strips and a sterile dressing.

POSTERIOR APPROACH

When performing a posterior spinal fusion, the posterior iliac crest is easily harvested. The decision to harvest the right or left crest should be based on which leg is most symptomatic. This provides the patient with at least one good leg to bear weight in the postoperative period.

Obtaining the graft through a separate incision or via a subfascial plane utilizing the same operative incision is ultimately based on surgeon preference. However, if the patient is immunocompromised or diabetic, a separate incision may offer increased protection against a potential deep wound infection. If the fusion extends to the sacrum or to the L5 body, a subfascial dissection avoids a second scar without compromising the surgical exposure of the crest (Fig. 21.4). To access the posterior crest, gently dissect the iliolumbar fascia from the overlying adipose tissue with a Bovie cautery pencil or blunt dissection with one's finger. The dissection proceeds until approximately 5 to 8 cm of crest is palpated beneath the iliolumbar fascia. Any defect in the fascia should be repaired.

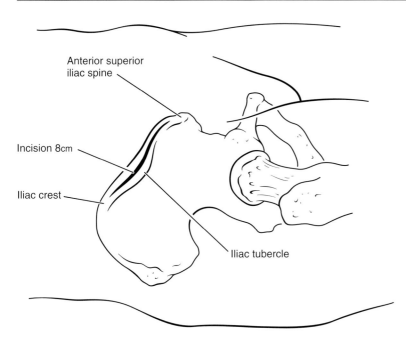

FIGURE 21.1. Make an 8-cm incision parallel to the iliac crest and centered over the tubercle. (From Hoppenfeld S, deBoer P, eds. *The pelvis in surgical exposures in orthopaedics: the anatomic approach,* 2nd ed. Philadelphia: JB Lippincott Co, 1994, with permission.]

If performing the harvest through a separate incision, palpate the posterior crest and sacrum. Plan on a 5- to 8-cm incision along the crest. The incision should be diagonally opposed to the primary spinal incision (Fig. 21.4). Sharply incise the skin and obtain hemostasis with a Bovie cautery pencil. Dissect through the adipose tissue until the iliolumbar fascia is located. Expose a 5- to 8-cm strip of the crest. If the dissection is carried more

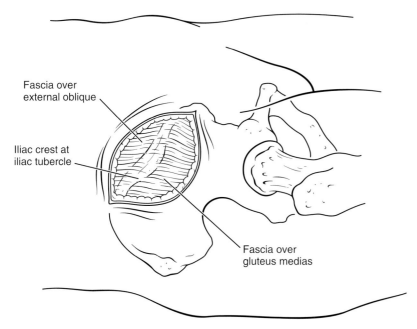

FIGURE 21.2. Retract the skin, identify the iliac crest, and incise the soft tissues overlying the crest down to bone. (From Hoppenfeld S, deBoer P, eds. *The pelvis in surgical exposures in orthopaedics: the anatomic approach,* 2nd ed. Philadelphia: JB Lippincott Co, 1994, with permission.]

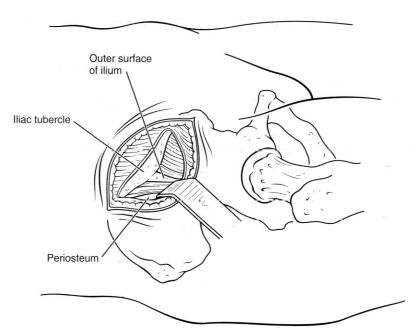

FIGURE 21.3. Remove the origins of the gluteus minimus and medius muscles subperiosteally from the outer cortex of the ilium. (From Hoppenfeld S, deBoer P, eds. *The pelvis in surgical exposures in orthopaedics: the anatomic approach,* 2nd ed. Philadelphia: JB Lippincott Co, 1994, with permission.]

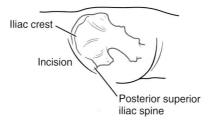

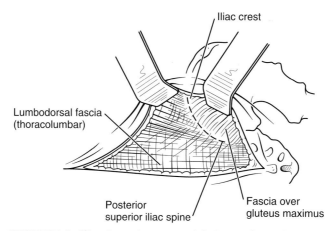

FIGURE 21.4. If lumbar spine surgery is being performed, extend the midline incision distally, retracting the skin laterally until the posterior superior iliac spine and crest can be palpated and seen. Incise the soft tissue overlying the crest down to bone. Make an 8-cm oblique incision, centered over the posterior superior iliac spine and in line with the iliac crest (*inset*). (From Hoppenfeld S, deBoer P, eds. *The pelvis in surgical exposures in orthopaedics: the anatomic approach,* 2nd ed. Philadelphia: JB Lippincott Co, 1994, with permission.]

anterolaterally, the cluneal nerves are subject to damage. Although it is not debilitating if the cluneal nerves are injured, they provide cutaneous sensation to the gluteal region.

One can utilize either approach, and the remainder of the procedure is similar. Incise the fascia overlying the crest in its midline. Because this is a true internervous plane, no muscle is denervated with this incision. Elevate the fascia from the posterior superior iliac spine. This is best accomplished with a Bovie. The fascia should be elevated from the sides of the ilium in a blunt fashion using a Cobb elevator. The exposure of the lateral wall of the ilium should not extend to the nearby sacroiliac joint caudally or to the sciatic notch inferiorly (Fig. 21.5).

After adequate subperiosteal dissection is completed, place a Taylor retractor to hold the gluteal muscles away from the exposed bone. One must be cognizant of the sciatic notch when placing the retractor. If the retractor is placed above the notch, the sciatic nerve and superior gluteal vessels are protected. Injury to the superior gluteal vessel at this level is catastrophic because the artery tends to retract into the pelvis, necessitating an emergent anterior approach to ligate the vessel.

An assistant can hold the Taylor retractor in place, or the surgeon can secure the retractor utilizing a 4 × 4 roll of Kerlix. The Kerlix is wrapped about the retractor, and a loop is dropped to the floor. The surgeon can stand on the loop to maintain exposure.

The bone is removed from the crest in a variety of ways. An osteotome or an AO gouge should be used to remove strips of corticocancellous bone. Every effort must be made to avoid violation of the inner wall of the ilium and the sacroiliac joint. Once the strips are removed, the remaining cancellous bone can be scraped from the ilium with a curette or Capner gouge.

Complete removal of cancellous bone from the inner table should minimize the bleeding. A small square of Gelfoam or other hemostatic agent can be placed into the wound. A drain for closure is optional. In our experience, we found that the use of Gelfoam with closure of the deep wound with a running no. 1 Vicryl is sufficient to avoid the use of a drain. The wound is closed in layers in standard fashion if the incision

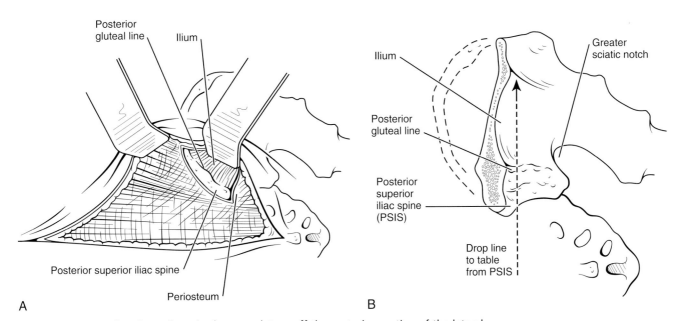

FIGURE 21.5. A: Subperiosteally, strip the musculature off the posterior portion of the lateral surface of the ilium. **B:** Proceeding down the outer surface of the ilium in the area of the posterior superior spine, the elevated posterior gluteal line can be seen and felt; pass subperiosteally up and over the line and then down its other side. Do not err by letting the line direct you outward from bone to muscle. If you draw an imaginary line from the posterior superior iliac spine perpendicular to the operating table and stay cephalad to it, you will avoid the sciatic notch and its contents. (From Hoppenfeld S, deBoer P, eds. *The pelvis in surgical exposures in orthopaedics: the anatomic approach,* 2nd ed. Philadelphia: JB Lippincott Co, 1994, with permission.]

was separate from the primary site. If one used a subfascial approach through the primary operative site, a few subcutaneous stitches to close the dead space are ideal.

The potential pitfalls are easily avoided with a thorough knowledge of the anatomy. Knowing where the sciatic notch lies is paramount to success. If this area of bone is violated while harvesting graft, the stability of the pelvis is reduced. Additionally, the superior gluteal artery hugs the superior arch of the sciatic notch. Injury to this vessel may be fatal because of the retraction of the artery into the pelvis. Injury to the sciatic nerve needs no explanation. Penetration into the sacroiliac joint results in significant morbidity due to the prolonged postoperative pain that results. Penetration of the inner wall of the ilium may result in injury to the bowels or vital organs.

Whether the graft is harvested from the anterior or posterior approach, morbidity results. Robinson and Wray (1) published a study addressing the associated postoperative morbidity associated with this surgery. The study of 105 patients showed that pain increased within the first 6 months and decreased after 12 months. Overall, 35% of patients complained of donor site pain. Patients tend to notice the defect more as time passes and the scar expands. Scar numbness and 10% cluneal nerve injury were reported. They did not find a significant difference in rehabilitation when the graft was harvested from the symptomatic side versus the nonsymptomatic side.

Regarding the void in the crest following harvest, no study has shown superior results in reconstituting the harvest site. Asano et al. (2) investigated the use of an apatite-glass ceramic in replacing the harvest-site void. They noted 98% incorporation of the ceramic via roentgenogram evaluation; however, they failed to biopsy the region to confirm histologic incorporation of the substitute. A study on the use of coral as a void filler proved unsuccessful after 2 years. No graft fully reconstituted, and only two of the seven grafts showed true bony ingrowth at 1 year (3). A resorbable copolymer that was noted to be successful in animals failed to provide similar results in humans. Roessler et al. (4) noted that computed tomographic evaluation up to 1 year later showed no successful regeneration of the crest site. Roesgen (5) performed a four-part study evaluating the results of crest reconstitution using hydroxylapatite, tricalcium phosphate, Kiel bone, and no filler. The biopsy results showed ingrowth of trabecular bone about the ceramics. Additionally, the smaller the ceramic size, the more complete and rapid the reconstitution. The Kiel bone failed completely, and the control filled with hard lamellar bone. Roesgen recommended using phosphate ceramics to fill defects. The search for a suitable graft filler is ongoing. Although the amount of potential graft provided by the crests is plentiful, it is also finite.

REFERENCES

1. Robinson P, Wray A. Natural history of posterior iliac crest bone graft donation for spinal surgery: a prospective analysis of morbidity. *Spine* 2001;26(13):1473–1476.
2. Asano S, Kaneda K, Satoh S, et al. Reconstruction of an iliac crest defect with a bioactive ceramic prosthesis. *Eur Spine J* 1994;3(1):39–44.
3. Vuola J, Bohling T, Kinnumen J, et al. Natural coral as bone-filling material. *J Biomed Mater Res* 2000;51(1):117–122.
4. Roessler M, Wilke A, Griss P, et al. Missing osteoconductive effect of a resorbable PEO/PBT copolymer in human bone defects: a clinically relevant pilot study with contrary results to previous animal studies. *J Biomed Mater Res* 2000;53(2):67–73.
5. Roesgen M. Regeneration capacity of the iliac crest after spongiosa removal in humans—induction by phosphate ceramics [in German]. *Unfallchirurgie* 1991;17(1):44–59.

22

HARVEST OF FIBULA SHAFT

SCOTT D. HODGES
JASON C. ECK

Anterior cervical discectomy and fusion is a well-established technique that can provide significant pain relief to patients with radicular symptoms. This technique has a reported successful single-level fusion rate of approximately 95%, with good to excellent clinical results in nonsmoking patients (1,2). However, when multiple levels are involved there is a significant increase in the rate of nonunion (3,4).

Several sources of bone graft are available to enhance spinal fusion. The most common include iliac crest, rib, and fibula strut graft. In cases of tumor, infection, trauma, and multiple-level degeneration, it may be necessary to reconstruct large anterior column defects. In these cases, in which bone graft is needed to span multiple segments and withstand compressive loading, the fibula is a useful option. Fibula strut graft provides a solid longitudinal ring of cortical bone that is the approximate size of the vertebral body and is capable of providing strong axial support until fusion is achieved.

A question that arises when using any bone graft is whether to use autograft or allograft. The advantages of fibular autograft versus allograft are similar to other sources of bone graft and are summarized in Table 22.1. Fernyhough et al. (4) reported on the results of 126 patients in a study comparing anterior multilevel cervical fusion rates when using autograft versus allograft. It was determined that patients receiving autograft had a significantly lower rate of pseudoarthrosis than patients receiving allograft (27% vs. 41%).

An additional issue related to the use of autograft fibula is the decision to use vascularized or nonvascularized graft. When using nonvascularized grafts, bone regeneration can occur either through osteogenesis or osteoconduction. Osteogenesis, or new bone formation, can be stimulated by osteoprogenitor cells and osteoblasts, which are transferred within the bone graft. This method is more common in cancellous bone. Alternatively, osteoconduction occurs when the osteoprogenitor cells are provided by the host bone; it is more common in cortical bone. During the healing process cortical bone is resorbed and gradually replaced by new bone. This bone turnover causes weakening of the graft before it eventually returns to its original strength.

When using vascularized fibular grafts, the peroneal (fibular) artery and vein are harvested with the diaphysis of the fibula. The peroneal artery and vein are then anastomosed with an artery and vein at the fusion site. In cervical spine fusion, the anastomosis

TABLE 22.1. ADVANTAGES OF AUTOGRAFT AND ALLOGRAFT

Autograft	Allograft
No risk of disease transmission	No donor site morbidity (neurovascular injury, infection, fracture, persistent pain, hematoma, etc.)
Improved rate and degree of graft incorporation	Reduced operative time
No conflict with patient's religious or emotional beliefs	No limit on quantity of graft material available

generally occurs between the peroneal artery and the superior thyroid artery, and between the peroneal veins and either the anterior cervical vein, external jugular vein, external carotid vein, or inferior thyroid vein (5,6). Vascularized bone grafts have the advantage of transferring viable osteocytes within the graft (7,8). This allows for more rapid integration of the bone graft. Because there is less bone turnover during the healing process, the graft is able to maintain its strength with fewer fractures. The strength and stiffness of vascularized grafts have been reported to be significantly greater than those of nonvascularized grafts between 6 weeks and 6 months postoperatively, but they return to similar levels after 1 year (8). The main disadvantages of vascularized fibular grafts are increased cost, a more technically demanding procedure, and the need for more preoperative studies to assess the vascular supply of the patient's lower extremity.

Although harvesting of bone graft is not generally a technically demanding procedure, there are significant risks of morbidity, including donor site pain and neurovascular injury. A thorough understanding of the proper preoperative planning, regional anatomy, surgical technique, and postoperative care can help reduce the morbidity associated with fibula graft harvest.

SURGICAL ANATOMY

The fibula is the lateral bone in the leg that lies posterolateral to the tibia (Fig. 22.1). Although the fibula serves little function in weight bearing, it does play a role in maintaining ankle stability and acts as a site for multiple muscle attachments. The head of the fibula is located proximally. The superior surface of the head has a facet for articulation with the inferior surface of the lateral tibial condyle. The shaft of the fibula varies consid-

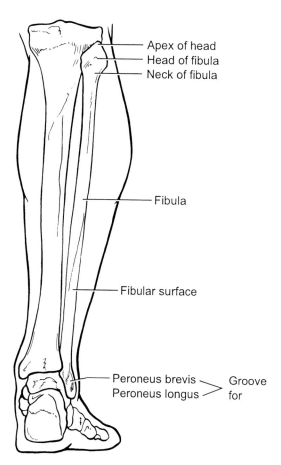

FIGURE 22.1. Posterior view of the bones of the leg.

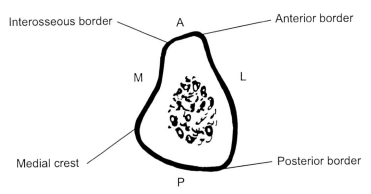

FIGURE 22.2. Cross-sectional view of the shaft of the fibula.

erably throughout its length, but in general it consists of four surfaces (anterior, lateral, posterior, and medial) and four crests (anterior, posterior, medial, and interosseous), as shown in Figure 22.2. The distal portion of the fibula forms the lateral malleolus, which articulates with the distal tibia and the talus.

The shaft of the fibula is an attachment site for multiple muscles of the leg, as shown in Figures 22.3 and 22.4. The muscles of the leg are located in three compartments (Fig. 22.5). The anterior compartment is located between the tibia and the anterior crural septum and contains the extensors. The posterior compartment is located between the tibia and the posterior crural septum and contains the flexors. The posterior compartment is further divided into superficial and deep posterior compartments by the intermuscular

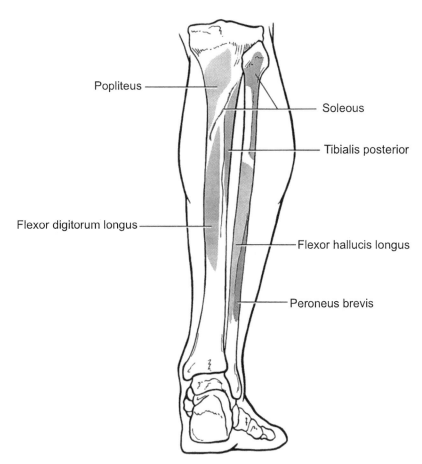

FIGURE 22.3. Posterior view of the fibula, showing muscle attachment sites.

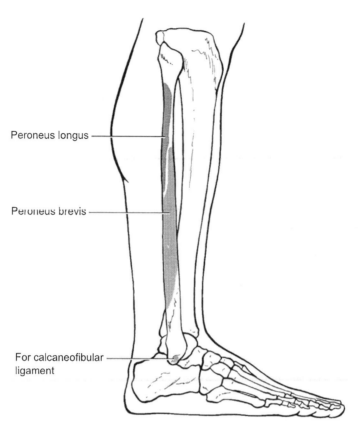

Peroneus longus ⎯

Peroneus brevis ⎯

For calcaneofibular ⎯
ligament

FIGURE 22.4. Lateral view of the fibula, showing muscle attachment sites.

septum. The lateral compartment is located between the anterior and posterior crural septa and contains the peroneal muscles. Table 22.2 lists the muscles found in each compartment of the leg.

The common peroneal nerve is one of the terminal branches of the sciatic nerve. It originates at the superior angle of the popliteal fossa and exits the fossa by passing superficial to the lateral head of the gastrocnemius muscle. It then crosses over the

TABLE 22.2. MUSCLES AND NEUROVASCULAR SUPPLY OF THE LEG ARRANGED BY COMPARTMENT

Compartment	Muscles	Nerve supply	Arterial supply
Anterior	Tibialis anterior, extensor hallucis longus, extensor digitorum longus, peroneus tertius	Deep peroneal nerve	Anterior tibial artery
Lateral	Peroneus longus, peroneus brevis	Superficial peroneal nerve	Muscular branches from peroneal artery
Superficial posterior	Gastrocnemius, soleus, plantaris	Tibial nerve	Posterior tibial artery
Deep posterior	Popliteus, flexor digitorum longus, flexor hallucis longus, tibialis posterior	Tibial nerve	Posterior tibial artery

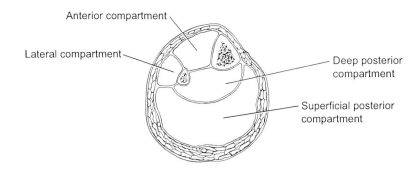

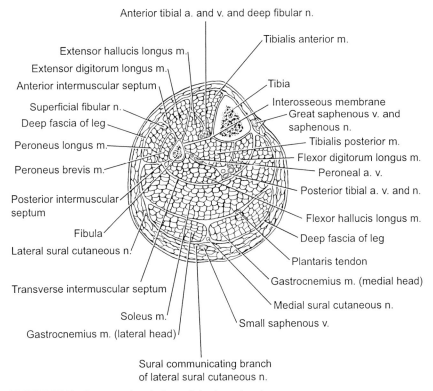

FIGURE 22.5. Cross-sectional view of the leg, showing compartments.

posterior aspect of the head of the fibula to the lateral surface of the neck of the fibula, where it continues to the superior portion of the peroneus (fibularis) longus muscle. The common peroneal nerve then divides to form the superficial and deep peroneal nerves (Fig. 22.6).

The deep peroneal nerve lays inferomedially to the fibula and deep to the extensor digitorum longus muscle. The deep peroneal nerve pierces the anterior crural intermuscular septum and descends in the anterior compartment. At the ankle joint, the deep peroneal nerve passes deep to the extensor retinaculum and divides into medial and lateral branches.

The other branch of the common peroneal nerve is the superficial peroneal nerve. It runs anterolateral to the fibula between the peroneus muscles and the extensor digitorum longus muscle. In the distal third of the leg, the superficial peroneal nerve pierces the deep fascia and becomes superficial. It continues past the ankle to supply the dorsum of the foot and digits.

The other, larger terminal branch of the sciatic nerve is the tibial nerve. The tibial nerve passes through the popliteal fossa and runs posterior to the popliteal artery and

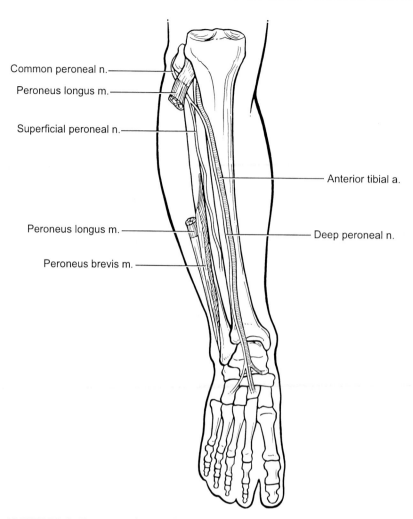

Common peroneal n.

Peroneus longus m.

Superficial peroneal n.

Anterior tibial a.

Peroneus longus m.

Deep peroneal n.

Peroneus brevis m.

FIGURE 22.6. Neurovascular supply of the anterior portion of the leg.

vein (Fig. 22.7). It descends distally, deep to the soleus muscle on the tibialis posterior muscle along with the posterior tibial artery and vein. At the ankle the tibial nerve divides to form the medial and lateral plantar nerves.

The arterial supply of the leg originates from the popliteal artery, which is a continuation of the femoral artery. At the inferior border of the popliteus muscle, the popliteal artery divides to form the anterior and posterior tibial arteries. The popliteal vein is also formed at the inferior border of the popliteus muscle by the union of the venae comitantes of the anterior and posterior tibial arteries.

The anterior tibial artery is the smaller of the branches of the popliteal artery. It passes anteriorly through the interosseous membrane and travels distally on its anterior surface between the extensor hallucis longus and tibialis anterior muscles. It supplies the muscles of the anterior compartment before entering the ankle joint as the dorsalis pedis artery.

The posterior tibial artery is the larger branch of the popliteal artery. It passes deep to the soleus muscle and gives off the peroneal artery. It then descends deep to the transverse crural septum to the ankle, where it divides into the medial and lateral plantar arteries. The peroneal artery runs along the medial surface of the fibula and supplies muscles of the posterior and lateral compartments. Additionally, the peroneal artery gives off the nutrient artery to the fibula. The location of the nutrient foramen

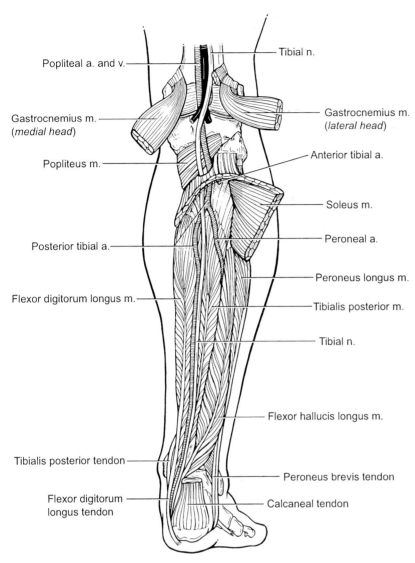

Popliteal a. and v.

Gastrocnemius m.
(*medial head*)

Popliteus m.

Posterior tibial a.

Flexor digitorum longus m.

Tibialis posterior tendon

Flexor digitorum
longus tendon

Tibial n.

Gastrocnemius m.
(*lateral head*)

Anterior tibial a.

Soleus m.

Peroneal a.

Peroneus longus m.

Tibialis posterior m.

Tibial n.

Flexor hallucis longus m.

Peroneus brevis tendon

Calcaneal tendon

FIGURE 22.7. Neurovascular supply of the posterior portion of the leg.

is important when harvesting a vascularized fibula graft. In most cases the fibula contains a single nutrient foramen, which enters on the posterior surface immediately proximal to the midpoint of the fibula shaft (9).

PREOPERATIVE PLANNING

No specific preoperative procedures are necessary when harvesting a nonvascularized fibula strut graft. However, it is necessary to adequately assess the patient's vascular anatomy prior to harvesting a vascularized graft. There remains some controversy over the appropriate method for preoperative vascular examination. A preoperative physical examination with evaluation of the distal pulses is routine. However, the need for routine arteriography is debated. This test provides useful information, including identification of vascular anomalies and peripheral vascular disease and measurements of vessel lengths and diameters. Studies have reported that preoperative arteriography resulted in a change in the operative plan in 11% to 16% of cases (10,11). However,

TABLE 22.3. REPORTED PREVALENCE OF CONGENITAL VASCULAR ANOMALIES PRECLUDING THE USE OF VASCULARIZED FIBULAR GRAFT

Anomaly	Prevalence (%)
Peroneal artery magna (absence or hypoplasia of both anterior and posterior tibial arteries)	0.2–7
Anterior tibial artery is absent or terminates in the leg	2–6
Posterior tibial artery is absent or terminates in the leg	4–5
Dorsalis pedis artery arises from two branches of equal size from the peroneal and anterior tibial arteries	1%
Peroneal artery is absent	<0.1

Data from Young DM, Trabulsy PP, Anthony JP. The need for preoperative leg angiography in fibula free flaps. *J Reconstr Microsurg* 1994;10:283–287; Kim D, Orron DE, Skillman JJ. Surgical significance of popliteal artery variants: a united angiographic classification. *Ann Surg* 1989;210:776–781; and Lippert H, Pabst R. *Arterial variations in man: classifications and frequency.* New York: JF Bergman Verlag, 1985.

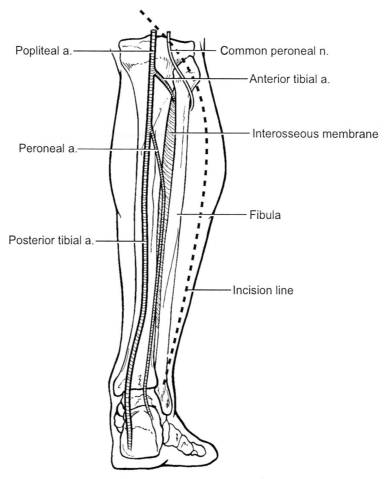

FIGURE 22.8. Posterior view of the leg, showing line of incision and key anatomic structures.

opponents argue that a thorough physical examination is sufficient in the majority of cases and that the cost and potential complications of routine arteriography are not justified (12,13). Long-term morbidity related to arteriography has been reported to be between 0.5% and 3.9% (14,15). Although arteriography is the gold standard for preoperative vascular assessment, others have reported on the ability of magnetic resonance imaging to provide comparable data more cost-effectively and with less morbidity (16,17).

Significant congenital vascular anomalies exist that would preclude the use of a vascularized fibular graft. Previous investigators have reported on the prevalence of these anomalies, as shown in Table 22.3 (11,18,19) Each of these anomalies may necessitate leaving the peroneal artery in order to allow for adequate blood flow to the foot.

NONVASCULARIZED GRAFT HARVEST TECHNIQUE

The patient is placed in a lateral decubitus position with a tourniquet placed at the upper thigh. The distal portion of the thigh and the entire leg, ankle, and foot are prepped and draped. Anatomic landmarks are identified, including the head of the fibula, the tendon of the biceps femoris, and the lateral malleolus. A lateral incision is made beginning one handbreadth above the head of the fibula. The incision is extended anteriorly in line with the biceps tendon, over the head and neck of the fibula, and distally to a location posterior to the lateral malleolus (Fig. 22.8). The length of the incision can be adjusted based on the length of graft being harvested. The plane separating the lateral and superficial posterior compartments is identified and dissected down to the fibula.

The head and neck of the fibula are identified and exposed. The posterior portion of the biceps femoris tendon is identified and dissected to allow exposure of the common peroneal nerve. The common peroneal nerve is identified and gently retracted anteriorly over the head of the fibula. This can be facilitated by cutting a portion of the peroneus longus muscle that attaches to the lateral surface of the head of the fibula. The plane between the lateral and superficial posterior compartments (i.e., between the peroneus muscles and the soleus muscle) is developed distally along the shaft of the fibula.

The shaft of the fibula is exposed by subperiosteal stripping of the muscles from both the anterior (peroneus muscles) and posterior (soleus and flexor hallucis longus muscles) surfaces of the fibula. The lateral compartment is gently retracted anteriorly and the superficial posterior compartment is gently retracted posteriorly to visualize the shaft of the fibula (Fig. 22.9). The interosseous membrane is dissected from its attachment to the medial aspect of the shaft of the fibula. The peroneal vessels lie just medial to the fibula and should be identified. Branches of these vessels should be cauterized during dissection. At this point the tourniquet should be released to identify any remaining bleeding vessels.

Once the shaft of the fibula has been isolated, a portion can be measured to the desired length and harvested. Care should be taken to leave at least 8 cm proximally to avoid injury of the common peroneal nerve and 6 cm distally to maintain ankle joint stability. Either a Gigli saw or an oscillating saw is used to make cuts at the proximal and distal ends of the shaft of the fibula. The isolated fibula shaft is then gently removed.

After the graft is harvested, the site should be inspected for any remaining bleeding, copiously irrigated, and closed primarily with suction drains. Care should be taken to avoid excessively tight closure, which has been reported to cause contracture of the flexor hallucis longus muscle (7). A posterior splint is applied with the foot in dorsiflexion for 5 to 7 days postoperatively.

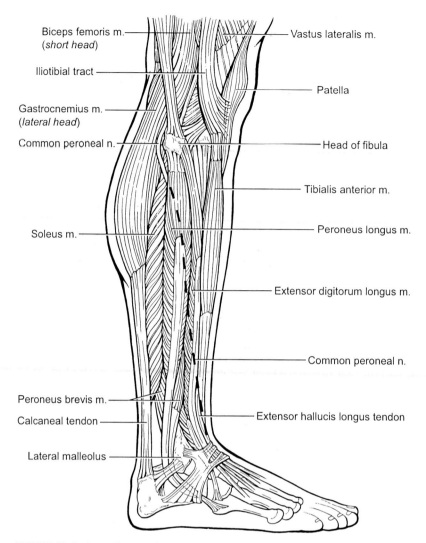

FIGURE 22.9. Lateral view of the leg, showing dissection of the fibula.

VASCULARIZED GRAFT HARVEST TECHNIQUE

The initial portion of the vascularized graft harvest is identical to the nonvascularized graft harvest. The patient is placed in a lateral decubitus position with a tourniquet placed at the upper thigh. The distal portion of the thigh and the entire leg, ankle, and foot are prepped and draped. Anatomic landmarks are identified, including the head of the fibula, the tendon of the biceps femoris, and the lateral malleolus. A lateral incision is made beginning one handbreadth above the head of the fibula. The incision is extended anteriorly in line with the biceps tendon, over the head and neck of the fibula, and distally to a location posterior to the lateral malleolus (see Fig. 22.8). The length of the incision can be adjusted based on the length of graft being harvested. The plane separating the lateral and superficial posterior compartments is identified and dissected to the fibula.

From this point the technique differs from the traditional nonvascularized graft harvest technique. The muscles of the lateral compartment are elevated from the fibula, leaving a cuff of muscle attached to the fibula. The intermuscular septum is identified, and the soleus muscle is then removed from the fibula. The fibula can then be encircled both proximally and distally and cut using either a Gigli saw or an oscillating saw. As

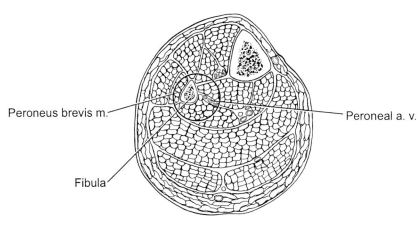

Peroneus brevis m.

Peroneal a. v.

Fibula

FIGURE 22.10. Cross-sectional view of the leg, showing dissection of the vascularized fibula graft.

with the nonvascularized graft, at least 8 cm of fibula proximally and 6 cm distally should be left in place. The muscles of the anterior compartment are then dissected from the fibula, again leaving a cuff of muscle attached.

The tourniquet is then deflated to aid in dissection of the vessels. The peroneal vessels can be palpated immediately anterior to the flexor hallucis longus muscle. The interosseous membrane is then divided while protecting the anterior tibial vessels and the deep peroneal nerve. The flexor hallucis longus and tibialis posterior muscles are then dissected, leaving a generous muscle cuff attached to the fibula containing the peroneal vessels (Fig. 22.10). Care should be taken to avoid injury to the posterior tibial vessels and tibial nerve.

The fibula with its muscle cuff and peroneal vessels is then retracted, and dissection of the proximal vascular pedicle is carried out. The peroneal vessels are carefully dissected proximally to the posterior tibial bifurcation and ligated. After the graft is removed, the site should be inspected for any remaining bleeding, copiously irrigated, and closed primarily with suction drains. A posterior splint is applied with the foot in dorsiflexion for 5 to 7 days postoperatively.

REFERENCES

1. Brodke DS, Zdeblick TA. Modified Smith-Robinson procedure for anterior cervical discectomy and fusion. *Spine* 1992;17:2427–2430.
2. Emery SE, Bolesta MJ, Banks MA, et al. Robinson anterior cervical fusion. Comparison of the standard and modified techniques. *Spine* 1994;19:660–663.
3. Emery SE, Rush J, Fisher S, et al. Three-level anterior cervical discectomy and fusion. *Spine* 1997; 22:2622–2624.
4. Fernyhough JC, White JI, LaRocca H. Fusion rates in multilevel cervical spondylosis comparing allograft fibula with autograft fibula in 126 patients. *Spine* 1991;16(suppl):561–564.
5. Asazuma T, Yamagishi M, Nemoto K, et al. Spinal fusion using a vascularized fibular bone graft for a patient with cervical kyphosis due to neurofibromatosis. *J Spinal Disord* 1997;10:537–540.
6. Minami A, Kasashima T, Iwasaki N, et al. Vascularized fibular grafts: an experience of 102 patients. *J Bone Joint Surg Br* 2000;82:1022–1025.
7. Davis OK, Mazur JM, Coleman GN. A torsional strength comparison of vascularized and nonvascularized bone grafts. *J Biomech* 1982;15:875–880.
8. Shaffer JW, Field GA, Goldberg VM, et al. Fate of vascularized and nonvascularized autografts. *Clin Orthop Rel Res* 1985;197:32–43.
9. McKee N, Haw P, Vettese T. Anatomic variations of the nutrient foramen in the shaft of the fibula. *Clin Orthop Rel Res* 1984;184:141–144.
10. Margiotta MS, Markowitz B, Shaw W. Routine angiography in free fibula flap reconstruction. *Plast Surg Forum* 1997;20:102–106.
11. Young DM, Trabulsy PP, Anthony JP. The need for preoperative leg angiography in fibula free flaps. *J Reconstr Microsurg* 1994;10:283–287.

12. Disa JJ, Cordeiro PG. The current role of preoperative arteriography in free fibula flaps. *Plast Reconstr Surg* 1998;102:1083–1088.
13. Jones NF. The need for preoperative leg angiography in fibula free flaps [Discussion]. *J Reconstr Microsurg* 1994;10:287–289.
14. Hawkins I. Mini-catheter techniques for femoral run-off and abdominal arteriography. *Radiology* 1972;116:199–203.
15. Hessel S, Adams P, Abrams H. Complications of angiography. *Radiology* 1981;138:273–281.
16. Manaster BJ, Coleman DA, Bell DA. Magnetic resonance imaging of vascular anatomy before vascularized fibular grafting. *J Bone Joint Surg Am* 1990;72:409–414.
17. Manaster BJ, Coleman DA, Bell DA. Pre- and postoperative imaging of vascularized fibular grafts. *Radiology* 1990;176:161–166.
18. Kim D, Orron DE, Skillman JJ. Surgical significance of popliteal artery variants: a united angiographic classification. *Ann Surg* 1989;210:776–781.
19. Lippert H, Pabst R. *Arterial variations in man: classifications and frequency.* New York: JF Bergman Verlag, 1985:60–63.

INTERBODY FUSION

ROBERT A. MCGUIRE, JR.

Once the decision to perform an interbody fusion has been made, success depends on several factors. First, the correct type of bone graft type must be selected. Next, the endplates must be prepared in such a manner as to provide good graft acceptance, with as large a contact surface area as possible to encourage the influx of neovascularization to assist in bone formation. Finally, the graft itself must be appropriately contoured and sized to provide a stable interbody fit.

For an interbody graft to be successful, there must be an osteoconductive matrix, which serves as scaffolding for bone growth; osteoinductive agents, which are chemical factors that induce bone formation; and osteogenetic cells, which are able to transform and initiate bone regeneration. In addition to these biological requirements for bone healing, the graft component must also provide structural support for assisting in spine stability.

Of the potential graft materials, cancellous autograft has by far the most bioactive capabilities but provides no structural integrity; therefore, it is not a good selection by itself for interbody grafting. Tricortical iliac crest bone graft, on the other hand, has a very osteoconductive, osteoinductive, and osteogenetic cell matrix as well as the ability to provide structural integrity to the spinal segment. Of the allograft materials, frozen allograft appears to be the best option when looking at potential osteoconductivity, osteoinductivity, and structural integrity. Freeze-dried allograft is another option, but does not appear to have quite the structural integrity overall that frozen allografts possess. Radiation-sterilized bone has a significant propensity for collapse during the healing process and is not recommended. In assessing the reasons for the significant difference of collapse and nonunion of allograft iliac crest compared with autogenous iliac crest, Zdeblick and Ducker (1) found that patients with collapse and nonunion had received irradiated allograft, which reinforces the suggestion not to use grafts sterilized in this manner.

Selection of the type of bone to be used depends on several criteria. The advantages of autograft are that it is histocompatible, with no propensity for disease transfer, and is able to retain viable cells to assist in formation of new bone. The disadvantages, however, are that it is in the body in limited quantity and that donor site morbidity consisting of infection, chronic pain, increased anesthetic time, and increased blood loss is possible. The advantages of allograft are the relatively unlimited supply of this material, the saving of harvest time, and the lack of donor site morbidity. The disadvantages of this material are its minimum biologic potential, an apparently increased rate in graft collapse with a potentially lower fusion rate, and possible immune response with potential disease transmission.

A study performed by Zdeblick and Ducker (1) looking at the outcomes of the different types of grafts revealed that freeze-dried iliac crest graft resulted in delayed union at 3 months of 37%, compared with 13% for iliac crest autograft. At 1 year, the nonunion rate for allograft was 22%, compared with 8% for the autograft. Graft collapse was 30% in the freeze-dried group, compared with 5% in the iliac crest autograft group. Comparison of multilevel nonunions revealed a rate of 63% for the freeze-dried group versus 17% for the autograft group. However, clinical success (measured in relief of arm and neck pain) was similar in the two groups.

An et al. (2) looked at tricortical allograft with the addition of demineralized bone matrix compared with autograft and found outcomes similar to those of the previously discussed study. This study revealed a nonunion rate of 46% in those patients treated with allograft, compared with 26% in those treated with autograft. Graft collapse occurred in 39% of the allograft group, compared with 24% in the autograft group. Again, clinical success when comparing the two types of graft was not significantly different. Young and Rosewasser (3), in their study comparing fibular allograft with autograft, found a similar outcome in fusion rates, with the allograft group's rate being 92% and the autograft group's rate being 88%. Again, similar clinical outcomes were noted.

Lofgrend et al. (4), evaluating the clinical success of this type of procedure, found clinical improvement regardless of the type of graft used and found that acceptable rates of union occurred with both autograft and allograft. The autograft group seemed to do better (although it was not statistically significant), but this group did have problems related to the graft site itself. In a meta-analysis of autograft versus allograft, Floyd and Ohnmeiss (5) looked at the literature and found four studies that were appropriate for this type of evaluation. One- and two-level fusions were evaluated, which resulted in a study group of 310 patients with 379 levels. They found that autograft results in higher radiographic union and lower incidence of collapse in both one- and two-level fusions, but they were unable to determine the superiority of autograft when compared with allograft. They did note that clinical results do not correlate with the radiographic outcome and concluded that the risks of graft site morbidity and patient preference should be considered in choosing the type of bone graft to be utilized when performing an interbody fusion.

TECHNIQUE

The patient is positioned supine with a bolster under the shoulders to provide extension and maintenance of cervical lordosis. If iliac crest bone autograft is to be used, the side of the pelvis selected is bolstered using a small hip roll to make the anterior margin of the iliac crest more prominent. The arms are then carefully padded and tucked to the side to facilitate radiographic exposure of the cervical spine (Fig. 23.1). After sterilely prepping

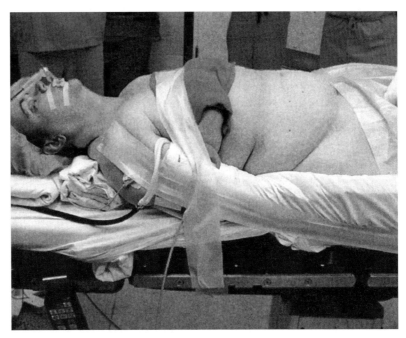

FIGURE 23.1. The patient is positioned in such a way as to protect soft tissues and facilitate radiographic visualization.

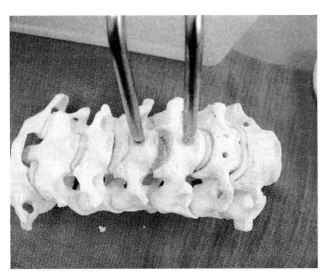

FIGURE 23.2. Placement of the distractor facilitates vertebral stability, allows visualization, and, if the pins are placed correctly, facilitates sagittal alignment correction.

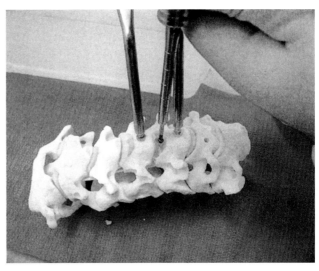

FIGURE 23.3. The high-speed drill allows the endplates to be safely contoured in an accurate manner, providing a good interface between the graft and endplate.

the surgical sites, the standard anterior medial approach is made to the cervical spine and the correct level identified radiographically. Disc space distractors are placed in the vertebral bodies (not in the disc spaces), which not only stabilizes the segment but also allows adequate visualization during the decompression phase of the procedure (Fig. 23.2).

Following the discectomy, the endplates are carefully prepared to accept the interbody graft (Fig. 23.3). It is imperative to leave a rim of cortical bone on each endplate if at all possible because this provides structural stability to maintain the normal alignment and disc height with the graft itself. Use of a high-speed burr facilitates the removal of the cartilaginous portion of the endplate as well as allowing the contouring of bone to be performed safely. If bone grafting alone is to be performed without internal fixation, a small shelf of bone should be left both posteriorly as well as anteriorly to provide mechanical blocks against graft migration. If anterior fixation is to be performed, then it is imperative to remove the bony osteophytes fully to allow the internal fixation device to sit flat upon the vertebral bodies. This not only provides a more stable bone–plate interface but also tends to lower the profile of the construct itself. If one does not remove these anterior osteophytes, there can be potential loss of stability of the construct because the fixation device sits proud and the full biomechanical advantage of the fixation screws could be potentially lost. It is also important to utilize as long a screw as possible in the vertebral bodies to enhance the structural integrity of the construct itself.

Once both endplates have been prepared, it is possible to correct kyphosis and realign the cervical spine appropriately. This can be done by cutting the grafts in a wedge shape to enhance the formation of lordosis. In inserting the graft, the cortical portion of the tricortical iliac crest graft should be turned so the anterior cortical margin is resting on the margin of the anterior aspect of the superior and inferior vertebral endplates themselves.

Graft Insertion

After harvesting the bone graft from the iliac crest, it is trimmed to the appropriate length so that when inserted it does not protrude into the spinal canal (Fig. 23.4). Utilizing the disc space distractor, the disc space is slightly overdistracted to allow the graft to be placed into position; once the graft is inserted just below the anterior margin of the vertebral bodies, the tension is relaxed, locking the graft into position (Fig. 23.5). If the

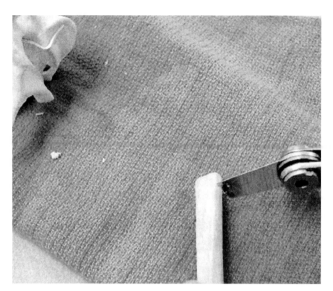

FIGURE 23.4. The oscillating saw, which minimizes microfracture, is used to cut the bone graft to the appropriate length.

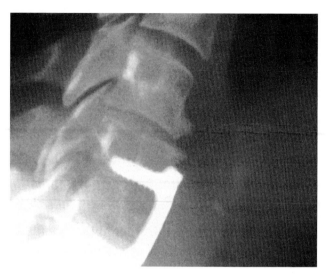

FIGURE 23.5. The iliac crest graft has been inserted and the level plated. No obvious gap exists between the vertebral endplate and the graft.

carpentry has been done correctly, the graft should fit tightly, with no obvious spaces between the graft and the vertebral endplates. The fit of the graft should be such that it is unable to be moved with manipulation using forceps.

If allograft has been selected, whether it be fibula or iliac crest, it is cut to the measured dimensions in exactly the same manner as previously described for autograft. Some companies provide templates for the allografts to ensure adequate endplate preparation so that the grafts fit correctly. These trial templates provide a method whereby the endplates can be machined so that the allograft does not have to be inserted more than once. The graft should fit quite easily into the interspace so as not to require vigorous tamping of the bone to seat it into position, which can result in microfractures and potential collapse of the graft.

If internal fixation is needed, then the device is now placed according to the manufacturer's recommendations.

GRAFT TECHNIQUES

Smith and Robinson (6) devised the technique of placing the bone graft with the cortical margin of the tricortical segment being placed anteriorly. This is probably the most common graft technique presently utilized (Fig. 23.6). Brodke and Zdeblick (7) modified the

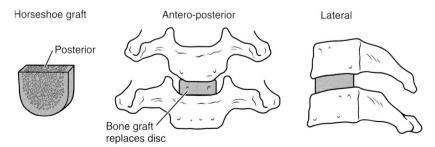

Horseshoe graft

Posterior

Antero-posterior

Bone graft replaces disc

Lateral

FIGURE 23.6. Smith-Robinson technique.

Smith and Robinson technique by turning the graft 180 degrees, pointing the cortical margin posteriorly. This modified technique has been noted to be quite successful in obtaining fusion and maintaining disc heights. The size of the graft utilized is quite critical to the ability to obtain a solid arthrodesis. An et al. (8) assessed the ideal thickness of the graft used in the Smith and Robinson technique and found that a graft that is approximately 2 mm larger than the preoperative baseline disc height provides the greatest improvement in the foraminal height and subsequent enlargement of foraminal areas as well as provides the optimal disc height to minimize graft collapse. There seems to be a significantly greater risk of nonunion when placing grafts that are more than 4 mm larger than the resting preoperative disc height (9).

Iliac crest graft strength is also important. The structural integrity of the construct depends on the ability of the graft to bear weight through the segment (10). Grafts taken from the anterior iliac crest have been shown to be significantly stronger than those grafts taken from the posterior superior iliac spine. The overall success rate with the Smith-Robinson technique seems to be quite good regardless whether the grafts are placed with the cortical margin anteriorly, cortical margins posteriorly, or the cortical margins based laterally. The key to success with this procedure is having good contact with the bone endplates and the graft itself.

The Keystone Technique

Simmons and Bhalla (11) modified a technique that had been initially described by McNabb, in which the graft is constructed in a trapezoidal fashion. The endplates are carefully prepared to receive this keyed-in graft, with the posterior margin of the graft being greater than the anterior margin (Fig. 23.7). The endplates are tapered so as to provide a ledge of bone posteriorly in both the upper and lower endplates of the affected segment. The graft is then cut to match this segment. The vertebral bodies are then distracted in such a way as to allow the graft to be inserted; then, with relaxation of the distraction, the graft is locked into position. This particular configuration prevents the graft from extruding anteriorly, and the shelves of bone posteriorly prevent migration into the canal. The authors of this technique suggest that an angle of bevel between 14 and 18 degrees is ideal for interlocking the graft in the interspace.

The Cloward Technique

Ralph Cloward (12) designed a special set of instruments that allow a dowel graft to be placed as the interbody spacer. The cylindrical drill hole (half being on the cephalad margin of the caudal vertebral endplate, and half being on the inferior endplate of the cephalad vertebrae) then accepts an iliac crest graft that has been cut with a special cylindrical saw through the iliac crest, providing a graft that has cancellous bone sandwiched between bicortical plates of bone on each end (Fig. 23.8). This bone dowel is slightly larger in diameter than the drill hole. The vertebral bodies are distracted slightly, and the graft

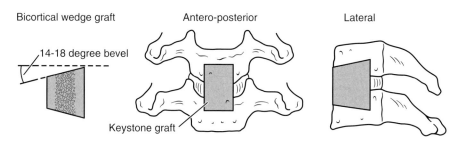

FIGURE 23.7. Keystone technique.

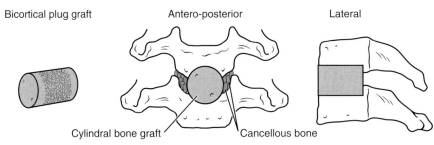

Bicortical plug graft   Antero-posterior   Lateral

Cylindral bone graft   Cancellous bone

FIGURE 23.8. Cloward technique.

is then tamped into position. This particular technique has been shown to allow migration of the dowel graft with kyphosis and subsequent pseudarthrosis. This particular technique is also the approach utilized in the newer dowel-type mechanical grafts.

CONCLUSION

The success of an interbody graft procedure depends on the selection of the bone graft and attention to detail during the carpentry phase of endplate preparation and graft harvesting to ensure a good uniform graft–endplate surface contact while providing stability of the construct, which ultimately aids in the healing process. If attention to these details is maintained, one can expect a high degree of success with interbody grafting.

REFERENCES

1. Zdeblick T, Ducker T. The use of freeze-dried allograft bone for anterior cervical fusions. *Spine* 1991;16:726–729.
2. An HS, Simpson JM, Glover JM, et al. Comparison between allograft plus demineralized bone matrix versus autograft in anterior cervical fusion. *Spine* 1995;20:2211–2216.
3. Young FY, Rosewasser RH. An early comparative analysis of the use of fibular allograft versus autologous iliac crest graft for interbody fusion after anterior cervical discectomy. *Spine* 1993;18:1123–1124.
4. Lofgrend H, Johannsson V, Olsson T, et al. Rigid fusion after Cloward operation for cervical disc disease using autograft, allograft or xenograft. *Spine* 2000;25:1908–1916.
5. Floyd T, Ohnmeiss D. A meta-analysis of autograft versus allograft in anterior cervical fusion. *Eur Spine J* 2000;9:398–403.
6. Smith GW, Robinson RA. The treatment of certain cervical-spine disorders by anterior removal of the intervertebral disc and interbody fusion. *J Bone Joint Surg Am* 1958;40:607–624.
7. Brodke DS, Zdeblick TA. Modified Smith-Robinson procedure for anterior cervical discectomy and fusion. *Spine* 1992;17:S427–S430.
8. An HS, Evanish CJ, Nowicki BH, et al. Ideal thickness of Smith-Robinson graft for anterior cervical fusion: a cadaveric study with computed tomographic correlation. *Spine* 1993;18:2043–2047.
9. Browner RS, Herkowitz HN, Kurz L. Effect of distraction on the union rate of Smith-Robinson type anterior cervical discectomy and fusion. Presented at the 20th annual meeting of the Cervical Spine Research Society, Palm Desert, California, 1992.
10. Smith MD, Cody DD. Load-bearing capacity of corticocancellous bone grafts in the spine. *J Bone Joint Surg Am* 1993;75:1206–1213.
11. Simmons E, Bhalla S. Anterior cervical discectomy and fusion. *J Bone Joint Surg Br* 1969;51:225–237.
12. Cloward RB. The anterior approach for ruptured cervical disc. *J Neurosurg* 1958;15:602–614.

ANTERIOR STRUT GRAFTS: TYPES OF GRAFTS AND METHODS OF INSERTION

HIEU T. BALL
RICK B. DELAMARTER

Restoration of anterior column biomechanics plays an essential role in the success of cervical reconstructive surgery. By producing the proper cervical lordosis and anterior column support in reconstructive and traumatic cases with an anterior strut graft, proper mechanical load on the anterior column is provided. With successful restoration of cervical lordosis, the middle and posterior columns of the cervical spine assume more physiologic load sharing, and long-term failure due to adjacent-level degeneration may be minimized. Proper maintenance of disc space height with strut grafts after discectomy and fusion procedures reduces foraminal stenosis that may be caused by cephalad-caudad stenosis. Anterior strut grafts provide support and biologic surface area upon which bony fusion may occur.

TYPES OF GRAFTS

Types of graft materials available include autogenous tricortical bone graft (iliac crest, fibula, and rib), allograft bone, and foreign materials such as titanium spacers and threaded cage devices (e.g., BAK-C, Harms) and polymethylmethacrylate (PMMA), which is sometimes used in tumor. This chapter focuses on bone products; foreign materials are addressed elsewhere in this book. The important decision regarding whether to use autogenous or allograft bone must take into account the number of levels being fused, the quality of the host and donor bone, body habitus (which may complicate harvest procedures), and medical comorbidities such as diabetes, malnutrition, osteoporosis, and the smoking status of the patient.

Autogenous bone graft may be harvested from the iliac crest, fibula, or rib. For most anterior cervical discectomy and fusion procedures, the appropriate-sized tricortical bone graft may be successfully obtained from the anterior iliac crest. Either a dual-bladed sagittal saw or osteotomes may be used to obtain the bone graft in a minimally traumatic fashion. For longer constructs, such as multilevel corpectomies or revision procedures, a large tricortical graft may be harvested from the iliac crest or from the patient's fibula (Fig. 24.1). Alternatively, long fibular allografts have been shown to be effective in multilevel corpectomies (Fig. 24.2). Each type of bone graft harvest carries its own risks and morbidities.

Anatomic considerations for anterior iliac crest graft harvesting are essential in obtaining acceptable graft material while causing the least pain at the donor site, the most common complication of iliac crest graft harvest. The anterior superior iliac spine (ASIS) must be identified and protected. The skin incision should be made distal and inferior to

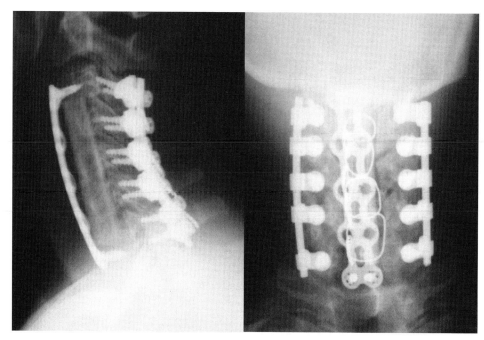

FIGURE 24.1. Plain radiographs of a patient who presented with acute cervical spondylotic myelopathy spanning four levels. The patient required an anterior-posterior C3 to C7 decompression with corpectomies and arthrodesis with a fibular allograft.

the prominence of the crest to avoid creating a scar on the contact surface of the crest as it rubs against clothing (Fig. 24.3). An avascular plane exists on the iliac crest, between the insertion of the abdominal oblique muscles and the hip abductors (Fig. 24.4). Incision through this plane directly down to the bony surface of the iliac crest minimizes bleeding and postoperative donor site pain. Subperiosteal exposure of the inner and outer table of the ilium protects the ilioinguinal and iliohypogastric nerves from injury due to sagittal saw or osteotome use. The graft should be taken at least 3 cm posterior to the ASIS in order to avoid damage to the lateral femoral cutaneous nerve, because it occasionally sends a branch lateral to the ASIS. Avoidance of the ASIS will also prevent injury to the origin of the sartorius and tensor fascia lata; by avoiding the ASIS, the likelihood of iatrogenic stress risers from the crest harvest is reduced, thus reducing the risk of avulsion fractures caused by the powerful muscle forces on the ASIS with normal daily activities.

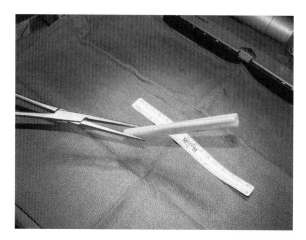

FIGURE 24.2. Fibular strut graft (allograft). This type of strut graft can be cut to appropriate dimensions for multilevel corpectomy.

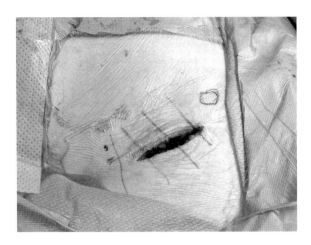

FIGURE 24.3. The incision for the autogenous iliac crest bone graft is placed distal and inferior to the prominence of the crest and several centimeters posterior to the anterior superior iliac spine, shown by the circle.

A dual-bladed sagittal saw allows precise graft sizing and lessens the risk of iatrogenic fracture sometimes caused by osteotomes, particularly in osteoporotic patients (Fig. 24.5). The autogenous tricortical structural graft can thus be efficiently harvested to uniform thickness (Fig. 24.6). Potential complications from iliac crest graft harvest include persistent donor site pain, lateral femoral cutaneous or cluneal nerve injury or neuroma formation, avulsion fractures to the ASIS, abdominal hernia, hematoma, and infection.

Autogenous fibular grafts can be obtained from the middle third of the fibula in order to avoid damage to the peroneal nerve in the proximal 10 cm of the fibula. Iatrogenic ankle instability can be caused by harvesting from the distal 10 cm of fibula. This type of graft provides an option for longer constructs that exceed 6 to 7 cm, and provides a uniform bone quality and diameter not found in iliac crest grafts of longer lengths because of anatomic thinning of the cancellous portion of the ilium in its superior and posterior portion as one moves away from the ASIS. Potential complications of fibular harvest involve neurovascular injury, compartment syndrome, ankle instability, and extensor hallucis longus weakness.

In any of the situations discussed previously, precut allograft spacers (Fig. 24.7) or long fibular allograft strut bone may be applied, utilizing the same principles of appropriate axial distraction during measurement and insertion to optimize compression across the graft once it is in place. Advantages to using allograft primarily concern avoidance of graft donor site morbidity. Disadvantages involve trends of poorer fusion rates and longer times to fusion, particularly when the arthrodesis spans two or more levels.

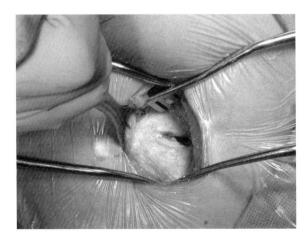

FIGURE 24.4. The incision through the deep fascia is performed along the avascular plane on the superior-lateral aspect of the iliac crest, between the insertion of the abdominal oblique muscles and the hip abductors. Pain, bleeding, and destruction of muscular anatomy can be avoided by staying within this plane, frequently seen as an aponeurotic "white line" of soft tissue.

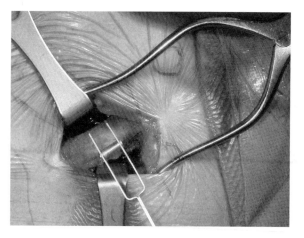

FIGURE 24.5. The iliac crest is subperiosteally exposed along its inner and outer cortical tables. A dual-bladed sagittal saw sized to the recipient disc space, under the appropriate annular distractive tension, is selected and provides a precisely cut tricortical autogenous strut graft for the cervical fusion.

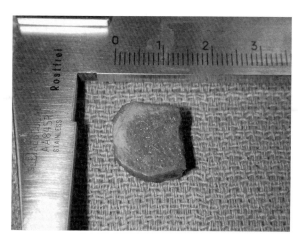

FIGURE 24.6. The tricortical autogenous strut graft is precisely measured, with particular attention paid to the diameter of the graft in order to avoid posterior impingement of the spinal cord by an oversized graft.

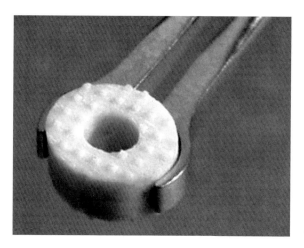

FIGURE 24.7. Precut allograft bone strut graft.

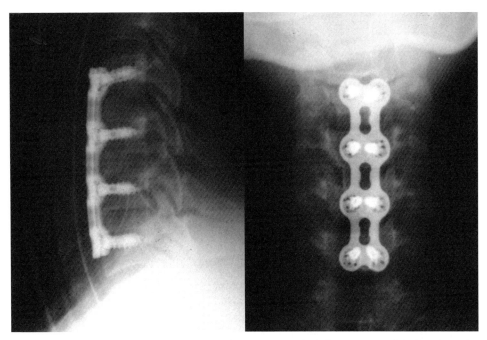

FIGURE 24.8. Radiographs of the three-level anterior cervical discectomy and fusion show the position of fusion in lordosis with appropriate distraction across the facet joints at each level.

METHODS OF INSERTION

Preparation of the recipient graft bed, proper sizing of the grafts, and successful insertion of anterior strut grafts under compressive load dictate the success of the fusion surgery. Anterior column annular tension and cervical lordosis during graft placement are critical to a successful arthrodesis (Fig. 24.8). Patient positioning at the beginning of the surgery on a flat table with a transverse roll placed behind the shoulders will help establish the lordosis for graft insertion. A head halter device, halo ring, or Gardner-Wells tongs applied to a strain gauge that measures up to 50 pounds of tension allow for a nonscrubbed assistant to apply axial force during graft measurement and graft insertion (Fig. 24.9).

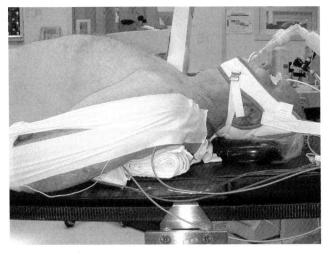

FIGURE 24.9. Patient positioning is essential in creating the proper degree of cervical lordosis. A head halter device allows gentle traction longitudinally. The shoulders are taped distally to allow for intraoperative imaging of the cervical spine by fluoroscopy or plain radiographs.

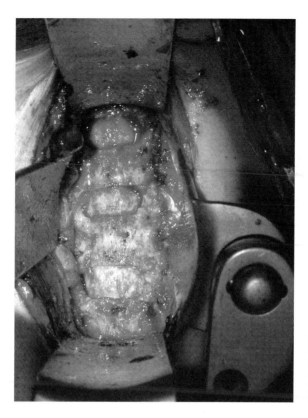

FIGURE 24.10. The autogenous tricortical strut grafts are properly fashioned to preserve the intervertebral distances and function as anterior column support for the cervical arthrodesis.

Intraoperative gradual, sequential axial traction of between 20 and 40 pounds can be applied as the space for the graft is measured. Once the proper-size graft is obtained, it can be placed under the same amount of traction to avoid crushing or "plowing" of the endplates during insertion, thus maintaining the appropriate compressive forces across the graft after traction is released in order to optimize fusion rates (Fig. 24.10). Preoperative measurements from the radiographs are helpful but frequently unreliable predictors of graft size; often, anterior and posterior osteophyte excision, discectomy, and endplate preparation with a high-speed drill such as a Midas Rex or Stryker TPS result in a disc space that must be measured intraoperatively under distraction for best accuracy.

Alternatively, distraction and lordosis during graft measurement and insertion may be achieved with local distraction pins placed in the superior and inferior vertebral bodies surrounding the disc space being measured. It is important to insert these pins at

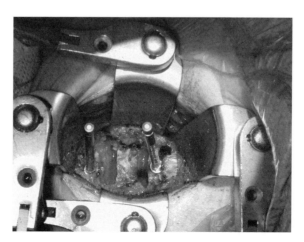

FIGURE 24.11. Cloward distraction pins are placed in the vertebral bodies to provide distraction across the disc spaces. Note that the pins are positioned in slight divergence, which will help produce lordosis when distraction is applied.

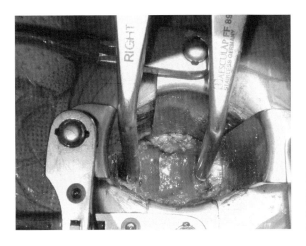

FIGURE 24.12. Distraction pins with gentle force applied will create the appropriate amount of annular tension and allow accurate sizing of the strut grafts.

divergent angles such that when they become parallel in the distractor, the appropriate amount of lordosis is achieved (Figs. 24.11 and 24.12). Drawbacks from this technique include compromise to the bone stock of the vertebral bodies where the final screws to secure the plate must be applied, cutout for the pins in osteoporotic bone with resultant loss of the lordosis from the divergent pin placement, imprecise measurement of the lordosis achieved, and imprecise measurement of the amount of distraction actually being applied across the disc space.

CONCLUSION

Anterior grafting for cervical spine decompression and fusion procedures can be done safely and effectively. Strict attention to important anatomic considerations and knowledge of potential complications from autogenous graft harvest will effectively reduce morbidity and significantly improve rates of successful fusion. Meticulous recipient bed endplate preparation, establishment of cervical lordosis, reconstruction of anterior column support with appropriate compressive tension across the graft, and rigid internal fixation will determine the success of any fusion procedure, whether autograft or allograft is utilized.

BIBLIOGRAPHY

Coventry MB, Tapper EM. Pelvic instability: a consequence of removing iliac bone for grafting. *J Bone Joint Surg Am* 1972;54:83–101.

Cowley SP, Anderson LD. Hernias through donor sites for iliac-bone grafts. *J Bone Joint Surg Am* 1983;65:1023–1025.

Ebraheim NA, Elgafy H, Xu R. Bone-graft harvesting from iliac and fibular donor sites: techniques and complications. *J Am Acad Orthop Surgeons* 2001;9(3):210–218.

Ebraheim NA, Yang H, Lu J, et al. Anterior iliac crest bone graft: anatomic considerations. *Spine* 1997; 22:847–849.

Gore DR. Arthrodesis rate in multilevel anterior cervical fusions using autogenous fibula. *Spine* 2001; 26:1259–1263.

Gore DR, Gardner GM, Sepic SB, et al. Function following partial fibulectomy. *Clin Orthop* 1987; 220:206–210.

Goulet JA, Senunas LE, DeSilva GL, et al. Autogenous iliac crest bone graft: complications and functional assessment. *Clin Orthop* 1997;339:76–81.

Grossman W, Peppelman WC, Baum JA, et al. The use of freeze-dried fibular allograft in anterior cervical fusion. *Spine* 1992;17:565–569.

Hacker RJ, Cauthen JC, Gilbert TJ, et al. A prospective randomized multicenter clinical evaluation of an anterior cervical fusion cage. *Spine* 2000;25:2646–2654.

Hu RW, Bohlman HH. Fracture at the iliac bone graft harvest site after fusion of the spine. *Clin Orthop* 1994;309:208–213.

Jones AA, Dougherty PJ, Sharkey NA, et al. Iliac crest bone graft: osteotome versus saw. *Spine* 1993; 18:2048–2052.

Kahn B. Superior gluteal artery laceration: a complication of iliac bone graft surgery. *Clin Orthop* 1979; 140:204–207.

Kurz LT, Garfin SR, Booth RE Jr. Harvesting autogenous iliac bone grafts: a review of the complications and techniques. *Spine* 1989;14:1324–1331.

Macdonald RL, Fehlings MG, Tator CH, et al. Multilevel anterior cervical corpectomy and fibular allograft fusion for cervical myelopathy. *J Neurosurg* 1997;86:990–997.

Majd ME, Vadhva M, Holt RT. Anterior cervical reconstruction using titanium cages with anterior plating. *Spine* 1999;24:1604–1610.

Massey EW. Meralgia paresthetica secondary to trauma of bone graft. *J Trauma* 1980;20:342–343.

Rupp RE, Podeszwa D, Ebraheim NA. Danger zones associated with fibular osteotomy. *J Orthop Trauma* 1994;8:54–58.

Schnee CL, Freese A, Weil RJ, et al. Analysis of harvest morbidity and radiographic outcome using autograft for anterior cervical fusion. *Spine* 1997;22:2222–2227.

Shin AY, Moran ME, Wenger DR. Superior gluteal artery injury secondary to posterior iliac crest bone graft harvesting: a surgical technique to control hemorrhage. *Spine* 1996;21:1371–1374.

Summers BN, Eisenstein SM. Donor site pain from the ilium: a complication of lumbar spine fusion. *J Bone Joint Surg Br* 1989;71:677–680.

Vail TP, Urbaniak JR. Donor-site morbidity with use of vascularized autogenous fibular grafts. *J Bone Joint Surg Am* 1996;78:204–211.

Xu R, Ebraheim NA, Yeasting RA, et al. Anatomic considerations for posterior iliac bone harvesting. *Spine* 1996;21:1017–1020.

ALTERNATIVE METHODS FOR FILLING VERTEBRAL BODY DEFECTS: CARBON FIBER SPACERS

GARY L. LOWERY
SAMIR KULKARNI

CARBON FIBER RECONSTRUCTION OF VERTEBRAL BODY DEFECTS

Reconstruction after anterior cervical corpectomy must accomplish several goals. It needs to maintain spinal alignment and prevent collapse of the remaining vertebral bodies into the reconstructed defect, leading to localized kyphosis (1–3). The reconstruction should also provide the appropriate environment for bony incorporation while maintaining sagittal balance over a patient's lifetime. These goals should be accomplished while minimizing patient morbidity.

Historically, either corticocancellous iliac crest struts or cortical fibular struts have been the most commonly used reconstruction materials, either autograft or allograft (4–8). Whitecloud and LaRocca (8) reported initial success with fibular strut grafts. After long-term follow-up, however, Fernyhough, White, and LaRocca (4) found high nonunion rates, namely 27% for autograft and 41% for allograft. Furthermore, autograft fibular harvest is associated with donor site morbidity of 5% to 10% (8). Autograft iliac crest often fails to fill large corpectomy defects, and there is an associated risk of donor site morbidity (9–11). Donor site morbidity also occurs with autograft fibula (11). Delayed union and nonunion are more common with allograft (fibula and iliac crest) than with autograft (4,12). Allograft has a low patient morbidity, but an increased nonunion rate compared with autograft (12) and has the theoretical possibility for transmission of infectious diseases (13,14).

Reconstruction with carbon fiber spacers and anterior cervical plating is proposed to overcome the shortcomings of more traditional procedures. This technique potentially meets all the requirements for a successful reconstructive procedure. The modular carbon fiber components can be selected to fit any anterior cervical reconstruction. The wedge-shaped construct helps to restore spinal alignment. More important, carbon fiber conduits can be filled with locally harvested cancellous autograft. Alternatively, cancellous bone can be harvested from the iliac crest through a less invasive procedure than that required for tricortical graft preparation. The use of cancellous allograft, bone mineral substitutes, or osteoinductive compounds is not precluded. Carbon fiber spacers provide a stable biomechanical environment for the biological process of bone healing to occur, which we call "biological enhancement of biomechanics."

Carbon fiber spacers provide excellent biomechanical support and allow early bone graft in-growth and maturation, while yielding a more accurate assessment of fusion than other methods of composite grafting. Carbon fiber has inherent biomechanical stability, both initially and long term. Cunningham et al. (15) have reported that the axial compressive capability of the carbon fiber reinforced cage is 10 times greater than that of autologous freeze-dried or fresh frozen iliac bone graft. This difference is even more noticeable for longer struts used for two-level reconstruction. A biomechanical comparison of iliac strut grafts, polymethylmethacrylate reconstruction, and carbon fiber composite cages packed with autograft by Shono et al. (3) revealed that the carbon fiber cage had good stiffness in axial compression and rotation and was the most rigid construct in the flexion-extension tests. Apart from the intrinsic biomechanical features of carbon fiber spacers, axial compression on the construct continually imparts the stresses to the bone in order for late bony maturation to occur. Wedged carbon fiber spacers help to avoid the problem of localized kyphosis after cervical reconstruction.

Supplementing the reconstruction with anterior or posterior plating, or both, provides additional mechanical stability, prevents migration of the construct, and promotes fusion.

SURGICAL TECHNIQUE

General endotracheal intubation is performed after placement of intravenous lines, intraarterial lines, and a Foley catheter. A roll under the neck and between the shoulder blades is often helpful to maintain a lordotic posture of the cervical spine. Slight distraction with head halter traction is beneficial to prevent abnormal cervical positioning, such as rotation, during cervical instrumentation. The neck is then sterilely prepared and draped in the usual fashion.

A standard left-sided approach is then performed. A transverse incision can be readily used for one- and two-level corpectomies, whereas more extensive soft tissue dissection is routinely required for corpectomies spanning three or four levels. A carotid incision minimizes soft tissue retraction when the procedure requires decompression of three

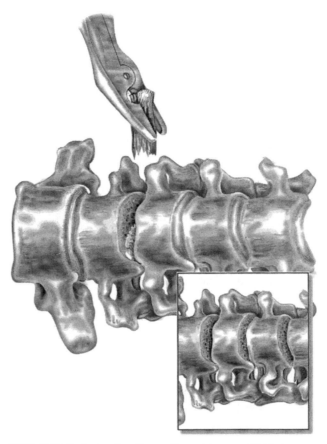

FIGURE 25.1. Excise the disc or discs with a no. 15 blade, rongeurs, and curettes. Identify the uncinate processes.

or more levels. Anterior cervical instrumentation and construct insertion are more safely performed through a carotid incision.

The appropriate disc levels to be excised are confirmed on x-ray or fluoroscopy. The disc spaces are excised with a no. 15 blade, and discal material is removed with pituitary rongeurs and curettes (Fig. 25.1). Punctate bleeding surfaces can easily be prepared with a curette or with light pressure using a high-speed burr. Care is taken to preserve the bony subchondral plate upon which the supportive carbon fiber conduit will rest. It is important to clearly identify the uncinate processes, since these serve as the anatomic landmarks for adequate central decompression and for nerve root decompression via anterior foraminotomies. Proper construct insertion and positioning of an anterior cervical plate also depend on identifying this anatomy.

When performing a corpectomy, a sagittal saw blade is used to make three vertical cuts in the vertebral body—one in the midline and one on either side of the midline—within the confines of the uncinate processes (Fig. 25.2). The vertebral cuts should not be made to penetrate more than 14 mm. Leksell rongeurs are then used to remove this bone, which is saved for the cancellous graft (Fig. 25.3).

This process is repeated for each level. Cancellous bone bleeding from the side walls can be controlled with bone wax (removed prior to reconstruction and grafting).

After harvesting of the local autograft is completed, a high-speed burr is used to further widen the subtotal corpectomy site. The uncinate process again serves as the limit for subtotal decompression. The width of the decompression should be approximately 15 to 16 mm to accommodate the construct. Keyhole foraminotomies and pedicle-to-pedicle decompression are easily performed. Resection of the posterior longitudinal ligament is dependent on the type of anterior compressive pathology.

A custom carbon fiber construct is assembled from various sizes (Fig. 25.4), and a trial implantation is performed with slight distraction (10 to 15 pounds traction). It is imperative not to overdistract the facets linearly. Although the compression on the

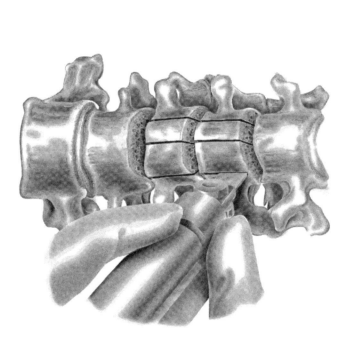

FIGURE 25.2. Make vertical cuts through the vertebral bodies with a sagittal saw.

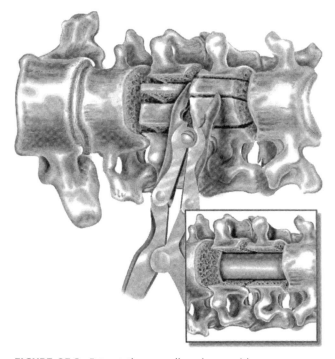

FIGURE 25.3. Extract the cancellous bone with rongeurs, curettes, and Kerrisons and save. Perform a wide decompression (15 to 16 mm), using the uncinate process as the limit and performing pedicle-to-pedicle decompression. Resect the posterior longitudinal ligament if necessary.

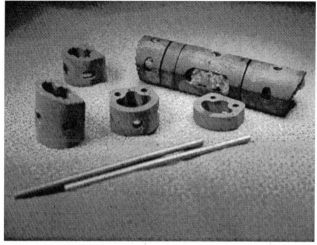

A

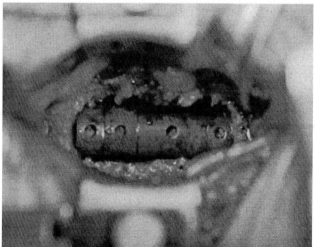

B

FIGURE 25.4. A custom carbon fiber is assembled from various sizes and filled with autograft.

construct is favored with increased distraction, this may prevent the posterior elements from sharing the load, which may cause subsequent settling. Either anterior cervical plating (neutralization) or posterior cervical plating (articular pillars) is considered mandatory for optimal stability of the reconstruction. Excessive settling of the construct predisposes the anterior cervical plate and screws to failure. The implant then has increased cyclical loading compared with the initial loads in neutralization. In addition, linear distraction unloads the facets and causes a kyphotic cervical posture. A combination of slight distraction with preservation of lordosis ("lordotic distraction" or "locking the facets") helps to maintain a normal cervical posture and minimizes the loads on the anterior construct.

Once the appropriate construct has been assembled, it is packed with the autologous cancellous bone saved from the corpectomy procedure. Again with minimal cervical distraction, the construct is gently pressed into the subtotal corpectomy defect (Fig. 25.5). The construct is pressed just past the anterior vertebral edge, and the distraction is released. The stability of the construct is tested prior to anterior cervical plate stabilization (Fig. 25.6).

Radiographic confirmation of appropriate construct position is necessary prior to and after anterior cervical plate stabilization (Fig. 25.7), which is required for optimal stabilization of the reconstruction. Whether or not to add posterior stabilization depends on

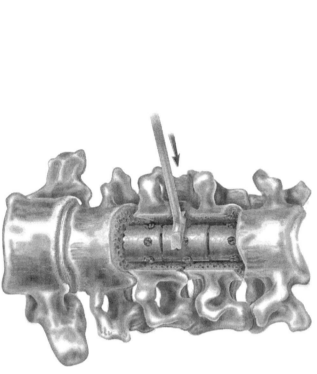

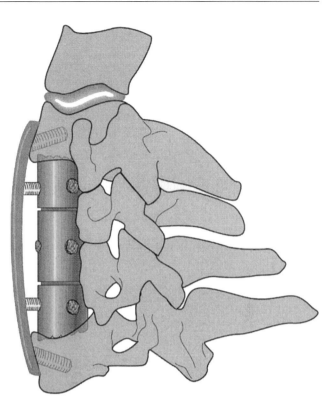

FIGURE 25.5. Adjust the cervical lordosis (lordotic distractor). Measure the corpectomy defect. Pack the conduit with autologous cancellous bone. Implant carbon fiber under slight distraction.

FIGURE 25.6. Release distraction. Check the stability of the conduit. Check position of the conduit with a lateral radiograph. Apply anterior cervical plate.

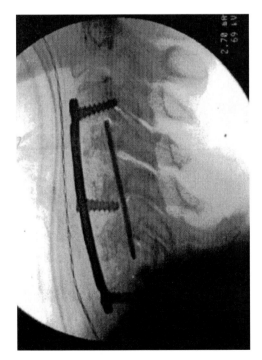

FIGURE 25.7. Check position of the plate with a lateral radiograph.

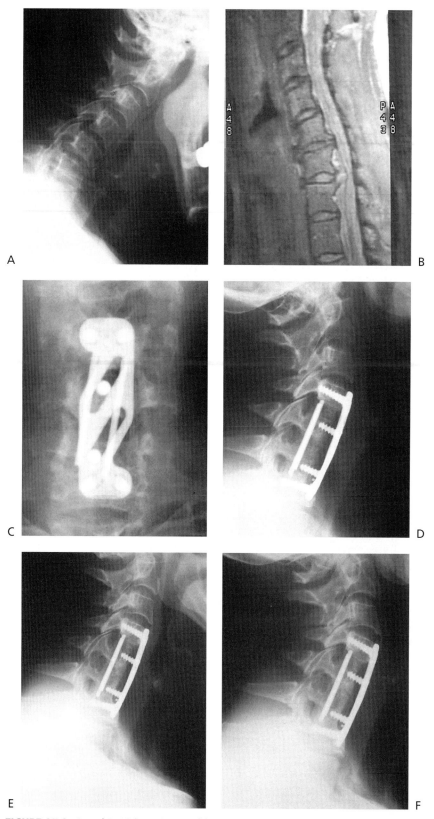

FIGURE 25.8. **A** and **B:** JG is a 43-year-old woman who had multilevel cervical stenosis secondary to spondylotic osteophytes. She underwent an anterior cervical corpectomy of C5 and C6 that was reconstructed with a carbon fiber strut and local autologous bone graft. Orion divergent plating was used from C4 to C7 to stabilize the construct. **C** and **D:** Within 5 months a solid fusion is seen on lateral radiographs. **E** and **F:** At last follow-up, 24 months after surgery, the patient is completely pain free. There is no motion on flexion/extension, and she appears to show mature graft.

the type of pathology, the number of levels reconstructed, and any preexisting dynamic instability. The wound is then irrigated and closed over a drain in a routine fashion.

Figure 25.8 presents a case example of a two-level corpectomy reconstruction with carbon fiber stabilized by anterior plating.

REFERENCES

1. Lowery GL. Anterior cervical osteosynthesis: Orion™ anterior cervical plate system. (1995) In: Hitchon PW, Treynalis VC, Rengachary S, eds. *Techniques in spinal fusion and stabilization.* New York: Thieme Medical Publishers, 1995:191–197.
2. Lowery GL. Three-dimensional screw divergence and sagittal balance: a personal philosophy relative to cervical biomechanics. *Spine* 1996;10(2):343–356.
3. Shono Y, McAfee PC, Cunningham BW, et al. A biomechanical analysis of decompression and reconstruction methods in the cervical spine. Emphasis on a carbon-fiber-composite cage. *J Bone Joint Surg Am* 1993;75(11):1674–1684.
4. Fernyhough JC, White JI, LaRocca H. Fusion rates in multilevel cervical spondylosis comparing allograft fibula with autograft fibula in 126 patients. *Spine* 1991;16:S561–S564.
5. Hanai K, Fujiyoshi F, Kamei K. Subtotal vertebrectomy and spinal fusion for cervical spondylotic myelopathy. *Spine* 1986;11:310–315.
6. Meding JB, Stambough JL. Critical analysis of strut grafts in anterior spinal fusions. *J Spinal Disord* 1993;6:166–174.
7. Swank ML, Lowery GL, Bhat AL, et al. Anterior cervical allograft arthrodesis and instrumentation: multilevel interbody grafting or strut graft reconstruction. *Eur Spine J* 1997;6(2):138–143.
8. Whitecloud TS, LaRocca H. Fibular strut graft in reconstructive surgery of the cervical spine. *Spine* 1976;1:33–43.
9. DePalma AF, Rothman RH, Lewinnek GE, et al. Anterior interbody fusion for severe cervical disc degeneration. *Surg Gynecol Obstet* 1972;134:755–758.
10. Kurz LT, Garfin SR, Booth RE. Harvesting autogenous iliac bone grafts: a review of complications and techniques. *Spine* 1989;14(12):1324–1331.
11. Younger EM, Chapman MW. Morbidity of bone graft donor sites. *J Orthop Trauma* 1989;3:192–195.
12. Brodke DS, Zdeblick TA. Modified Smith-Robinson procedure for anterior cervical discectomy and fusion. *Spine* 1992;17:S427–S430.
13. Scarborough NL. Allograft bones and soft tissues: current procedures for banking allograft human bone. *Orthopedics* 1992;15(10):1161–1167.
14. Scarborough NL, White EM, Hughes JV, et al. Allograft safety: viral inactivation with bone demineralization. *Contemp Orthop* 1995;31(4):257–261.
15. Cunningham BW, Brantigan J, Shono Y, et al. Reconstruction of anterior spinal column defects utilizing a carbon fiber reinforced composite. *Trans Orthop Res Soc* 1992;17:168.

ALTERNATIVE METHODS FOR FILLING VERTEBRAL BODY DEFECTS: CERAMICS

NOBORU HOSONO
KAZUO YONENOBU
KEIRO ONO

Various materials have been used over the years to replace collapsed vertebrae affected by metastasis. Autogenous bone graft was the first applied. Incorporation of the grafted bone was made difficult by either postoperative irradiation or local tumor recurrence. Polymethylmethacrylate (bone cement) was subsequently widely used to reconstruct collapsed vertebrae (1–3). Bone cement can be molded to a desired shape, and its solidity is not affected by irradiation or tumor recurrence (4). Establishment of spinal stability just after treatment is ensured by replacement surgery with bone cement. However, bone cement is not a durable material either, and unfortunately fatigue fracture of the implanted cement has been occasionally reported (5).

Accordingly, thirty years ago Keiro Ono developed a new ceramic prosthesis as a solid spacer to replace the affected vertebrae (Fig. 26.1). This spacer is composed of alumina glass ceramic, a bioinert material that provokes little tissue reaction in neighboring tissues. Biomechanical testing has proved that its strength is sufficient against compression, bending, and rotational stresses.

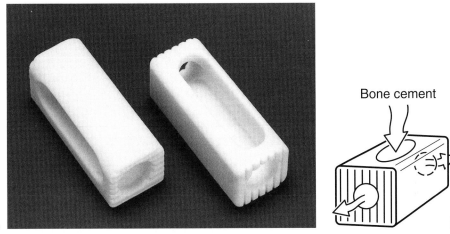

FIGURE 26.1. **A:** Alumina glass ceramics have three windows, one for bone cement packing and two for anchoring to the adjacent vertebrae. **B:** Bone cement is packed with pressure from the anterior window and pushed out from upper and lower portals.

INDICATIONS

When the main metastatic lesion is within the vertebral body of the cervical spine, replacement surgery with ceramics is indicated under the following circumstances.

■ *Pathological fracture or impending fracture of the vertebral body.* Most spinal metastases chiefly affect the vertebral bodies,and osteolytic metastasis can result in vertebral collapse (Fig. 26.2). Computed tomographic (CT) scans are usually more useful than plain radiographs in delineating bony destruction, especially in the lower cervical spine, where the contour of the vertebrae are concealed by the shoulder on a lateral view. In general, half or more trabecular destruction on CT scans is an indication of vertebral collapse. Magnetic resonance imaging is also indispensable; it well detects bone marrow changes suggesting metastatic deposits, because sound vertebral bodies adjacent to an affected body are mandatory for replacement surgery.

■ *Persisting symptoms that resist conservative therapy.* Although more than 85% of all skeletal metastases can be successfully controlled by irradiation (6,7), well-differentiated thyroid cancer, lung cancer (except small cell carcinoma), renal cell carcinoma, and some malignancies are well known to show little sensitivity to radiotherapy (8,9). Even narcotic agents can have no effect on the symptoms caused by pathological fractures. Replacement surgery is indicated when these kinds of conservative therapy have failed to relieve symptoms.

■ *Emergency situations and occult primaries.* When there is rapidly progressive paresis due to vertebral metastasis, replacement surgery is indicated as an emergency operation, despite the higher risks compared with elective surgeries. We cannot expect early recovery with radiotherapy even for the radiosensitive tumors.

When the source of skeletal metastasis remains unknown despite a thorough search for the primary lesion, replacement surgery is also indicated to provide a good tumor specimen as well as to stabilize the spine.

CONTRAINDICATIONS

Replacement surgery is generally not indicated in patients who have a short (6 or fewer months) life expectancy, which is often difficult to accurately predict and remains one of the largest problems in the treatment of spinal metastases. Progressive primary tumor, visceral organ metastases, multiple skeletal metastases, bone marrow insufficiency, and hypercalcemia may suggest a poor prognosis. Metastases of vital organs alone are not contraindications if their function is sufficiently maintained. However, multiple skeletal

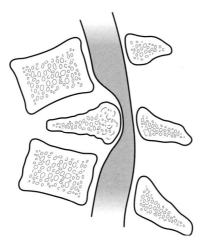

FIGURE 26.2. Angular deformity caused by pathological fracture of the affected vertebra. The spinal cord is severely compressed by tumor and bony fragments.

metastases make the patient bedridden, and it is of no use to perform vertebral replacement in such patients. The performance status of each patient is an important issue to evaluate. Patients with infections or a prolonged bleeding time are contraindicated for surgery.

For successful replacement, metastatic tumor expansion should be restricted to two consecutive vertebrae, with adjacent vertebrae grossly free of metastasis. Replacement of three consecutive vertebral bodies compromises the stability of the spine: The stress is too great for the long prosthesis to be effectively anchored with bone cement.

PREPARATION FOR THE SURGERY

Preoperative evaluation of candidates should be completed to ensure a sound anesthesia and surgery. Blood analysis that includes blood cell count, chemistry, and coagulation function is performed. Drugs that may affect coagulation function should be washed out before surgery. Evaluation of respiratory function is sometimes difficult in a patient with a halo vest. Chest x-ray and arterial blood gas analysis replace it. Pathological or impending fracture of the cervical spine is sometimes well treated with an immediate application of a halo vest before surgery. For general anesthesia, endoscopic intubation is safer and preferable for a patient in a halo vest.

OPERATIVE TECHNIQUES

The approach used for vertebral replacement surgery is the same as the conventional anterior approach to the cervical spine. Dissection goes between the trachea and carotid sheath. Preoperative embolization of feeder arteries is often impracticable because of the risk of vertebral artery obstruction. After the anterior aspect of the vertebral body is exposed, the level of the lesion is confirmed radiologically. A self-retaining retractor is applied between the edge of longus colli muscles, and then the intervertebral discs are curetted first above and below the lesion to orient the width and depth of the affected vertebrae. Resection of the affected vertebrae should be done as quickly as possible because undesirable bleeding continues throughout the curettage and never stops until the lesion is totally resected. Bone wax is good for bleeding from the cancellous bone, and hemostatic agents such as thrombin, collagen fleece, oxidized cellulose, and gelatin are sometimes useful for controlling bleeding from the epidural space. Forceps and rongeur are usually sufficient to resect the lesion. The spreader hooked to the edge of the adjacent vertebrae facilitates further curettage and correction of any angular deformity (Fig. 26.3). The posterior longitudinal ligament

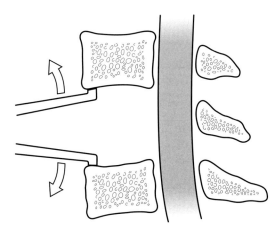

FIGURE 26.3. The spreader hooked to the edge of the adjacent vertebrae facilitates further curettage and correction of any angular deformity.

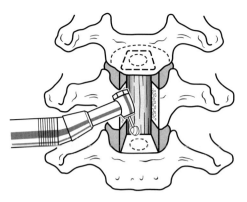

FIGURE 26.4. After confirming a proper position of a trial on x-ray, the surface of the endplates of both adjacent vertebrae is marked through the upper and lower portals of a trial with a curved curette. Thus the anchoring holes are correctly made after removal of a trial prosthesis. The holes are further deepened using a dental burr on an air drill. The anchoring holes must be wider than the portals of the prosthesis because the long-term mechanical stability depends on the amount of anchoring cement.

can be saved if tumor mass does not invade the epidural space. One must be cautious not to injure the dura, which is sometimes invisible under massive bleeding.

After excision of the impinging bone, discs, and tumor, a trial prosthesis is introduced into the cleaned-out space while an assistant applies a proper distraction force on the cervical spine using a halo ring attached to the skull. Too much force on the potentially unstable spine might result in excessive and dangerous distraction. Radiologic control is essential to confirm the correction of preexisting deformity and positioning of the prosthesis. Straight alignment is best for the replaced segment to ensure mechanical stability. The centers of the endplates of both adjacent vertebrae are marked through the upper and lower portals of a trial, and anchoring holes are further deepened after removal of a trial prosthesis using a dental burr on an air drill (Fig. 26.4). A ceramic prosthesis of the appropriate size is then introduced into the spread space, and bone cement is packed with pressure through the anterior window until it fills the prosthesis and then the anchor holes in the adjacent vertebrae (Fig. 26.5). Bone cement pushed out from the upper and lower portal tightly stabilizes a prosthesis between the disease-free vertebrae.

A ceramic prosthesis can be a good barrier against thermal damage of the dura from polymerization of the cement. However, irrigation around the prosthesis with cold saline

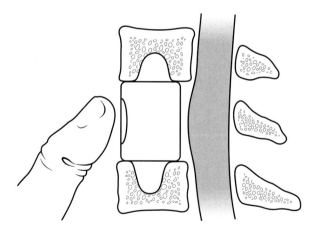

FIGURE 26.5. After placement of a ceramic prosthesis, bone cement is packed with pressure, which tightly connects a prosthesis with the adjacent vertebrae. A ceramic prosthesis can be a good barrier of dura against the thermal damage from polymerization of the cement. However, irrigation around the prosthesis with cold saline is recommended for protection of surrounding tissues from thermal damage. Care should be taken not to leak the bone cement. Strict hemostasis and clear vision of the operating field are mandatory to check for accidental and critical leaks. Too aggressive compression during packing cement should be avoided.

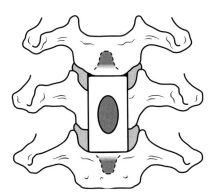

FIGURE 26.6. Anterior view after fixation of a prosthesis. Strong fixation of the prosthesis could be tested by the push-pull method.

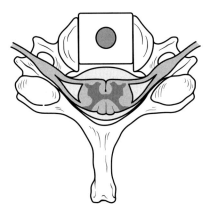

FIGURE 26.7. Decompression of the spinal cord is confirmed on an axial image.

is recommended for protection of surrounding tissues from thermal damage. Fixation of the prosthesis can be tested by the push-pull method (Figs. 26.6 and 26.7). After rinsing with much saline, a closed drainage tube is put into the wound.

OPERATIVE COMPLICATIONS

Hoarseness is one of the most notorious complications associated with an anterior approach to the cervical spine. Direct injury to the recurrent laryngeal nerve can occur, especially on the right side, where the recurrent laryngeal nerve is, on rare occasions, aberrant and curves at a higher level than on the left side. Thus, the left-sided approach is usually preferred. Prolonged retraction and vigorous dissection can be a cause of damage to the nerve. The self-retaining retractor should be taken off every 1 hour to avoid this morbidity. Intubation is also a possible cause of laryngeal edema. Hoarseness due to irritation of the trachea or larynx by retraction or intubation usually subsides within a few days with use of antiinflammatory drugs.

Injury to the esophagus is known as the most serious complication. If the operator realizes the esophagus has been perforated during the surgery, the perforation should be tightly repaired in two layers. The silicon drainage is kept in the wound until there is no leak of saliva. During that period, the patient has to refrain from eating and drinking. Injury to the esophagus, however, may not always be identified during the surgery. Unrealized injury can lead to mediastinitis and more serious, sometimes fatal complications.

DISLODGEMENT OF PROSTHESIS

When dislodgement of the prosthesis unfortunately occurs due to tumor involvement to an adjacent vertebra, posterior stabilization with pedicle or lateral mass screwing is an emergency measure. When displacement of the prosthesis causes obstruction of the esophagus, repositioning or removal of the prosthesis is indicated.

POSTOPERATIVE CARE

Ambulation is allowed a few days after the operation. The initial stability of the prosthesis is good enough to exclude the necessity of a neck collar. After the wound is healed, irradiation is established to the lesion in the amount of approximately 30 Gy. Dysphagia and sore throat may occur as a complication of concomitant radiation to the esophagus.

OUTCOME OF REPLACEMENT SURGERY WITH CERAMICS

Our own experience with replacement surgery with ceramics has already been published (10). From 1972 to 1993, 27 prostheses were used in 27 patients to replace cervical vertebrae affected by metastatic tumor. Fifteen patients were male and 12 were female. The average age at surgery was 53.2 years (range, 34–75 years), and the average follow-up period was 19.5 months. Twenty-two patients eventually died after a follow-up period ranging from 2 to 84 months, while 4 patients remain alive after a follow-up period of 9 to 84 months. The final outcome was unknown for the remaining patient. The primary tumor was thyroid cancer in five patients, lung cancer in four, gastrointestinal cancer in four, breast cancer in two, and so on. A single vertebral body was resected in 25 patients, and two consecutive vertebral bodies were removed in 2 patients (Fig. 26.8).

Clinical outcome was assessed by evaluating the ability to walk and the severity of paresis and pain before and after the procedure. Ambulation was graded as follows: gait without support, gait with a cane, or nonambulatory due to severe spinal pain or motor weakness of the lower extremities. Paresis was graded as absent, incomplete, or complete. Pain was graded as absent (no analgesics needed), moderate (analgesics needed), or severe (uncontrolled by analgesics, including narcotics). Radiographic follow-up was done at 3-month intervals to detect local tumor recurrence. The incidence of local recurrence was investigated in relation to the primary lesion.

Twelve patients could walk without support both before and after surgery. Of the remaining 15 patients, 13 (87%) showed improvement in ambulation, and 10 (91%) of the 11 nonambulatory patients became ambulatory.

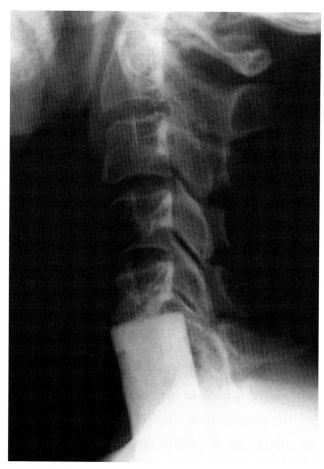

FIGURE 26.8. The consecutive two vertebrae are replaced with our ceramic prosthesis.

Ten patients were neurologically normal both before and after surgery. Six (43%) of the 14 patients with incomplete paresis were normalized postoperatively. The remaining 8 patients still had incomplete paresis after surgery, but 7 (88%) of them showed significant improvement of muscle power. Two (67%) of the 3 patients with complete paresis showed improvement. Thus, 15 (88%) of the 17 patients with preoperative paresis demonstrated improvement.

All of the 25 patients with pain showed significant alleviation of pain, and 18 (72%) became pain free.

Worsening of clinical symptoms did not occur in any patient. Local recurrence was observed in seven patients (26%), where three had thyroid cancer as a primary tumor. The relatively high recurrence rate in thyroid cancer was attributed to the good prognosis and long follow-up period (37.4 months).

COMPLICATIONS

There were no serious complications in our series. In three patients, additional surgery was required due to mechanical loosening of the prosthesis or local recurrence.

Operative death, neurologic deterioration, infection, and tumor dissemination have not been encountered so far.

REFERENCES

1. Cross GO, White HL, White LP. Acrylic prosthesis of the fifth cervical vertebra in multiple myeloma. *J Neurosurg* 1971;35:112–114.
2. Dunn EJ. The role of methyl methacrylate in the stabilization and replacement of tumors of the cervical spine. *Spine* 1977;2:15–24.
3. Scoville WB, Palmer AH, Samra K, et al. The use of acrylic plastic for vertebral replacement or fixation in metastatic disease of the spine. Technical note. *J Neurosurg* 1967;27:274–279.
4. Murray JA, Bruels MC, Lindberg RD. Irradiation of polymethyl-methacrylate: *in vitro* gamma radiation effect. *J Bone Joint Surg Am* 1974;56:311–312.
5. McAfee PC. Failure of methylmethacrylate stabilization of the spine. In: Sherk HH, ed. *The cervical spine,* 2nd ed. Philadelphia: JB Lippincott Co, 1989:838–850.
6. Gilbert HA, Kagan AR, Nussbaum H, et al. Evaluation of radiation therapy for bone metastases: pain relief and quality of life. *Am J Roentg* 1977;129:1095–1096.
7. Schoker JD, Brady LW. Radiation therapy for bone metastasis. *Clin Orthop* 1982;169:38–43.
8. Fossa SD, Kjolseth I, Lund G. Radiotherapy of metastases from renal cell. *Eur Urol* 1982;8:340–342.
9. Harrington KD. *Orthopaedic management of metastatic bone disease.* St. Louis: Mosby, 1988:83–94.
10. Hosono N, Yonenobu K, Fuji T, et al. Vertebral body replacement with a ceramic prosthesis for metastatic spinal tumors. *Spine* 1995;20:2454–2462.

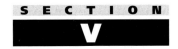

METHODS OF
FIXATION/STABILIZATION

OVERVIEW OF FIXATION: BASIC BIOMECHANICS

JEFFREY D. COE

Some of the most significant preoperative decisions that the cervical spinal surgeon can make are whether to use internal fixation and, if so, what type and via what surgical approach (1). The factors that must be considered in making these decisions include the underlying pathology; the stability of the cervical spine as a consequence of both the primary pathology and the contemplated neural decompression or bone resection (or both) required to treat the underlying disorder; the bone mineral density of the cervical spine; the age and general health of the patient; and any relevant anatomic variations (1–6). The implications of the race between osseous healing (union of a fracture or spinal fusion) and failure of fixation vary between patients based on these factors. For example, consider a young patient who has sustained an unstable fracture or dislocation of the cervical spine and an elderly patient with metastatic disease involving the cervical spine with spinal cord compression from a pathologic fracture. In the former case the ultimate goal is the development of a solid, durable fusion, in contrast to the latter case, in which immediate stability is more important than osseous union (3,7–13). This chapter provides an overview of these topics, with particular emphasis on the biomechanics and anatomic features that are important in surgical decision making.

INSTABILITY OF THE CERVICAL SPINE

The criteria for instability have been well established in both the upper (occiput to C2 level) and mid- to lower (i.e., C2 to T1 level) cervical spine (14). The most important soft tissue structures affecting the C1–2 level are the transverse ligament; the dentate, apical, and alar ligaments; and the joint capsules (Fig. 27.1). The transverse ligament is the primary stabilizing ligament, whereas the dentate, apical, and alar ligaments are considered secondary stabilizers. The landmark biomechanical studies by Fielding and co-workers (15) indicated that more than 3 mm of anterior translation of C1 on C2 represented failure of the transverse ligament. Most important, with this level of displacement, the secondary stabilizers are incapable of preventing additional displacement under significant loads that would result in failure of an intact transverse ligament.

Table 27.1 lists the criteria for upper cervical spine instability as defined by White and Panjabi based on this and other biomechanical studies (14). By these criteria, a patient who has sustained a deceleration injury with radiographic evidence of 5 mm of atlantoaxial translation between flexion and extension would be considered to have an unstable spine and to have sustained a significant injury of the transverse ligament, most likely a complete rupture.

In the subaxial cervical spine, White and Panjabi (14) and others have performed biomechanical studies to define instability at these levels. These investigators have developed a checklist (Table 27.2) to determine the diagnosis of instability in the subaxial cervical spine. Not only are these criteria biomechanical, radiographic, and anatomic; but

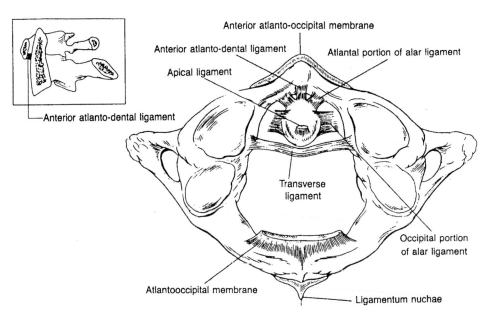

FIGURE 27.1. Top view of the C1–2 joint. Schematic of the major ligaments involved in the clinical stability of the upper cervical spine. (From Clark CR, Ducker TB, Dvorak J, et al., eds. *The cervical spine*, 3rd ed. Philadelphia: Lippincott–Raven, 1998, with permission.)

TABLE 27.1. CRITERIA FOR INSTABILITY OF C0 TO C2

>8° axial rotation of C0 to C1 to one side
>1 mm C0 on C1 translation
>7 mm overhang of C1 to C2 (total right and left, on
   anteroposterior radiograph)
>45° axial rotation of C1 to C2 to one side
>4 mm C1 on C2 translation
<13 mm from posterior body of C2 to posterior ring of C1
Avulsed transverse ligament

From Clark CR, Ducker TB, Dvorak J, et al., eds. *The cervical spine*, 3rd ed. Philadelphia: Lippincott–Raven, 1998, with permission. Data from White AA, Panjabi MM. *Clinical biomechanics of the spine*, 2nd ed. Philadelphia: JB Lippincott Co, 1990.

TABLE 27.2. CHECKLIST FOR THE DIAGNOSIS OF CLINICAL INSTABILITY IN THE MIDDLE AND LOWER CERVICAL SPINE

Element	Point value
Biomechanical considerations	
Anterior elements destroyed or unable to function	2
Posterior elements destroyed or unable to function	2
Positive stretch test	2
Radiographic criteria[a]	4
Flexion-extension radiographs	
Sagittal plane translation > 3.5 mm or 20%	2
or	
Resting radiographs	
Sagittal plane displacement > 3.5 mm or 20%	2
Relative sagittal plane angulation > 11°	2
Other considerations	
Developmentally narrow spinal canal (sagittal diameter 13 mm; Pavlov's ratio < 0.8)	1
Abnormal disc narrowing	1
Spinal cord damage	2
Nerve root damage	1
Dangerous loading anticipated	1

From Clark CR, Ducker TB, Dvorak J, et al., eds. *The cervical spine*, 3rd ed. Philadelphia: Lippincott–Raven, 1998, with permission.
[a]See Fig. 27.2.

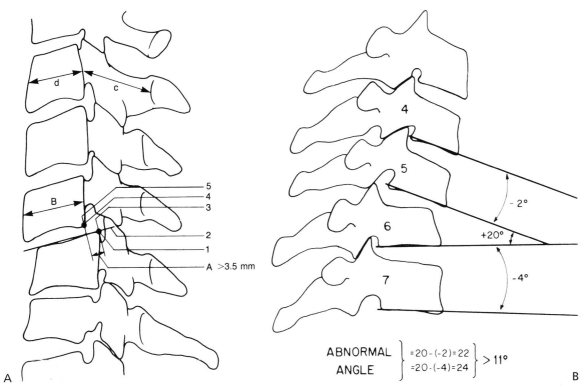

FIGURE 27.2. A unilateral facet dislocation at C5–6 with 4 mm of translation (2 points), 11 degrees of angulation compared with the C4–5 and C6–7 motion segments (2 points), and a unilateral C6 nerve root injury (1 point) would be considered unstable, with a total score of 5 points. (From Clark CR, Ducker TB, Dvorak J, et al., eds. *The cervical spine,* 3rd ed. Philadelphia: Lippincott–Raven, 1998, with permission.)

they also take into account neurologic injury as an indicator of the severity of the injury and therefore the presence of instability. For example, a patient with a ligamentous injury that has resulted in 5 mm of translation (2 points), more than 11 degrees of angulation relative to adjacent (ostensibly uninvolved) segments (2 points), and a nerve root injury (1 point) would be considered unstable by these criteria (as is often seen in a unilateral facet dislocation) (Fig. 27.2).

FIXATION TO THE SKULL

Described techniques of skull fixation include wires passed through tunnels drilled into the skull or passed completely through burr holes in the skull, affixing bone graft, rods, or plates; unicortical or bicortical screws to which plates or rods are fixed; and rod/hook systems that create a claw between burr holes and the foramen magnum (6,16–18). Although biomechanical studies have indicated that the most rigid fixation involves bicortical screws affixed to rods or plates, unicortical screws when applied to the more midline (thicker) bone of the occiput can be nearly as secure and have been proved to be clinically effective (17,19). Wire techniques have been shown in several clinical studies to be sufficiently effective, provided there is appropriate supplemental posterior postoperative immobilization (usually a halo vest) (18,20,21).

The most common indication for fixation of the cervical spine through the skull is rheumatoid disease (16,18,20–22). Other indications include tumor, congenital abnormalities, and revision surgery. Special considerations with regard to rheumatoid disease include bone mineral density and secondary deformity, as well as patient tolerance to postoperative immobilization (16,18,20–22). With regard to tumor, the extent of osseous resection required to provide tumor control may demand an extraordinarily rigid construct, particularly if postoperative immobilization is to be avoided in these patients, who usually have a shortened life expectancy as a consequence of their disease.

Occipitocervical trauma sufficient to result in cervical instability is most often lethal as a consequence of spinal cord injury resulting in respiratory failure and early death (unless resuscitation is immediately carried out). These injuries are nearly always ligamentous, although associated fractures often occur. Most of these patients are young and therefore have normal bone mineral density; thus, there is a wide choice of options for internal fixation. Occiput fixation is rarely required for degenerative indications or primary deformity (16,18,20–22).

C1–2 FIXATION: WIRES, MAGERL SCREWS, C1–2 SCREWS, AND ANTERIOR ODONTOID SCREWS

The C1–2 level is perhaps the most technically challenging motion segment to stabilize in the cervical spine. The traditional wiring techniques of Brookes and Gallie nearly always require halo immobilization and are biomechanically inferior to the transarticular C1–2 screw technique developed by Magerl (23,24). Particular concerns of C1–2 instability involve its multidirectional nature; that is, most often there is translational and rotational instability, which makes the traditional wiring techniques less favorable compared with the transarticular screw method (25,26). One of the major biomechanical benefits of the transarticular screw technique is the "truss" formed by the oblique screws, which resists translation of C1 on C2 (Fig. 27.3).

In both trauma and rheumatoid arthritis patients, the Magerl screw method has been shown to be a safe and technically feasible fixation option (25–27). Computed tomographic (CT) scanning with multiplanar reconstruction, however, is necessary to ensure that the planned screw trajectory does not cross the path of the vertebral artery (25,26). Frameless stereotactic techniques can provide helpful imaging in these cases.

More recently, Harms and Melcher (28) have described a technique of C1–2 stabilization using C1 lateral mass screws and C2 pars/pedicle screws with favorable clinical results (Fig. 27.4). So far, however, there are no published biomechanical studies comparing the stability of this technique with other methods of C1–2 stabilization.

C1–2 fusion results in a significant loss of cervical rotation (approximately 50%); therefore, techniques of stabilizing odontoid fractures to allow primary fracture healing

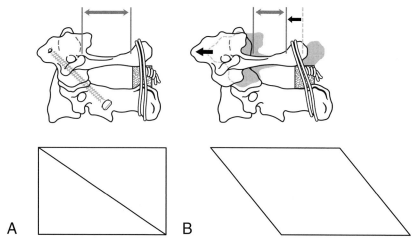

FIGURE 27.3. A: Transarticular screws cross the C1–2 facet joints obliquely, resisting anterior-posterior translation of these joints and, particularly when combined with a traditional posterior wiring, providing a very stable construct. **B:** Posterior wiring alone, without the truss formed by the transarticular screw, is more susceptible to translational instability.

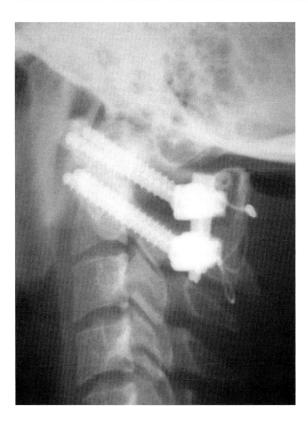

FIGURE 27.4. Lateral radiograph of a patient with traumatic C1–2 instability stabilized with a rod-screw construct using C1 lateral mass screws and C2 pars/pedicle screws.

have been developed, obviating the need for fusion of the C1–2 level. These techniques involve placement of either one or two screws into the base of C2 from an anterior approach, transfixing the fractured odontoid process using a lag-compression technique (29–31). Several studies have demonstrated the clinical feasibility of this technique, with most investigators indicating that single-screw fixation is usually sufficient to allow healing in most cases (29–31).

POSTERIOR FIXATION: PEDICLE SCREWS, LATERAL MASS SCREWS, AND WIRES

Posterior fixation of the subaxial cervical spine has traditionally involved wiring techniques, usually spinous process wiring or variations thereof—for example, the triple-wire technique of Bohlman and its variations (32–35). Sublaminar wiring has also been in wide use; however, biomechanical studies have shown that the spinous process wiring techniques are just as effective as sublaminar wiring in stabilizing the cervical spine. Moreover, because the spinal canal is not violated with spinous process wiring techniques, they pose a lower risk of neurologic injury than sublaminar wiring. At least one animal study has demonstrated that neuropathologic changes can occur with the passage or the presence of sublaminar wires in narrow spinal canals (36).

More recently, posterior screw fixation techniques, including lateral mass screws (used primarily from C3 to C6) and pedicle screws (used primarily at C2 and C7) have been developed (37–40). Plates or rods can be used to create the construct. Three different lateral mass screw placement techniques have been described (Table 27.3). The Roy-Camille technique (41) involves a more or less anterior-posterior screw trajectory with slight lateral angulation. The technique of Magerl (41), as well as the modification described by An (38), involves a superior and lateral screw trajectory in order to minimize the risk of injury to the exiting nerve roots or vertebral arteries. Some risk of neurovascular injury remains with any

TABLE 27.3. START POINTS AND TRAJECTORIES FOR LATERAL MASS SCREWS

Method	Lateral	Cephalad	Start point
Roy-Camille (41)	10°	0°	Center of lateral mass
Magerl (41)	25°	40°–60°	1–3 mm medial to midpoint of lateral mass
An (38)	30°	15°	1 mm medial to midpoint of lateral mass

of these screw techniques, however. Biomechanical studies have shown lateral mass screw fixation to be very effective in stabilizing the cervical spine, and to be perhaps somewhat more stable to torsion than interspinous wire fixation (32,34,42–51).

Abumi has been a proponent of pedicle screw fixation in the subaxial cervical spine and has published his surgical technique (16,37). Most surgeons in the United States, however, find cervical pedicle screw placement extremely challenging and do not place pedicle screws except at the C2 and C7 levels, where lateral mass screw fixation is anatomically challenging.

Despite the risks involved, screw-rod and screw-plate techniques are more feasible than wiring techniques over very long segments. Moreover, if a complete midline decompression (laminectomy) is required, spinous process wiring techniques cannot be used, leaving facet wiring as the only feasible wiring method (52). Although widely used clinically, it should be noted that there are no screw-rod and screw-plate devices approved by the Food and Drug Administration specifically for use in the cervical spine: All of these "approved" devices have been approved as general-use "bone screw" and rod or plate devices only. Screw fixation techniques lend themselves particularly well to multilevel (rheumatoid deformity and tumor) fusion in which fixation to the skull or thoracic spine or both is required (16,40). In general, however, wiring techniques are quite suitable for nearly all single-level fusions and most two-level fusions in which laminectomy is not performed (33,35).

ANTERIOR FIXATION: GRAFT ALONE VERSUS PLATES AND GRAFTS (STATIC VS. DYNAMIC)

The increasing trend has been to use anterior plate fixation in the majority of anterior cervical fusions for nearly all indications (8,13,46,53–56). Anterior cervical plating began with the use of plates originally designed for use in the appendicular skeleton (7). Subsequently, plates were specifically designed for use in the cervical spine and evolved from plates that required bicortical fixation (necessitating screw penetration of the spinal canal) to plates that secured or "locked" the screw to the plate, preventing screw back-out and allowing for very secure unicortical fixation (8,9,57–61). Anterior cervical plates have been shown to enhance biomechanical stability and promote fusion in animals (32,34,36,57,58,61). Used for a variety of clinical indications, anterior cervical plates have also been shown to be effective in promoting fusion in many human clinical studies (8–12,60,62).

Although several biomechanical studies have shown a significant superiority of posterior stabilization over anterior stabilization for certain types of traumatic instability (flexion-distraction injuries) of the cervical spine, many clinical studies have shown that anterior fusion with plate fixation has been extremely successful clinically in this patient population (8,10–12,19,32,62–64). Moreover, studies by Garvey et al. (10) and Goffin et al. (22) have shown that anterior plate fixation, even in trauma cases, results in radiographic and clinical adjacent segment degeneration in a large percentage of patients over time. In degenerative cases, despite the trend for the use of plates in single-level fusion, there has been no evidence that the union rate for one-level fusions (in contrast to multilevel fusions) is enhanced by plate stabilization (56,62,65).

Multilevel corpectomy for myelopathy, tumor, or trauma has been shown by Vaccaro et al. (66) to have a significant risk of early construct failure. They reported a 50% graft/plate dislodgement rate in patients undergoing three-level corpectomies and a 9.1% graft/plate dislodgement rate in patients undergoing two-level corpectomies ($p < .05$).

Saunders et al. (67), however, have shown a relatively low rate of graft complications (9.7%) in four-level corpectomy cases even when plate fixation is not used. Biomechanically, DiAngelo and colleagues (43,44) have shown that anterior plate fixation actually reverses the loads on multilevel corpectomy grafts as compared with unplated specimens; that is, the graft is unloaded in flexion and loaded in extension in the plated specimens, in contrast to the unplated specimens, where they are loaded in flexion and unloaded in extension, since the cervical plate acts as an anterior tension band or hinge (Fig. 27.5). These findings have been confirmed by other investigators (68).

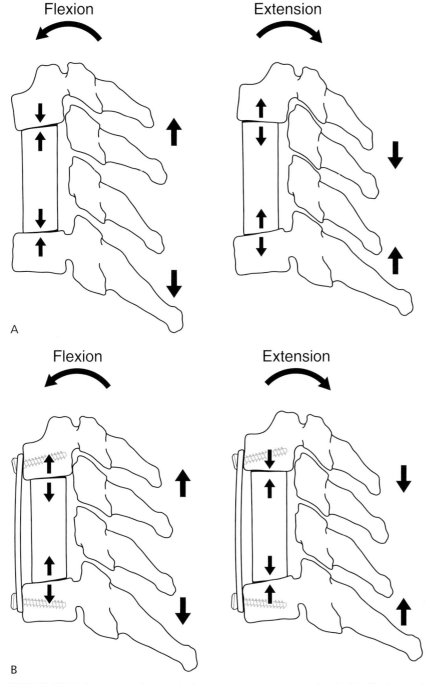

FIGURE 27.5. A: An anterior cervical corpectomy construct is loaded in flexion and unloaded in extension. **B:** The addition of an anterior cervical plate, functioning as a tension band, reverses the loading pattern, with the graft now being unloaded in extension and loaded in flexion.

One strategy that has been utilized to obviate plate and graft failure in corpectomy patients is to use a junctional or buttress plate at one or both (usually lower) ends of the corpectomy construct, thereby allowing subsidence without plate loosening (69). Clinical experience with this technique, however, has been mixed, and fatal respiratory complications associated with graft/plate dislodgement have been reported (70).

One of the most recent developments in anterior stabilization of the cervical spine has been the development of "hybrid" or dynamic anterior cervical plates (or devices) that allow screw rotation or cephalocaudad screw-plate translation or both, thereby permitting graft settling as the fusion matures (71). These plates ostensibly allow greater load sharing between the graft and the plate, potentially resulting in a higher union rate compared with static plates. Examples of these devices include the PEAK plate (DePuy Acromed, Cleveland, OH), the Atlantis plate (Medtronic Sofamor Danek, Minneapolis, MN), the dynamic DOC device (DePuy Acromed), the ABC plate (Aesculap, San Francisco, CA), and the Premier plate (Medtronic Sofamor Danek). The early clinical experience with these devices has been favorable, and biomechanical studies have shown that the graft unloading seen in static plate stabilization in flexion is reduced (72–74).

SPECIAL CONSIDERATIONS: OSTEOPENIC BONE AND ANATOMIC VARIATIONS

Osteopenic bone is an extremely common challenge to spinal surgeons with regard to internal fixation and stabilization. In certain disease processes (e.g., rheumatoid arthritis and tumor), osteopenia can be predicted. Occasionally the surgeon is surprised to find a relatively young and ostensibly healthy patient in whom the tactile feedback of screw insertion indicates a low insertional torque and therefore, in all likelihood, poor holding power. Polymethylmethacrylate has been shown to increase the holding power of pedicle screws in the lumbar spine (75). However, little has been written on the use of these strategies in the cervical spine. Polymethylmethacrylate has been used to supplement wire fixation; however, this technique has been condemned except in the case of tumor (76). Even in tumor cases, polymethylmethacrylate is recommended for use only when loaded in compression (i.e., corpectomy constructs) (3).

Some studies have demonstrated that sublaminar hooks (in the thoracolumbar spine) are superior to pedicle screws in resisting pull-out (77). The pull-out strength can be improved by cross-linking the construct (78). Cross-links are rarely utilized in the cervical spine, however. The most common strategies to avoid bone–implant interface failure involve the use of multiple fixation points, sometimes using different fixation techniques in the same construct, such as wires and screws (1,17,18,23).

Anatomic variations may also present a particular challenge to cervical fixation. Examples include an absent posterior arch of C1 (either congenital or postsurgical), which precludes the use of wires for C1–2 stabilization. A tortuous vertebral artery may intrude sufficiently into one or both of the C2 pars interarticulares so as to preclude transarticular or pars/pedicle screw placement. Fortunately, if this condition is unilateral, a single transarticular C1–2 screw combined with posterior wiring has been shown to be clinically effective. Curylo et al. (53) have shown that a tortuous vertebral artery can be a hazard (and a potential impediment to fixation) even with the anterior approaches to the cervical spine. Fortunately, vertebral artery injury, while certainly a spectacular complication to be avoided, usually does not result in permanent sequelae if handled appropriately at the time of injury (79).

SUMMARY

Cervical spine surgeons contemplating surgical treatment options for all cervical spinal disorders must take into account the biomechanical, anatomic, physiologic (e.g., bone mineral density), and pathologic factors of each particular case when making their choice with regard to the use of and type of internal cervical spinal fixation. The subsequent chapters in this section address these specific issues in regard to anterior cervical plating, transarticular (Magerl) screw fixation, posterior wiring techniques, posterior lateral mass plating, occipitocervical fixation, cervicothoracic fixation, and cervical pedicle screw fixation.

REFERENCES

1. Abraham D, Herkowitz H. Indications and trends in use in cervical spine fusions. *Orthop Clin North Am* 1998;29:731–744.
2. Brockmeyer D, Apfelbaum R, Tippets R, et al. Pediatric cervical spine instrumentation using screw fixation. *Ped Neurosurg* 1995;22:147–157.
3. Davis RF, Zeidman S, North RB, et al. Metastatic disease of the cervical spine: review of 23 cases with a protocol for surgical intervention. Paper presented at the 18th annual meeting of the Cervical Spine Research Society, November–December 1992, Palm Desert, CA.
4. Ebraheim N, Rollins JR Jr, Xu R, et al. Anatomic consideration of C2 pedicle screw placement. *Spine* 1996;21(6):691–695.
5. Jones EL, Heller JG, Silcox DH, et al. Cervical pedicle screws versus lateral mass screws. Anatomic feasibility and biomechanical comparison. *Spine* 1997;22(9):977–982.
6. Schultz KD, Petronio J, Haid RW, et al. Pediatric occipitocervical arthrodesis. A review of current options and early evaluation of rigid internal fixation techniques. *Pediatr Neurosurg* 2000;33(4):169–181.
7. Bohler J, Gaudernak T. Anterior plate stabilization for fracture dislocation of the lower cervical spine. *J Trauma* 1980;20:203–205.
8. Caspar W, Barbier DD, Klara PM. Anterior cervical fusion and Caspar plate stabilization for cervical trauma. *Neurosurgery* 1989;25:491–502.
9. Caspar W, Pitzen T, Papavero L, et al. Anterior cervical plating for the treatment of neoplasms in the cervical vertebrae. *J Neurosurg* 1999;90(suppl 1):27–34.
10. Garvey TA, Eismont FJ, Roberto LJ. Anterior decompression, structural bone grafting, and Caspar plate stabilization for unstable spine fractures and/or dislocations. *Spine* 1992;17(suppl):431–435.
11. Goffin J, Plets C, van den Bergh R. Anterior cervical fusion and osteosynthetic stabilization according to Caspar: a prospective study of 41 patients with fracture and/or dislocations of the cervical spine. *Neurosurgery* 1989;25:865–871.
12. Goffin J, van Loon J, Van Calenbergh F, et al. Long-term results after anterior cervical fusion and osteosynthetic stabilization for fractures and/or dislocations of the cervical spine. *J Spinal Disord* 1995;8:500–508.
13. Ripa DR, Kowall MG, Meyer PR Jr, et al. Series of ninety-two traumatic cervical spine injuries stabilized with anterior ASIF plate fusion technique. *Spine* 1991;16:S46–S55.
14. Panjabi MM, Dvorak J, Sander A, et al. Cervical spine kinematics and clinical instability. In: Clark CR, Ducker TB, Dvorak J, et al., eds. *The cervical spine,* 3rd ed. Philadelphia: Lippincott–Raven Publishers, 1998:53–77.
15. Fielding JW, Cochran GVB, Lawsing JF, et al. Tears of the transverse ligament of the atlas: a clinical and biomechanical study. *J Bone Joint Surg Am* 1976;58:400–407.
16. Abumi K, Tadaka T, Shono U, et al. Posterior occipitocervical reconstruction using cervical pedicle screws and plate-rod system. *Spine* 1999;24(14):1425–1434.
17. Grob D, Dvorak J, Panjabi M, et al. Posterior occipitocervical fusion. A preliminary report of a new technique. *Spine* 1991;16(suppl 3):S17–S24.
18. McAfee PC, Cassidy JR, Davis RF, et al. Fusion of the occiput to the upper cervical spine. A review of 37 cases. *Spine* 1991;16(suppl 10):S490–S494.
19. Sutterlin CE III, Bianchi JR, Kunz DN, et al. Biomechanical evaluation of occipitocervical fixation devices. *J Spinal Disord* 2001;14(3):185–192.
20. McAfee PC, Bohlman HH, Ducker TB, et al. One-stage anterior cervical decompression and posterior stabilization. A study of one hundred patients with a minimum of two years of follow-up. *J Bone Joint Surg Am* 1995;77:1791–1800.
21. Wertheim SB, Bohlman HH. Occipitocervical fusion. Indications, technique, and long-term results in thirteen patients. *J Bone Joint Surg Am* 1987;69(6):833–836.
22. Goffin J, Geusens E, Vantomme N, et al. Long-term follow-up after interbody fusion of the cervical spine. Paper presented at the 28th annual meeting of the Cervical Spine Research Society, November 2000, Charleston, SC.
23. Henriques T, Cunningham BW, Olerud C, et al. Biomechanical comparison of five different atlantoaxial posterior fixation techniques. *Spine* 2000;25(22):2877–2883.
24. Montesano PX, Juach EC, Anderson PA, et al. Biomechanics of cervical spine internal fixation. *Spine* 1991;16:S10–S16.

25. Haid RW Jr. C1-C2 transarticular screw fixation: technical aspects. *Neurosurgery* 2001;49(1):71–74.

26. Song GS, Theodore N, Dickman CA, et al. Unilateral posterior atlantoaxial transarticular screw fixation. *J Neurosurg* 1997;87(6):851–855.

27. Eleraky MA, Masferrer R, Sonntag VK. Posterior atlantoaxial facet screw fixation in rheumatoid arthritis. *J Neurosurg* 1998;89(1):8–12.

28. Harms J, Melcher RP. Posterior C1-C2 fusion with polyaxial screw and rod fixation. *Spine* 2001; 26(22):2467–2471.

29. Apfelbaum RI, Lonser RR, Veres R, et al. Direct anterior screw fixation for recent and remote odontoid fractures. *J Neurosurg* 2000;93(suppl 2):227–236.

30. Henry AD, Bohly J, Grosse A. Fixation of odontoid fractures by an anterior screw. *J Bone Joint Surg Br* 1999;81(3):472–477.

31. Jenkins JD, Coric D, Branch CL Jr. A clinical comparison of one- and two-screw odontoid fixation. *J Neurosurg* 1998;89(3):366–370.

32. Coe JD, Warden KE, Sutterlin CE, et al. Biomechanical evaluation of cervical spinal stabilization methods in a human cadaveric model. *Spine* 1989;14:1222–1231.

33. Rogers WA. Fractures and dislocations of the cervical spine: an end-result study. *J Bone Joint Surg Am* 1957;39:341.

34. Sutterlin CE III, McAfee PC, Warden KE, et al. A biomechanical evaluation of cervical spinal stabilization methods in a bovine model. Static and cyclical loading. *Spine* 1988;13:795–802.

35. Weiland DJ, McAfee PC. Posterior cervical fusion with triple-wire strut graft technique: one hundred consecutive patients. *J Spinal Disord* 1991;4(1):15–21.

36. Zdeblick TA, Becker PS, McAfee PC, et al. Neuropathologic changes with experimental spinal instrumentation: transpedicular versus sublaminar fixation. *J Spinal Disord* 1991;4(2):221–228.

37. Abumi K, Itoh H, Taneichi H, et al. Transpedicular screw fixation for traumatic lesions of the middle and lower cervical spine: description of the techniques and preliminary report. *J Spinal Disord* 1994;7(1):19–28.

38. An HS, Gordin R, Renner K. Anatomic considerations for plate-screw fixation of the cervical spine. *Spine* 1991;16(suppl 10):S548–S551.

39. Harris BM, Hilibrand AS, Nien YH, et al. A comparison of three screw types for unicortical fixation in the lateral mass of the cervical spine. *Spine* 2001;26(22):2427–2431.

40. Ludwig SC, Kramer DL, Vaccaro AR, et al. Transpedicle screw fixation of the cervical spine. *Clin Orthop* 1999;359:77–78.

41. Heller, JG, Carlson GD, Abitbol JJ, et al. Anatomic comparison of the Roy-Camille and Magerl techniques for screw placement in the lower cervical spine. *Spine* 1991;16(suppl 10):S552–S557.

42. Do Koh Y, Lim TH, Won You J, et al. A biomechanical comparison of modern anterior and posterior plate fixation of the cervical spine. *Spine* 2001;26(1):15–21.

43. DiAngelo DJ, Foley KT, Vossel KA, et al. Anterior cervical plating reverses load transfer through multilevel strut-grafts. *Spine* 2000;25:783–795.

44. Foley KT, DiAngelo DJ, Rampersaud YR, et al. The *in vitro* effects of instrumentation on multilevel cervical strut-graft mechanics. *Spine* 1999;24:2366–2376.

45. Kotani Y, Cunningham BW, Abumi K, et al. Biomechanical analysis of cervical stabilization systems. An assessment of transpedicular screw fixation in the cervical spine. *Spine* 1994;19(22):2529–2539.

46. McCullen GM, Garfin SR. Spine update: cervical spine internal fixation using screw and screw-plate constructs. *Spine* 2000;25:643–652.

47. Richman JD, Daniel TE, Anderson DD, et al. Biomechanical evaluation of cervical spine stabilization methods using a porcine model. *Spine* 1995;20:2192–2197.

48. Schultz KD Jr, McLaughlin MR, Haid RW Jr, et al. Single-stage anterior-posterior decompression and stabilization for complex cervical spine disorders. *J Neurosurg* 2000;93:214–221.

49. Swank ML, Sutterlin CE III, Bossons CR, et al. Rigid internal fixation with lateral mass plates in multilevel anterior and posterior reconstruction of the cervical spine. *Spine* 1997;22(3):274–282.

50. Ulrich C, Arand M, Nothwang J. Internal fixation on the lower cervical spine—biomechanics and clinical practice of procedures and implants. *Eur Spine J* 2001;10(2):88–100.

51. Ulrich C, Woersdoerfer O, Kalff R, et al. Biomechanics of fixation systems to the cervical spine. *Spine* 1991;16(suppl 3):S4–S9.

52. Robinson RA, Southwick WO. Surgical approaches to the cervical spine. Instructional course lecture, American Academy of Orthopedic Surgeons, St. Louis, 1960.

53. Curylo LJ, Mason HC, Bohlman HH, et al. Tortuous course of the vertebral artery and anterior cervical decompression: a cadaveric and clinical case study. *Spine* 2000;25:2860–2864.

54. Geer CP, Papadopoulos SM. The argument for single-level anterior cervical discectomy and fusion with anterior plate fixation. *Clin Neurosurg* 1994;80:963–970.

55. Isomi T, Panjabi MM, Wang JL, et al. Stabilizing potential of anterior cervical plates in multilevel corpectomies. *Spine* 1999;24:2219–2223.

56. Wang JC, McDonough PW, Endow KK, et al. Increased fusion rates with cervical plating for two-level anterior cervical discectomy and fusion. *Spine* 2000;25:41–54.

57. Chen IH. Biomechanical evaluation of subcortical versus bicortical screw purchase in anterior cervical plating. *Acta Neurochir (Wien)* 1996;138:167–173.

58. Clausen JD, Ryken TC, Traynelis VC, et al. Biomechanical evaluation of Caspar and cervical spine locking plate systems in a cadaveric model. *J Neurosurg* 1997;84:1039–1045.

59. Hollowell JP, Reinarts J, Pintar FA, et al. Failure of Synthes anterior cervical fixation device by fracture of the Morscher screws. A biomechanical study. *J Spinal Disord* 1994;7:120–125.

60. Lowery GL, McDonough RF. The significance of hardware failure in anterior cervical plate fixation. Patients with 2- to 7-year follow-up. *Spine* 1998;23:181–186.

61. Spivak JM, Chen D, Kummer FJ. The effect of locking fixation screws on the stability of anterior cervical plating. *Spine* 1999;15:334–338.

62. Connolly PF, Esses SI, Kostuik JP. Anterior cervical fusion: outcome analysis of patients fused with and without anterior cervical plates. *J Spinal Disord* 1996;9:202–206.

63. Grubb MR, Currier BL, Shih JS, et al. Biomechanical evaluation of anterior cervical spine stabilization. *Spine* 1998;15:886–892.

64. Kirkpatrick JS, Levy JA, Carillo J, et al. Reconstruction after multilevel corpectomy in the cervical spine. A sagittal plane biomechanical study. *Spine* 1999;24:1186–1190.

65. Wang JC, McDonough PW, Endow KK, et al. The effect of cervical plating on single-level anterior cervical discectomy and fusion. *J Spinal Disord* 1999;12:467–471.

66. Vaccaro AR, Falatyn ST, Scuderi GJ, et al. Early failure of long segment anterior cervical plate fixation. *J Spinal Disord* 1998;11:410–415.

67. Saunders RL, Pikus HJ, Ball P. Four-level corpectomy. *Spine* 1998;23:2455–2461.

68. Wang JL, Panjabi MM, Isomi T. The role of bone graft force in stabilizing the multilevel anterior cervical spine plate system. *Spine* 2000;25:1649–1654.

69. Vanichkachorn JS, Vaccaro AR, Silveri CP, et al. Anterior junctional plate in the cervical spine. *Spine* 1998;23:2462–2467.

70. Riew KD, Sethi NS, Devney J, et al. Complications of buttress plate stabilization of cervical corpectomy. *Spine* 1999;24:2404–2410.

71. DiAngelo DJ, Foley KT, Liu W, et al. Biomechanical testing of a translational anterior cervical plate with a constrained anterior cervical plate. Paper presented at the 29th annual meeting of the Cervical Spine Research Society, November–December 2001, Monterey, CA.

72. Apfelbaum RI, Dailey AT, Barbera J. Clinical experience with a new load-sharing anterior cervical plate. Paper presented at the 27th annual meeting of the Cervical Spine Research Society, November–December 1999, Seattle, WA.

73. Epstein NE. The management of one-level anterior cervical corpectomy with fusion using Atlantis hybrid plate: preliminary experience. *J Spinal Disord* 2000;13:324–328.

74. Zdeblick TA, Herkowitz HN. Translational cervical plating: early clinical results. Paper presented at the 29th annual meeting of the Cervical Spine Research Society, November–December 2001, Monterey, CA.

75. Wittenberg RH, Lee KS, Shea M, et al. Effect of screw diameter, insertion technique, and bone cement augmentation of pedicular screw fixation strength. *Clin Orthop* 1993;296:278–287.

76. McAfee PC, Bohlman HH, Ducker TB, et al. Failure of stabilization of the spine with methylmethacrylate. A retrospective analysis of twenty-four cases. *J Bone Joint Surg Am* 1986;68(8):1145–1157.

77. Coe JD, Warden KE, Herzig MA, et al. Influence of bone mineral density on the fixation of thoracolumbar implants. A comparative study of transpedicular screws, laminar hooks, and spinous process wires. *Spine* 1990;15(9):902–907.

78. Dick JC, Jones MP, Zdeblick TA, et al. A biomechanical comparison evaluating the use of intermediate screws and cross-linkage in lumbar pedicle fixation. *J Spinal Disord* 1994;7(5):402–407.

79. Smith MD, Emery SE, Dudley A, et al. Vertebral artery injury during anterior decompression of the cervical spine. A retrospective review of ten patients. *J Bone Joint Surg Br* 1993;75:410–415.

28

ANTERIOR CERVICAL PLATING

THOMAS A. ZDEBLICK

INDICATIONS AND CONTRAINDICATIONS

Anterior cervical plates were first introduced in the early 1980s. Since then their popularity has soared and the controversy surrounding their use has diminished. Although once controversial, most surgeons would now agree that anterior cervical plating increases the fusion rate in multilevel anterior cervical fusions (1–11). In addition, anterior plating is indicated for trauma, nonunion repair, corpectomies, and cervical deformity (12). Traumatic conditions that are amenable to anterior cervical plating include burst fracture, hyperextension with disc space disruption, subluxation, and facet dislocation following a reduction. Although anterior plating has been used in the face of disc space infection, some authors would argue that this remains a contraindication. Other contraindications include inappropriate vertebral body size, severe osteoporosis, and inadequate exposure.

SURGICAL TECHNIQUE

Patients are positioned supine with the head in neutral position, resting on a well-padded horseshoe headrest. For corpectomies or in traumatic conditions, in-line tong traction is utilized. The arms are pulled caudally and taped in place at the patient's sides. I prefer a transverse skin incision and a left-sided approach for all anterior cervical fusion procedures. For procedures involving three levels or more, an oblique incision may be utilized. Rarely, for very long fusions I've used two separate transverse skin incisions. Transverse or oblique incisions are more cosmetic and allow more than adequate exposure. Following the skin incision, the platysma is incised in line with the incision; alternatively, its fibers may be split. Subplatysmal blunt dissection identifies the sternocleidomastoid muscle. Standard blunt dissection is carried out in a plane keeping the trachea and esophagus medially and the sternocleidomastoid muscle and carotid sheath laterally. The appropriate spinal level is confirmed with a needle in the disc space and a radiograph.

Appropriate anterior spinal exposure is key in performing anterior cervical plating. The longus colli muscle should be carefully elevated 2 to 3 mm on either side of the vertebral bodies (Figs. 28.1 and 28.2). In general, a sulcus at the midportion of the vertebral body will be located at the corner of the vertebral margins. With large anterior osteophytes, the longus colli muscle will need to be retracted over these osteophytes laterally. It is this medial margin of the longus colli muscle that helps orient the surgeon to the midline of the vertebral body. A discectomy is then performed at each level to be involved in the fusion (Fig. 28.3). At each level, the uncovertebral joints need to be exposed laterally. This will help orient the surgeon to the midline. Appropriate decompression either with discectomy or corpectomy is then performed. Appropriate bone grafting either with separate discectomy-type grafts or with a strut corpectomy graft is then performed. The details of the decompression and grafting procedures are outlined elsewhere

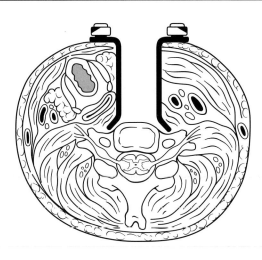

FIGURE 28.1. After the vertebral column has been exposed, the longus colli muscle is elevated and the "slotted foot" medial/lateral self-retaining retractor blades are securely positioned.

in this book. However, care must be taken to ensure that the inferior end of a strut graft is positioned as far inferiorly as is safely possible. If the inferior end of the strut is left near the anterior cortex, it is more prone to anterior displacement with or without vertebral body fracture. If this were to occur, plate displacement might result, with construct failure.

Once the bone grafts are in place, anterior plating can begin. The first step, and one that is very important, is to smooth all of the anterior surfaces of the cervical spine. I use a large rongeur to remove significant anterior osteophytes from the affected disc space levels (Fig. 28.4). In addition, a burr is used to smooth out these ridges on either side of each endplate, as well as any prominences of the graft. I've used the phrase "gardening of the spine" to describe the need to ensure that a smooth surface on the anterior aspect of all vertebral bodies is obtained. A common complication is to leave a prominence anteriorly, which forces the plate to rock back and forth on this prominence. This will lead to a plate that is proud and may lead to later dysphagia.

The appropriate plate length must now be selected. Preoperative templates are available and may occasionally be helpful. The ideal plate length should be the shortest plate that just spans the fused levels. My preference is to begin the superior screws 1 to 2 mm

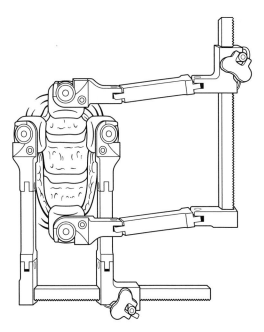

FIGURE 28.2. Longitudinal retractors may be used to maximize the exposure.

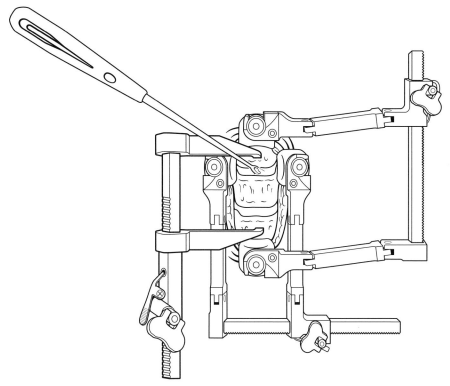

FIGURE 28.3. Discectomies are completed at each level. Pituitaries, curettes, and Kerrisons may be used to remove the disc material and cartilage to expose the posterior longitudinal ligament and to locate the uncovertebral joints bilaterally at each level.

above the junction of the bone graft and endplate. Similarly, the inferior screws must begin as close to the junction of the graft and endplate as possible (Fig. 28.5).

Once the correct plate length is selected, contouring may be necessary to ensure that the plate follows the lordotic curvature of the spine (Fig. 28.6). The plate must remain centered at each level to be fused. This is often difficult because of the unilateral side of the surgical approach. The landmarks that I use to help center the plate include palpating the sternal notch and palpating the prominence of the anterior ring of C1 and the odontoid. Using these two landmarks, one can usually maintain a vertical position of the plate. The plate is then held temporarily in position with small fixation pins (Fig. 28.7). If plate length or position is not definite, anteroposterior or lateral x-rays or both can be obtained at this time to ensure correct plate length and position. Alternatively, fluoroscopy may also be used.

The screw holes of the most superior and inferior vertebral bodies can then be drilled. I prefer to drill to a length that is approximately 80% to 90% of the depth of the vertebral body. Most typically, this length is between 15 and 17 mm (13). I do not typically obtain

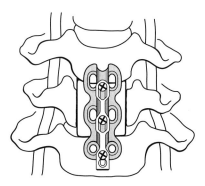

FIGURE 28.4. Soft tissue and anterior osteophytes are removed from the adjacent vertebral bodies so that the plate may sit evenly on the anterior cortex. Position the plate so that the superior screw slots are close to the inferior endplate. This will ensure that as settling occurs and the plate effectively shifts upward, there is adequate vertebral body height to accommodate the shift.

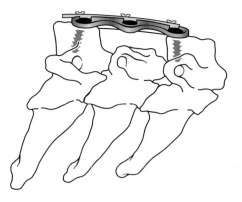

FIGURE 28.5. The inferior screw holes should be placed close to the superior endplate, angled away from the bone graft. This ensures good screw purchase. This will allow for placement of the fixed bone screws in the center of the vertebra. The edge of the plate should not interfere with the adjacent unfused disc spaces.

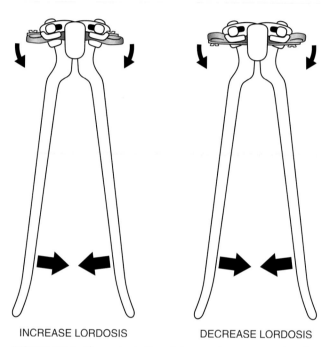

INCREASE LORDOSIS   DECREASE LORDOSIS

FIGURE 28.6. If required, the plate may be contoured to increase the amount of lordotic curvature or decrease the amount of lordotic curvature using the plate bender. A gradual bend should be made over the entire length of the plate, and abrupt changes in curvature should be avoided.

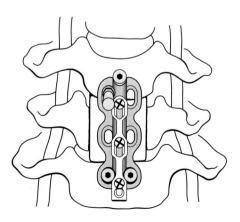

FIGURE 28.7. After the plate length has been selected and placed on the anterior cervical spine, a plate holding pin can be placed in the plate to provide temporary fixation while drilling and placing bone screws.

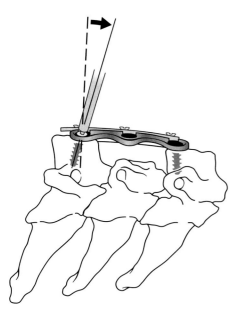

FIGURE 28.8. A single drill guide is utilized to place the bone screws in the fixed holes of the plate. Appropriate drill and screw angles are shown.

bicortical purchase, although this has some mechanical advantage, particularly in osteoporotic bone (14). Ideal screw trajectories are obtained by angulating away from the bone graft approximately 10 to 12 degrees and triangulating medially approximately 10 degrees. This "triangulation" is safe and increases the pull-off strength. Most plating systems come with single- or double-barreled guides to help ensure proper drill trajectory (Figs. 28.8 and 28.9).

Screws are then placed. I prefer to place the two inferior screws first and then to use the two superior screws in a compression mode (Fig. 28.10) (15). For nondynamic or

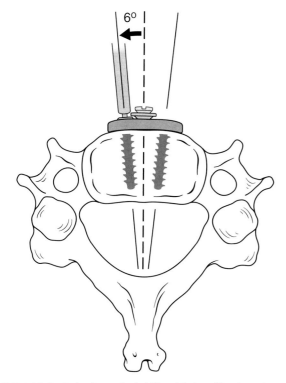

FIGURE 28.9. A single or dual drill guide is utilized to place the bone screws in the fixed holes of the plate. Appropriate drill and screw angles are shown.

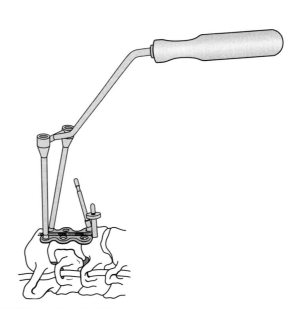

FIGURE 28.10. Final tightening of all screws is done sequentially so that the plate is evenly applied to the anterior cortical surface of the spine.

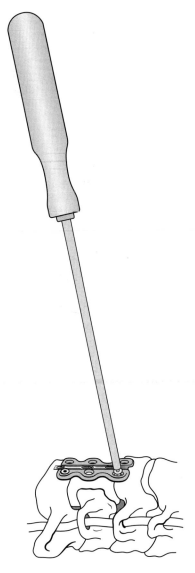

FIGURE 28.11. Once all of the bone screws have been securely seated in the plate, the locking washer should be translated into the locked position. Once the washer is in the locked position covering the bone screw heads, the locking screwdriver is engaged into each locking screw and tightened. The locking screw mechanism is now firmly secured. Note: A variety of locking mechanisms exist, and the surgeon should be familiar with the specific technique for the selected plate.

nontranslational plates, the screws can be placed with an initial single screw superiorly and a diagonally opposite screw inferiorly. This allows the surgeon some leeway in plate alignment. The remaining superior and inferior screws are then placed. Once the two superior and two inferior screws are placed, intermediate screws may be placed as well (for multilevel discectomies). For corpectomies, I do not place a screw in the strut graft. There are no biomechanical studies that prove that this screw is helpful, and it may create a stress riser within the graft (16,17). Once all screws are in place, a final radiograph is taken to ensure appropriate screw placement. The locking mechanisms may then be fully secured (Fig. 28.11).

COMPLICATIONS

Most plate complications are secondary to poor exposure or poor spine preparation. Hoarseness or dysphagia may be secondary to plate prominence. This may be due to prominent anterior osteophytes that lift the plate off the spinal surface or to inappropriate plate contour. Care should be taken to ensure that the plate is closely approximated to the vertebral body at each level. Losing orientation to the midline may cause a plate to be placed extremely laterally. This may then bring the vertebral artery foramen into danger. Appropriate midline orientation techniques include longus colli retraction, establishment of the uncovertebral joints, palpation of the odontoid prominence, and palpation of the sternal notch.

Other complications include poor screw purchase. This may be secondary to poor bone quality or inadequate screw length. If screw purchase is not obtained on a screw's first pass, a loose screw should never be left in place. Either a larger-diameter screw must be used or, occasionally, a vertebroplasty can be performed with methylmethacrylate to enhance screw purchase. Adjacent-level degeneration may occur above or below a fusion. Plate impingement or screw penetrating may increase this tendency, as may sagittal alignment (18,19). Finally, hardware failure may occur if fusion does not occur. Appropriate attention must be paid to endplate preparation and bone graft placement so that arthrodesis is the successful end result. Without successful arthrodesis, hardware failure may be inevitable.

REFERENCES

1. Bolesta MJ, Rechtine GR, Chrin AM. Three- and four-level anterior cervical discectomy and fusion with plate fixation: a prospective study. *Spine* 2000;25(16):2040–2044.
2. Bose B. Anterior cervical instrumentation enhances fusion rates in multilevel reconstruction in smokers. *J Spinal Disord* 2001;14(1):3–9.
3. Caspar W, Geisler FH, Pitzen T, et al. Anterior cervical plate stabilization in one- and two-level degenerative disease: overtreatment or benefit? *J Spinal Disord* 1998;11(1):1–11.
4. Connolly PJ, Esses SI, Kostuik JP. Anterior cervical fusion: outcome analysis of patients fused with and without anterior cervical plates. *J Spinal Disord* 1996;9(3):202–206.
5. Grob D, Peyer JV, Dvorak J. The use of plate fixation in anterior surgery of the degenerative cervical spine: a comparative prospective clinical study. *Eur Spine J* 2001;10(5):408–413.
6. Kaiser MG, Haid RW Jr, Subach BR, et al. Anterior cervical plating enhances arthrodesis after discectomy and fusion with cortical allograft. *Neurosurgery* 2002;50(2):229–236.
7. Sasso RC, Ruggiero RA Jr, Reilly TM, et al. Early reconstruction failures after multilevel cervical corpectomy. *Spine* 2003;28(2):140–142.
8. Wang JC, McDonough PW, Endow KK, et al. Increased fusion rates with cervical plating for two-level anterior cervical discectomy and fusion. *Spine* 2000;25(1):41–45.
9. Wang JC, McDonough PW, Endow K, et al. The effect of cervical plating on single-level anterior cervical discectomy and fusion. *J Spinal Disord* 1999;12(6):467–471.
10. Zaveri GR, Ford M. Cervical spondylosis: the role of anterior instrumentation after decompression and fusion. *J Spinal Disord* 2001;14(1):10–16.
11. Zdeblick TA, Cooke ME, Wilson D, et al. Anterior cervical discectomy, fusion, and plating. A comparative animal study. *Spine* 1993;18(14):1974–1983.
12. Tribus CB, Corteen DP, Zdeblick TA. The efficacy of anterior cervical plating in the management of symptomatic pseudoarthrosis of the cervical spine. *Spine* 1999;24(9):860–864.
13. Lu J, Ebraheim NA, Yang H, et al. Anatomic bases for anterior spinal surgery: surgical anatomy of the cervical vertebral body and disc space. *Surg Radiol Anat* 1999;21(4):235–239.
14. Chen IH. Biomechanical evaluation of subcortical versus bicortical screw purchase in anterior cervical plating. *Acta Neurochir* 1996;138(2):167–173.
15. Epstein NE. Anterior dynamic plates in complex cervical reconstructive surgeries. *J Spinal Disord Techniques* 2002;15(3):221–227.
16. Foley KT, DiAngelo DJ, Rampersaud YR, et al. The *in vitro* effects of instrumentation on multilevel cervical strut-graft mechanics. *Spine* 1999;24(22):2366–2376.
17. Rapoff AJ, O'Brien TJ, Ghanayem AJ, et al. Anterior cervical graft and plate load sharing. *J Spinal Disord* 1999;12(1):45–49.
18. Eck JC, Humphreys SC, Lim TH, et al. Biomechanical study on the effect of cervical spine fusion on adjacent-level intradiscal pressure and segmental motion. *Spine* 2002;27(22):2431–2434.
19. Troyanovich SJ, Stroink AR, Kattner KA, et al. Does anterior plating maintain cervical lordosis versus conventional fusion techniques? A retrospective analysis of patients receiving single-level fusions. *J Spinal Disord Techniques* 2002;15(1):69–74.

METHODS OF FIXATION AND STABILIZATION: MAGERL SCREWS

DIETER GROB

BIOMECHANICAL ASPECTS OF ATLANTOAXIAL SCREW FIXATION

The goal of atlantoaxial fusion is to eliminate relative motion between the atlas and axis. The principal physiologic motion in this segment is axial rotation; additional lesions such as fractures and ligamentous injuries or deficiency of the dens cause transverse instability. Because the shape of the bones is not suitable to provide intrinsic stability except posterior dislocation of the atlas with intact dens, any valuable implant has to provide multidirectional stability. As shown by several *in vitro* tests, Magerl screws show equal or superior stability than conventional posterior atlantoaxial fusion techniques (1–3). The immediate reliable stability provided by atlantoaxial screws eliminates the risk of loosening of posterior wire or cable fixation (1) and promotes bony ingrowth of the graft (Fig. 29.1).

Transarticular screws in occipitocervical fixation techniques are an important contribution to stability by eliminating atlantoaxial rotation. In addition, the screws provide reliable integration of the atlas into the construct by firmly fixing both lateral masses. Conventional posterior techniques rely on the quality and integrity of the posterior arch of the atlas, which can be fixed by wires. This augmentation of stability provided by the atlantoaxial screws allows short fixation (e.g., occiput to C2), whereas other constructs need minimum extension of the fixation down to C4-5 to achieve a sufficient lever arm (4).

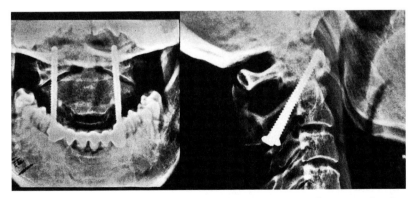

FIGURE 29.1. Anteroposterior and lateral view of transarticular screw fixation of C1-2. Note the strictly sagittal orientation of the screws in the anteroposterior view. In the lateral view, the tip of the screws is projected over the superior half of the anterior arch of the atlas. The bone graft is fixed posteriorly with nonabsorbable suture.

INDICATIONS

Degenerative Osteoarthritis

Painful osteoarthritis of the atlantoaxial facets represents a standard indication for monosegmental fixation with transarticular screws (5). In cases where inclusion of the atlantooccipital joints is required, the screw fixation might be integrated into an occipital fixation system (4).

Rheumatoid Arthritis

Instability due to destruction of the osteoligamentous complex of C1-2 produces multidirectional instability, which may be stabilized by transarticular screw fixation. Appropriate positioning in a halo and intraoperative manipulation allow fixation in anatomically reduced position (Fig. 29.2). Atlantoaxial fusion at an early stage of the disease prevents neurologic damage and progression of the upward migration of the dens into the foramen magnum (6). Preoperative evaluation with CT or MRI of the local anatomy is mandatory.

Trauma

Fractures of the ring of the atlas may be stabilized with transarticular C1-2 screws. In the presence of lateral dislocation, reduction with halo traction or intraoperative manipulation has to precede screw fixation. Unstable posterior ring of the atlas requires bony reconstruction (7) or intraarticular grafting with autologous bone graft (8). Dens fractures with contraindications for anterior screw fixation can be stabilized by atlantoaxial fusion. Pseudarthrosis of the dens with atlantoaxial instability is managed by posterior transarticular screw fixation (9).

Congenital Anomalies

Occipitocervical anomalies or os odontoideum can be stabilized by posterior fusion using the atlantoaxial transarticular screw technique. Preoperative exclusion of bony or vascular anomalies is mandatory.

Symptomatic instability of the bifid posterior arch of the atlas requires bony reconstruction of the atlas with bone graft (7) and posterior transarticular screw fixation.

Infection or Tumor

Instability due to bony deficiency in tumors or infection requires adequate reconstruction and may be combined with transarticular screw fixation.

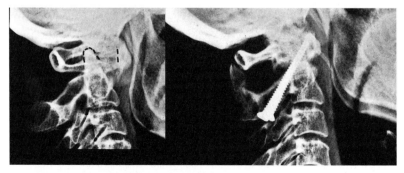

FIGURE 29.2. Atlantoaxial screw fixation in rheumatoid arthritis. **Left:** Severe C1-2 instability in lateral flexion view with atlantodental distance of 14 mm. **Right:** 48 months after atlantoaxial transarticular screw fixation: Solidly fused bone graft posteriorly and anatomically reduced C1-2 segment.

Osseous resection of metastasis may create instability of the occipitocervical junction. Transarticular screws represent a valuable adjunct to the stability of occipitocervical fusion.

Pediatric Indications

Atlantoaxial rotatory subluxations in children may require surgical stabilization (10). Using appropriately sized screws after anatomic study of the isthmus of C2, transarticular screw fixation may be applied in pediatric patients (11).

Atlantoaxial Screw Fixation as a Diagnostic Procedure

In rare cases of soft tissue injuries, occult ligamentous instability may cause pain (12). If imaging is unable to detect the injury but facet injection provides a positive result with pain relief, temporary internal fixation of the atlantoaxial segment might be considered. The screws are inserted without bone graft in a primary surgery. If the patient is able to give a positive response to the fixation with reduced pain, grafting is performed in a second intervention after 7 to 10 days. If no pain reduction is noted, the screws are removed through stab incisions without any further surgery.

SURGICAL TECHNIQUE

For safe drilling, anatomy and the dimension of the pedicle of C2 have to be verified preoperatively by computed tomographic (CT) scans with sagittal biplanar reconstruction or by magnetic resonance imaging.

Anesthesia in cases of instability of the atlantoaxial segment is ideally performed by insertion of the bronchial tube with fiberoptic guidance. This technique avoids an extended position of the head and the risk of neurologic compromise by atlantoaxial dislocation during the procedure. The use of intraoperative neuromonitoring allows the detection of intraoperative damage of the cord. During surgery, the anesthetist and monitor are situated at the feet of the patient.

Positioning

Positioning of the patient is a crucial factor for correct screw placement. The arms are positioned along the chest. The posterior iliac crest is sterilely draped for graft harvest. A straight subaxial cervical spine and flexed position in the atlantooccipital joint allow sufficient lowering of the drill in the cervicothoracic area to obtain an ideal screw position. This may be best achieved by a skull fixation that permits rotation around a transverse axis at the suboccipital area.

Approach

Through a posterior midline incision from the occiput to the midcervical spine (approximately 10–12 cm), the nuchal ligament is divided longitudinally, taking care to stay exactly in the midline to reduce hemorrhage.

The prominent spinous process of C2 serves as orientation. The muscle insertions are preserved by mobilizing the muscles bilaterally with a fragment of bone of the bifid spinous process, separated with the oscillating saw (13). These can be reattached at the spinous process at the end of the procedure.

The laminae of C2 are subperiosteally dissected. Landmarks to be brought into view are the C2-3 facet joint and the inner border of the isthmus of C2. This area of maximal width of the spinal canal can be identified by following the contour of the inner curve of the lamina and pedicle subperiosteally by detaching the atlantoaxial membrane until its most lateral point. If intraarticular bone grafting is planned, subperiosteal dissection is continued ventrally on the surface of the isthmus until the insertion of the joint capsule is reached. This may be incised and the facet brought into view.

Screw Insertion

Computer-generated image guidance (14,15) and other tools (16) have recently been developed to facilitate screw insertion. With adequate validation of accuracy, these devices may help the surgeon in the future to place transarticular screws with increased precision and safety. At present, however, the standard technique relies first of all on the surgeon's knowledge of the anatomy and the assistance of intraoperative imaging with the C-arm.

The correct position of the screw has to be checked continuously in two planes:

1. *Frontal plane:* The screw position in the frontal plane (i.e., lateral/medial) is checked directly in the operative field. The most important landmark is the inner border of the isthmus of C2. The trajectory of the drill has to pass 2 to 4 mm laterally from this curved line, representing the lateral border of the spinal canal. The drill has to be oriented strictly sagittal in order to stay intraosseous between the vertebral artery laterally and the spinal canal medially and not to miss the lateral mass of the atlas anteriorly. The entry point of the drill is situated 2 to 3 mm cranial to the lower margin of the lamina of C2, respecting the cortical layer of the C2 lamina (Fig. 29.3).
2. *Lateral plane:* The screw position in the sagittal plane is controlled in the accordingly positioned C-arm. The picture in the monitor has to show a strict lateral view of the atlas and axis. If there is a fixed rotation between C1 and C2, a simultaneous lateral view of atlas and axis is not possible, and the drilling has to respect this accordingly. The trajectory of the drill in the monitor has to pass from the entry point at the lamina of C2, cross the atlantoaxial facet in its posterior third, and end in the upper half of the lateral, oval-shaped projection of the anterior ring of the atlas (see Fig. 29.1). To achieve an ideal position of the drill, percutaneous drilling and screw insertion with extra-long drill bits and screwdriver may be necessary.

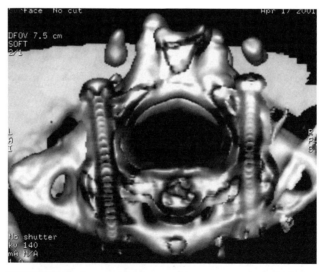

FIGURE 29.3. Computed tomographic reconstruction after C1-2 screw fixation. Note the strictly sagittal orientation of the screws. The screws pass close to the medial border of the isthmus of C2 in a safe distance to the vertebral artery.

With these landmarks, the position of the screw is defined. In addition to this, the tap drilling technique, in which the tip of the drill is advanced only 1 or 2 mm at a time before pulling back, allows one to verify the intraosseous position of the drill throughout the drilling procedure by feeling the resistance of bone. As soon as no bony resistance to the drill is felt, the drilling procedure must be immediately stopped in order to avoid possible damage to the vertebral artery. The application of this technique might be difficult in the presence of soft bone, as encountered sometimes in rheumatoid patients.

Bone Graft

For mechanical reasons, the bone graft is an essential part of the three-point stability of the construct and should not be omitted.

The technique for bone grafting corresponds to the traditional technique of the Gallie procedure (17). After harvesting a monocortical or bicortical graft from the posterior iliac crest, the bed of the graft is carefully prepared. Special attention has to be paid to the decortication of the posterior arch of the atlas, since frequently only a minimal amount of cancellous bone providing a viable bed for the graft is found. The cortical layer of the spinous process of C2 is removed, and the bone graft is positioned between the arch of the atlas and the spinous process of C2 and fixed with wire or nonabsorbable suture.

In certain cases there is a deficiency of the posterior ring of the atlas. In this situation, the fixation of the bone graft has to be modified. To reestablish stability, the graft has to be fixed firmly with 2.7-mm cortical screws bilaterally to the remaining parts of the atlas (7) (Figs. 29.4 and 29.5). As an alternative, grafting may be performed directly into the decorticated facet joint. This technique does not provide three-point stability and requires a postoperative halo fixation.

Postoperative Care

Correctly performed transarticular screw fixation with bone graft does not require extensive postoperative fixation. A simple soft collar worn out of bed for 2 months is sufficient. If there is doubt about the radiologic incorporation of the graft, this period may be extended. This primary stability of the construct with simple aftertreatment has proved to be of essential benefit to otherwise disabled patients such as those with rheumatism.

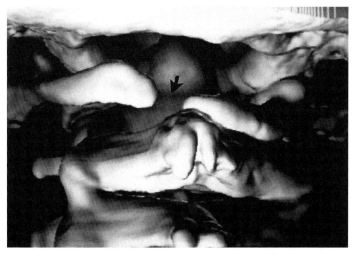

FIGURE 29.4. Bifid posterior arch of the atlas (*arrow*). This situation complicates the fixation of the posterior bone graft.

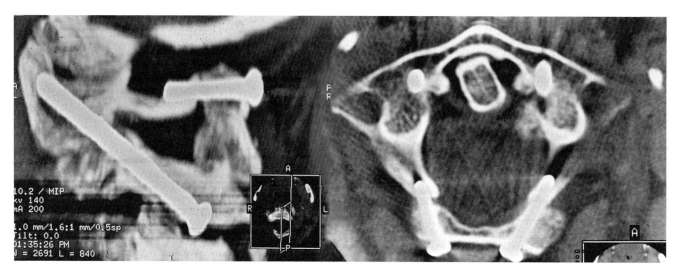

FIGURE 29.5 Graft fixation to the posterior part of the atlas with 2.7-mm cortical screws and transarticular screw fixation.

DIFFICULTIES AND PITFALLS

Altered Anatomy of C2

Preoperative CT reveals the details of the anatomy, which are essential to insert the screws safely. The lateral reconstruction of the isthmus of C2 allows measuring the dimensions necessary for the screws (usually 3.5-mm cortical screws). In rheumatoid patients, significant bone erosion might be detected. No transarticular screw insertion should be attempted unless sufficient bone stock is present on at least one side. Unilateral screw placement provides satisfactory fusion rates (18) but requires rigid postoperative fixation for 2 months.

Asymmetric Vertebral Artery

Angiography of the vertebral artery is not performed routinely in our practice and is done only in cases with symptoms indicating vascular pathology. If there is unilateral vertebral artery hypoplasia, screw insertion should be restricted to unilateral insertion on the same side.

Screw Positioning in the Lateral Plane

The positioning of the patient is of utmost importance. Maximal flexion in the atlanto-occipital joint and extension of the subaxial cervical spine bring the anatomy into a favorable position in relation to the thoracic cage. This allows lowering the drill for ideal screw position. In obese patients or in patients with marked upper thoracic kyphosis, this might be impossible and the technique of screw insertion has to be abandoned in favor of simple grafting techniques with wire or pedicular screws in the axis and atlas.

Screw Positioning in the Frontal Plane

Care has to be taken not to deviate from a strictly sagittal screw insertion. This might occur when the separate stab incision for the drill is not properly placed and the soft tissue hinders the drill orientation.

Since the bony spinal canal allows ample space for the cord, perforation of the cortical bone of the isthmus on the medial side is less hazardous than screw positioning too far lateral, where the vertebral artery is fixed in the vertebral foramen. This justifies the positioning of the screw in the most medial possible part of the isthmus.

SALVAGE PROCEDURES

Screw Insertion

If difficulties arise with proper bilateral screw insertion, unilateral positioning of a correctly placed screw is tolerable. This provides satisfactory fusion rate with rigid postoperative fixation if bone graft is added in the midline.

If malposition of a screw is detected intraoperatively, the screw should be removed and the fixation restricted to unilateral instrumentation.

Injury of the Vertebral Artery

Massive hemorrhage after drilling through the isthmus may indicate injury of the vertebral artery. As a precautionary measure, the contralateral screw should not be inserted (unless already done). Hemostasis is attempted first by inserting the screw in the drill hole. Close supervision of the blood pressure and neurologic situation indicates adequate compression or continuous bleeding. In the latter case, clamping of the vessel may be attempted, but significant removal of bone might be necessary for a successful procedure.

Hemorrhage out of the drill hole might also originate from the venous plexus surrounding the vertebral artery. In this case, insertion of the screw usually provides adequate hemostasis.

Reinstrumentation after Failed Fusion

If bony integration of the graft fails to occur, the screws eventually break at the level of the atlantoaxial joint or turn loose. Persisting instability and pain indicate refixation of the C1-2 segment. A meticulous study of the anatomy and the screw position within the isthmus of C2 has to be performed in order to detect possible alternative positioning options for the screws.

The same posterior midline approach may be used as for the primary intervention. The screws are removed. If they are loosened and the isthmus of C2 is of appropriate size, the 3.5-mm screw may simply be replaced by a 4.5-mm cortical screw. After breakage, the posterior fragment is removed and a 3.5-mm screw is replaced, passing the fragment in the atlas medial or lateral according to the anatomy. Extensive removal of scar tissue and decortication of the graft bed is mandatory for successful osteointegration of the new iliac bone graft.

RESULTS

A series of 54 patients with rheumatoid arthritis and atlantoaxial instability has been stabilized with C1-2 screw fixation. They were controlled retrospectively after a mean follow-up period of 6 (range 2–13) years. The surgical dates revealed a mean operation time of 78 (range 50–145) minutes and a mean blood loss of 250 cm^3. Neck pain at follow-up was 2 on a visual analogue scale (0–10), compared with 6 preoperatively. Seventy-nine percent of the patients responded that they would repeat the same surgery if found in the same situation, whereas 16% were not sure about the answer to this question and 5% responded negatively. Seventy-eight percent declared themselves satisfied with the outcome; 18% indicated a satisfactory result, and 3% a bad result.

Radiologic examination in this group of patients with rheumatoid arthritis revealed a reduction of the anterior atlantodental interval from an average of 9.3 mm preoperatively to 3.6 mm postoperatively. A radiologically solid fusion could be observed in 47 patients.

Six of the remaining 7 patients showed broken screws as a sign of delayed union, but only 2 of them had persistent instability and pseudarthrosis (3.9%). No other serious complication was observed in this series.

SUMMARY AND CONCLUSIONS

Fusion of the atlantoaxial segment is indicated in the presence of instability. Clinically, this instability may appear as persistent neck pain or as myelopathy as a consequence of repeat (micro)trauma of the cord. Conventional wiring techniques are simple to perform but implicate a considerable rate of pseudarthrosis, especially in unfavorable conditions such as rheumatoid arthritis. Transarticular atlantoaxial screws provide superior stability and a reduced rate of pseudarthrosis. Insertion of the screws requires meticulous study of the anatomic situation of the isthmus of C2 with CT scans or magnetic resonance imaging. The operative technique is delicate, but connected to a low complication rate if the surgeon follows the instructions and is knowledgeable about the local anatomy. The screw has to be placed in relation to the medial border of the isthmus of C2 in a sagittal orientation. The inclination is controlled with the C-arm. Successful osteointegration of the iliac bone graft is related to the grafting technique with decortication and graft positioning.

REFERENCES

1. Crawford NR et al. Differential biomechanical effect of injury and wiring at C1-C2. *Spine* 1999; 24(18):1894–1902.
2. Crisco JJ et al. Bone graft translation of four upper cervical spine fixation techniques in a cadaveric model. *J Orthop Res* 1991;9:835–846.
3. Grob D et al. Biomechanical evaluation of four different posterior atlantoaxial fixation techniques. *Spine* 1992;17(5):480–490.
4. Grob D et al. Posterior occipito-cervical fusion. *Spine* 1991;16(suppl 3):S17–S24.
5. Dvorak J, Wälchli B. Kopfschmerzen beim Zervikalsyndrom. *Therapeutische Umschau* 1997;54(2).
6. Grob D. Atlantoaxial immobilization in rheumatoid arthritis: a prophylactic procedure? *Eur Spine J* 2000;9:404–409.
7. Floyd T, Grob D. Translaminar screws in the atlas. *Spine* 2000;25(22):2913–2915.
8. Magerl F, Seemann P. Stable posterior fusion of the atlas and axis by transarticular screw fixation. In: Kehr P, Weidner A, eds. *Cervical spine.* Strasbourg: Springer Verlag, 1986:322–327.
9. Jeanneret B, Magerl F. Primary posterior fusion C1/C2 in odontoid fractures: indications, technique and results of transarticular screw fixation. *J Spinal Disord* 1992;5(4):464–475.
10. Subach BR et al. Current management of pediatric atlantoaxial rotatory subluxation. *Spine* 1998; 23(20):2174–2179.
11. Grob D. Atlantoaxial instability in odontoid hypoplasia. A long term follow up after atlantoaxial screw fixation. Presented at the 17th annual meeting of the Cervical Spine Research Society, Turin, Italy, 2001.
12. Dvorak J et al. Functional evaluation of the spinal cord by magnetic resonance imaging in patients with rheumatoid arthritis and instability of upper cervical spine. *Spine* 1989;14(10):1057–1064.
13. Yonenobu K, Ono K. Laminoplasty. In: Ono K, Dvorak J, Dunn E, eds. *Cervical spondylosis and similar disorders.* Singapore: World Scientific, 1998:501–522.
14. Dickman C, Sonntag V. Posterior C1-C2 transarticular screw fixation for atlantoaxial arthrodesis. *Neurosurgery* 1998;43:275–280.
15. Wigfield C, Bolger C. A technique for frameless stereotaxy and placement of transarticular screws for atlantoaxial instability in rheumatoid arthritis. *Eur Spine J* 2001;10:264–268.
16. Goffin J et al. Three-dimensional computed tomography-based, personalized drill guide for posterior cervical stabilization at C1-C2. *Spine* 2001;15(26):1343–1347.
17. Gallie WE. Fractures and dislocations of the cervical spine. *Am J Surg* 1939;46A:495–499.
18. Grob D et al. Complications of atlanto-axial fusion with transarticular screw-fixation. *J Bone Joint Surg Br* 1993;75(suppl II):178.

30

WIRE FIXATION OF THE LOWER CERVICAL SPINE

PAUL A. ANDERSON

Wire fixation of the cervical spine is a safe and effective means to stabilize an unstable condition and to promote fusion. This fixation has been utilized for both the C1–2 articulation and in the subaxial cervical spine. Hydra first placed an interspinous wire loop of silver around the spinous processes in 1892 in an infant who had a birth injury. Rogers (1) popularized a technique using stainless steel wire placed through drill holes in the spinous process in 1942. Bohlman (2) modified Rogers' technique, adding two wires that hold plates of bone graft to the spinous processes. Southwick (3) devised a technique to posteriorly stabilize laminectomized spines using wire placed into the facets that are tightened around struts of bone graft.

For patients with atlantoaxial instability, Gallie (4) recommends placement of a wire sublaminarly under the posterior atlantal arch and then looped around the spinous process of C2. An **H**-shaped bone graft is compressed onto the C1 and C2 lamina when the wire is tightened. Brooks and Jenkins (5) reported successful outcomes in patients treated by four wires under both the C1 and C2 laminae, which when tightened compress wedges of bone graft between the C1 and C2 laminae. In the early 1990s, titanium cable was introduced that allows controlled tightening, compatibility with magnetic resonance imaging (MRI), and increased resistance to breakage (6).

The advantages of wire fixation are ease of application; safety, because it avoids placement of instruments or implants into the spinal canal or neuroforamen; an efficacy reported to be greater than 95%; low cost; and use of implants that are approved by the Food and Drug Administration (FDA). Limitations of wire fixation exist when there are fractured or insufficient laminae and spinous processes, facet fractures, or multiple-level injuries and when a significant component of the injury is from axial compression.

The goal of treatment of patients with cervical spine disease is to protect the neural structures, stabilize and reduce deformities and dislocations, and create an environment for maximal neurologic recovery. In patients with fracture and dislocation, this process begins with closed reduction. The need for decompression is then assessed clinically and by neuroimaging. In unstable fractures, posterior fusion is frequently warranted. This chapter reviews the techniques of closed reduction of cervical fractures and dislocations, and posterior wire fixation of the atlantoaxial and subaxial cervical spine. The indications for surgery, relevant biomechanics, and specifics of these common techniques are discussed.

CLOSED REDUCTION OF CERVICAL FRACTURE AND DISLOCATIONS

Animal studies and anecdotal human cases have shown that immediate reduction is the best treatment for acute spinal cord injuries due to fracture or dislocation of the cervical spine. This is best accomplished by placement of a cranial tong device and then awake closed reduction using traction weights. However, the technique should only be applied with a rigid protocol to minimize chances for neurologic deterioration (7,8). In patients who are neurologically intact, further considerations are in order before proceeding with reduction. Eismont et al. (9) have identified the potential for displacement of herniated disc material into the epidural dural space, with subsequent cord compression and worsening in patients with cervical facet dislocations. Patients at risk are those undergoing open reduction, those with a significant loss of disc heights, or those whose prereduction MRI demonstrates that the intervertebral disc lies posterior to the cranial vertebral body. Therefore, in patients with facet dislocations who are neurologically intact, magnetic resonance imaging should be obtained before reduction. If a disc herniation is present, then an anterior discectomy is indicated before attempts at reduction are made.

The closed reduction technique has proved safe if governed by a rigid protocol. Grant et al. (8) prospectively documented successful reduction in 97% of 122 patients.

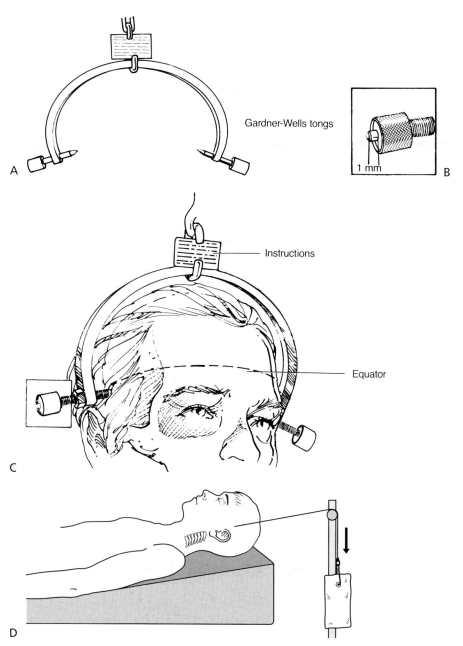

FIGURE 30.1. Application of traction weight using cranial tongs.

Only one patient had neurologic worsening 6 hours after reduction. Cotler et al. (10) similarly utilized a protocol involving application of up to 70% body weight in 39 patients, without neurologic worsening. Gardner-Wells tongs are preferred over the halo ring because they are simple to use, can be applied rapidly, and are effective. MRI-compatible sets using titanium pins and carbon fiber or aluminum bars are now available, although these hold less traction weight than stainless steel units (11). In patients with difficult fracture patterns, Rushton et al. (12) recommend the use of two tongs to better control reduction moments. Tong traction is contraindicated in patients with skull fractures or distractive injuries such as atlantooccipital dislocations, and in infants with open cranial sutures.

Surgical Technique: Closed Reduction Protocol

The tongs are connected to 5 to 10 pounds (2–5 kg) of weight using a rope and pulley (Fig. 30.1). The direction of tension is initially along the long axis of the patient but may be adjusted to help with reduction. After the traction weight is applied, a neurologic examination is repeated and a lateral radiograph is obtained. Neurologic function is carefully assessed, including the motor and sensory level. Complaints of increasing radicular pain or onset of paresthesias may herald neurologic worsening. The radiographs are reviewed for signs of overdistraction and reduction. Weights of 5 to 10 pounds (2–5 kg) are sequentially added only if no adverse neurologic changes occur and there are no signs of overdistraction. Overdistraction is best judged between the facet articulations and disc spaces. Disc height should not exceed 7 to 8 mm. However, in bilateral facet dislocations, an increased disc height may be required to overcome the slope and height of the superior facets before reduction can be achieved. Relaxation of the patient with anxiolytics or narcotics can be helpful to reduction. The use of C-arm fluoroscopy facilitates the speed of reduction.

The cycle of adding traction weight, repeating neurologic examination, and checking radiographs continues until reduction is achieved. Once achieved, traction weights can usually be reduced. Placing towels under the skull or thorax, changing the angle of applied traction, or gently manipulating the tongs may facilitate unlocking of facets and aid reduction. However, we do not recommend manipulative reductions. In cases of failed reduction, surgery is recommended after neural imaging.

ATLANTOAXIAL WIRE FIXATION

The strong posterior arches of the atlas and axis and the relatively large spinal canal usually allow safe placement of sublaminar wires for stabilization. Two wire techniques with many modifications have been developed. The Gallie technique is generically a sublaminar C1 wire that is looped around or through the spinous process of C2 and tightened over an **H**-shaped bone graft. In the Brooks technique, multiple sublaminar wires are placed under both the C1 and C2 laminae. These are tightened over wedge-shaped corticocancellous grafts that are compressed between the posterior arches. Both of these techniques (and their modifications) are highly effective, although a postoperative halo vest is usually required.

Indications and Contraindications

The Gallie and Brooks techniques are indicated to stabilize and achieve arthrodesis of unstable C1–2 articulations secondary to conditions such as trauma, inflammatory diseases, congenital anomalies such as os odontoideum, some destructive lesions, and osteoarthrosis of C1–2. Contraindications are fractures or missing posterior C1 or C2 arches, spinal stenosis at C1–2, or malreduction where wire passage could injure the neural elements.

Benefits and Limitations

The benefits of wire fixation of the atlantoaxial articulation are the relative ease of the techniques, good clinical results in up to 90% to 95% of cases, low cost, FDA approval of implants, and the minimal risk to neurologic or vascular structures. The limitation of wire fixation compared with other atlantoaxial stabilization techniques is the insufficient stability of the construct, so that a postoperative halo brace is required. Also, tightening of the posterior wire can induce retrolisthesis and malalignment when the odontoid is fractured or missing. The stabilization effect of these wire techniques is compromised by osteoporotic bone graft; therefore, results are poorer in groups such as patients with rheumatoid arthritis.

Preoperative Considerations

Preoperative evaluation must include a neuroimaging study to evaluate the bony structure and to determine if spinal canal stenosis is present. Spinal stenosis can result from malalignment, pannus formation, hematoma, or congenital small posterior arches. Spinal stenosis is a clear contraindication to sublaminar wire passage. In these cases, decompression of the lamina of C1 or C2 may be required and other techniques of C1–2 stabilization used. Congenitally immature posterior arches or atlantal spina bifida occulta are common anomalies that may prevent adequate wire stabilization.

Biomechanical Considerations

Atlantoaxial wire techniques require adequate bone stock of the C1 and C2 laminae as well as the bone graft to achieve sufficient stability. Similar to wire fixation in the subaxial cervical spine, the wires restore a posterior tension band. These constructs do not adequately control anterior translation; therefore, postoperative immobilization in a halo brace is required. Rotation is minimally controlled by the Gallie technique, but is significantly improved using the Brooks technique. In choosing an atlantoaxial technique, the biomechanics of injury, the relevant biomechanical strengths of fixation, and the type of postoperative immobilization should be considered. The surgical risks increase proportionally with improvement in biomechanical strength.

Numerous biomechanical studies have compared the Gallie technique, the Brooks method, and other stabilization techniques such as C1–2 transarticular screws. Hanley and Harvell (13) found that the Brooks technique was twice as stiff in extension and flexion and five times as stiff in rotation compared with the Gallie technique. Montesano et al. (14) and Grob and Crisco (15,16) compared the two wire techniques to the Magerl transarticular screw method. The Gallie technique was associated with significant increased motion in flexion, extension, and rotation compared with the Brooks or Magerl techniques. The Brooks technique was similar to the Magerl method in resisting these forces. However, the Magerl technique was significantly better at limiting anteroposterior shear.

Instruments

Few special instruments are required. A small suture passer (as used in Bankart shoulder repair) is helpful for safe sublaminar wire passage. Currently, we recommend titanium or multistrand polyethylene cable. Special instruments for tensioning and crimping of cables will be required. In the standard techniques, 18- or 20-gauge stainless steel wire is used. Lateral fluoroscopy is not required.

Anesthesia and Positioning

The patient is positioned prone with the head held in a Mayfield device as described in Chapter 1 (Fig. 30.2). A lateral radiograph is obtained to assess alignment and to identify if adequate space is present between the occiput and C1 to allow wire passage. If needed,

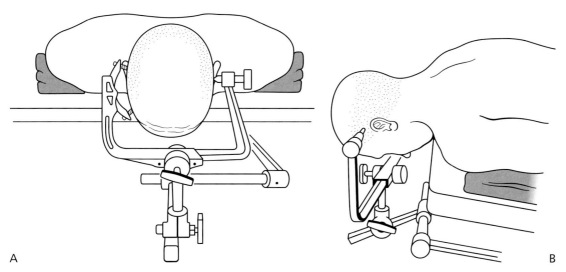

FIGURE 30.2. Prone positioning using Mayfield head-holding device. The pins are positioned at or below the skull equator and tightened to 60 to 80 pounds. The patient is turned prone, with the surgeon holding the head. Transverse rolls are placed under the patient's chest and pelvis to allow ventilation. The head is maintained in a neutral position, and radiographs are obtained to check alignment. **A:** Cranial view. **B:** Lateral view.

the head position is corrected. The skin from the skull inion to T1 and the iliac crest is prepared and draped sterilely.

Alternatively, the patient may be positioned in a halo vest. Halo vest placement and anatomic alignment are best achieved before surgery. In this case, the patient undergoes an awake nasotracheal intubation and is simply turned prone. The posterior shell and bars may be removed to allow access to the posterior neck, although we have usually been able to perform surgery with the vest intact.

Surgical Techniques

Gallie C1–2 Fusion

A midline incision is performed from the occiput to the caudal aspect of C2. The laminar arch of C1, spinous process of C2, and C2 lamina are exposed subperiosteally. Limit dissection to no more than 1.5 cm from the midline on the posterior C1 arch to prevent injury to the vertebral artery. Avoid penetration of the thin atlantoaxial membrane between the laminae.

To create a safe passage for the sublaminar wires, subperiosteally dissect on the cranial and caudal surfaces of the C1 lamina with 4–0 angled curettes to create a subperiosteal envelope. A suture passer is placed under the lamina and a no. 1 suture is grasped and pulled through (Fig. 30.3A). An 18- or 20-gauge wire is looped and tied to the end of the suture on the caudal side of the C1 posterior arch. The wire loop is bent in a small semicircle and gently pulled under the C1 lamina from the caudal to the cranial direction (Fig. 30.3B). The wire loop is pulled caudally and placed under the C2 spinous process (Fig. 30.3C). The arms of the wire are pulled laterally about 1 cm.

A 3 cm by 4 cm by 1 cm bone graft is harvested from the posterior iliac crest. It is contoured by notching on its caudal surface for the spinous process of C2 and on its inner surface to allow a close approximation to the curved C1 lamina (Fig. 30.3D). Additional notches are placed laterally for the wires. The graft is checked for fit and modified as needed. The C1 and C2 laminae and spinous process of C2 are lightly decorticated with a high-speed burr. The **H**-shaped graft is located onto the laminae, and the free ends of the wire are tightened over the graft (Fig. 30.3E). This should compress the graft down onto the laminae. A lateral radiograph is obtained to check alignment and position of the graft and wire. Carefully assess the alignment because retrolisthesis can

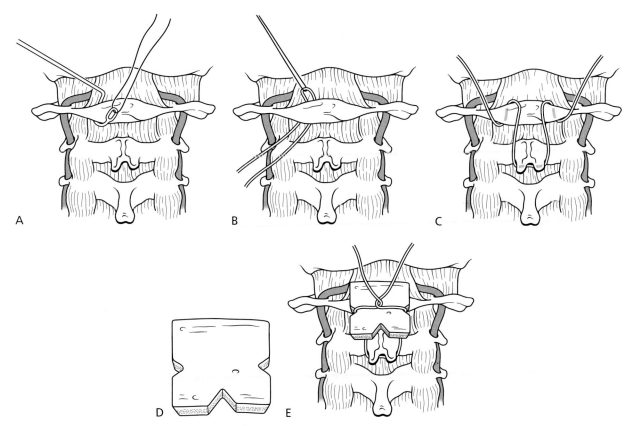

FIGURE 30.3. Gallie technique. **A:** A suture passer is placed under the C1 lamina and grasps a no. 1 suture, which is pulled under the lamina. **B:** A loop of 18-gauge wire is bent into a small semicircle, tied to the suture, and pulled under C1 from the caudal to cranial direction. **C:** The wire loop is passed under the C2 spinous process, and the arms at C1 are spread laterally. **D:** An iliac corticocancellous graft (3 cm by 4 cm by 1 cm) is harvested and notched inferiorly for the C2 spinous process. The cranial inner surface is contoured to match the curvature of the C1 lamina. Lateral notches stabilize the wire. **E:** The free wire ends are tightened, compressing the graft onto the C1 and C2 laminae.

occur in posteriorly unstable conditions. Additional cancellous bone graft is placed between any exposed bone on the laminae of C1 and C2.

The muscles and fascia are closed in two layers. It is important to repair the short occipital rotator muscles and the ligamentous nuchae to the spinous process of C2. The subcutaneous tissue and skin are closed using routine methods.

A modification of the Gallie technique is to place one wire sublaminarly at C1 and a second through the C2 spinous process. A loop of 18- or 20-gauge wire is passed under the C1 lamina from a cranial to caudal direction using the suture method. The free ends of the wire are passed inside the loop and then are tensioned, taking up the slack. This creates a tight loop around the C1 arch with two free ends of wire. A 3-mm hole is placed over each side at the base of the spinous process with a burr. The holes are connected with a Lewin clamp or towel clip. A second 18- or 20-gauge wire is passed through the hole in C2, under the C2 spinous process, and back through the hole to exit on the side opposite from where it was initially inserted. An **H**-shaped graft as described for the Gallie technique is harvested, contoured, and placed onto the decorticated C1 and C2 laminae. On each side, the free ends of the C1 and C2 wires are tightened, securing the graft to the laminae.

Brooks C1–2 Fusion

This section describes a modification of the Brooks method using multistrand cable and crimps. Positioning and exposure is performed as described previously for the Gallie technique. The interspace between C2 and C3 is additionally exposed. This may require the removal of a small amount of the caudal C2 lamina, which is normally shingled over the C2–3 interspace. This can be accomplished using a burr or 3-mm Kerrison rongeur. The C2–3 epidural space is entered using angled curettes. Removal of a small amount of the ligamentum flavum with Kerrison rongeurs facilitates wire passage. Subperiosteal dissection along the cranial laminar surface of C2 and both the cranial and caudal surfaces of C1 creates avenues for sublaminar wires.

Starting at the C2–3 interspace, a wire passer is placed in a cranial direction under the C2 lamina. A no. 1 suture is grasped at C1–2 and pulled under C2 using the suture passer. With a similar technique, a suture is passed under the C1 lamina (Fig. 30.4A). The suture at C2–3 is tied to the malleable lead of a titanium cable. It is pulled cranially under the C2 lamina and out the C1–2 interspace. The same cable is tied to the C1 sublaminar suture at C1–2 and pulled under the C1 arch from the caudal to cranial direction (Fig. 30.4B). The process is repeated once on the same side and twice on the oppo-

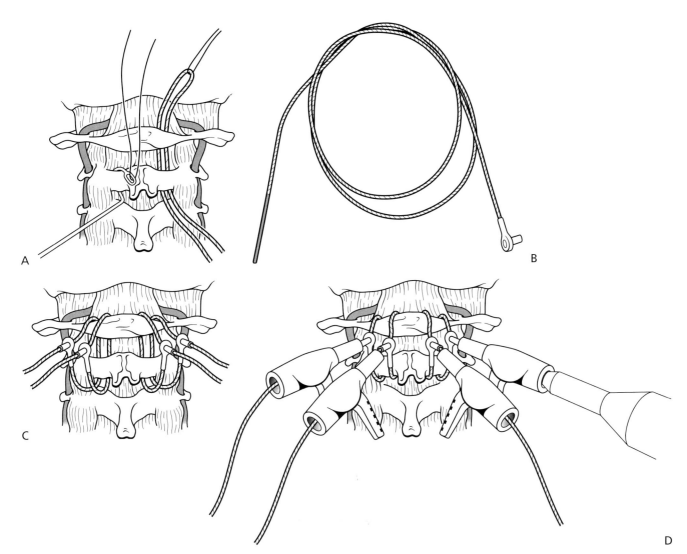

FIGURE 30.4. Brooks C1–2 arthrodesis technique. **A:** Sutures are placed under both C1 and C2. This requires removal of a small amount of the C2 spinous process and lamina to gain access to the C2–3 interspace. **B:** Titanium cable with soft malleable leader and crimp. **C:** The titanium cable is pulled under the C2 lamina and then under the C1 lamina, using the suture tied to the malleable leader on the cable. The process is repeated until four cables, two on each side, are placed. **D:** Two corticocancellous grafts are placed between the spinous processes and secured by cable tensioning. Temporary crimping devices are applied. Tension is applied with a calibrated tensioning device. *Continued.*

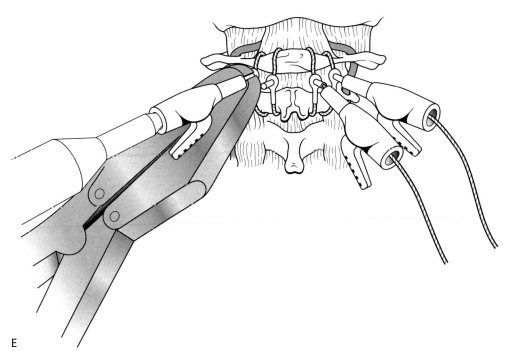

FIGURE 30.4. *(continued)* **E:** After an equal amount of tension is applied to all cables, the crimps are compressed.

site side, ending with four cables (two on each side) under both the C1 and C2 arches (Fig. 30.4C).

Triangular-shaped corticocancellous grafts are harvested from the posterior iliac crest. They are sized and shaped to wedge tightly between the C1 and C2 laminae. These grafts are checked for fit and modified as needed. The C1 and C2 laminae are lightly decorticated with a burr. The grafts are located, and then the free ends of the cables are passed through the crimp. Temporary crimping devices are placed onto all cables (Fig. 30.4D).

Creating equal tension on all four cables requires care because overtensioning one may loosen the tension on others. To accomplish this task, the free end of one cable is placed into the tensioning instrument. Progressively increased tension is applied and then locked using the temporary crimping devices. The tensioner is moved to the opposite side and back and forth until all cables have equal tension of 25 to 35 pounds (100–140 N). At this point, the crimps are compressed using the crimping tool (Fig. 30.4E). Excess cable is sectioned and removed. All cables are checked for adequate tension. A lateral radiograph is obtained to evaluate alignment. Retrolisthesis can occur due to excessive tensioning of the posterior wires. Additional cancellous bone graft is placed at any exposed bony surfaces on C1 or C2. Closure is as described for the Gallie fusion.

Postoperative Management of C1–2 Wire Techniques

Patients may be placed in cervicothoracic braces or the halo vest for 10 to 12 weeks. We prefer the latter time period for patients with anteroposterior instability or poor bone quality.

WIRE FIXATION OF THE SUBAXIAL CERVICAL SPINE (C2–T1)

In the subaxial spine (C2–T1), wires can anchor to the spinous processes, in the facets, and under the lamina. Common spinous process techniques are the Rogers technique (1) and the triple-wire technique of Bohlman (2). Facet techniques are used less frequently now that lateral mass screw fixation is available, but can be used to stabilize spines with fractured or missing laminae (3). Sublaminar wire fixation is rarely indicated, except in some patients with rheumatoid arthritis, and is potentially dangerous; therefore, it will not be discussed.

Indications

Posterior wire fixation of C2-T1 is indicated for unstable spines in patients with intact laminae and spinous processes. Fracture types include unilateral or bilateral facet dislocations, facet fracture dislocations, fracture separations of the lateral masses, posterior ligamentous injury, and some bursting fractures with posterior osteoligamentous injury. It is also indicated as an adjunct to anterior surgery following trauma or other destructive processes. Posterior wiring is indicated as an adjunct to multilevel anterior fusions, management of pseudoarthrosis, treatment for instability adjacent to a fused segment, and for patients with subaxial subluxation from rheumatoid arthritis. Posterior interspinous wire fixation is contraindicated in patients with fractured spinous processes or laminae at the levels to be stabilized and for patients who require posterior decompression.

Multilevel facet wire fixation is indicated when the laminae or spinous processes or both are fractured or missing. The technique described by Southwick (3) uses long rib or iliac struts that lie over on the lateral masses and are stabilized with multiple facet wires. In most cases, this is not a stable construct and requires postoperative halo vest bracing. Rotationally unstable injuries can be stabilized by a facet wire that is looped around the caudal spinous process, as advocated by Edwards et al. (17). This wire is called the oblique wire.

Benefits and Limitations

Posterior wire stabilization of C2-T1 has been proved to be highly reliable, safe, low cost, and well tolerated by patients (1,18). The implants are readily available, utilize standard equipment, and are FDA approved. Wire stabilization is less effective in certain injury patterns such as extension and axial loading. Wire fixation may require additional levels if the spinous processes are fractured or small. Compared with plate stabilization, wire fixation requires more rigid postoperative bracing.

Biomechanical Considerations

Most unstable cervical conditions involve hyperflexion with the center of rotation within the disc or at the anterior longitudinal ligament. Under this injury pattern, posterior wiring has a biomechanical advantage over anterior plates because the location of implant application is at the spinous process, which increases the moment arm two- to threefold. Biomechanically, interspinous wire fixation restores the normal tension band of the nuchal ligament complex. Also, prevention of the spreading of the spinous processes limits coupled rotational movements and therefore resists displacement in unilateral facet dislocations. However, standard wire constructs fail to resist extension, although modification such as that described by Bohlman minimizes this limitation.

Many biomechanical studies have demonstrated that wire fixation increases motion segment stiffness to two to three times normal (19–22). Posterior wire fixation is, in general, similar in stiffness to the anterior plate, but is significantly less stiff than lateral mass plate stabilization. The type and size of wire or cable also influence the stability of fixation (23,24). Weis et al. (23) compared stainless steel wire, cable, titanium wire and cable, polyethylene cable, and anterior cervical plate. They found that multistrut cable was preferable to monofilament wire and that wire fixation was intermediate in strength to anterior plate fixation and posterior lateral mass fixation.

Despite the positive effects of fixation on the biomechanics, loosening of implants and pull-out or fracturing of the spinous processes can occur, with resultant loss of stability and potential for deformity and nonunion. Therefore, in the majority of patients, postoperative immobilization in an orthosis should be prescribed.

Preoperative Considerations

Preoperatively, patients should be imaged to determine if decompression is required. Additionally, the status of the posterior elements is assessed to determine if wire stabilization is feasible. Decompression of depressed laminal fracture or foraminotomy can be accomplished during posterior fusion, although these may require extension of the construct to more levels. Alternative techniques should be considered under these conditions. Reduction should be attempted by closed means preoperatively, as discussed earlier.

Instrumentation and Imaging

Standard operative instruments are required, including a 3-mm high-speed burr. A Lewin clamp or large towel clip is needed to complete formation of a hole in the spinous process. The surgeon can choose 18- or 20-gauge stainless steel wire, multiple strands of 22-gauge wire twisted into a cable, or stainless steel, titanium, or polyethylene cable. Cables require special crimps, tensioning devices, and crimping tools. Lateral fluoroscopy is not required. A turning frame that allows maintenance of traction is advantageous in patients with acute injuries.

Anesthesia and Positioning

Patients with unstable spines undergo an awake nasotracheal intubation and are positioned prone using a turning frame while maintaining traction (Fig. 30.5A). After a neurologic check, the patient is placed under general anesthesia and a lateral radiograph is obtained. Repositioning of the head and neck is performed as needed. In cases where a reduction will be required, spinal cord monitoring is performed. The neck and iliac crest are prepared with antiseptic and draped sterilely.

Surgical Techniques

Rogers Interspinous Wire

A midline incision is made over the levels where arthrodesis is to be achieved. Subperiosteal dissection of the spinous processes, laminae, and lateral masses is performed. If possible, a cuff of soft tissue between the spinous processes is maintained. A lateral radiograph with a marker over the facet joint or a spinous process confirms the level.

After exposure, the base of the spinous processes is inspected. A 3-mm hole is placed in the base of the spinous processes on each side just above the spinal canal (Fig. 30.5B,C). The hole is completed with a Lewin clamp or towel clip. Careful selection of the location of the hole at the base of the spinous process is required to avoid placement of wire into the spinal canal but allow adequate bone stock for fixation.

An 18- or 20-gauge stainless steel wire or multistrand cable is passed through the cranial spinous processes from one side through to the opposite side (Fig. 30.5D). It is passed over the cranial edge of the spinous process and back through the hole to the opposite side. The wire or cable is now passed through the caudal spinous process, around the caudal edge of that spinous process, and back through the spinous process (Fig. 30.5E). The two free ends are now aligned on the same side. Corticocancellous plates of graft are placed under the wires as the free ends of the wire are twisted and tightened (Fig. 30.5F). In the case of cable, tension of 30 to 40 pounds is applied and then the crimp is compressed. A lateral radiograph is obtained to check alignment and position of

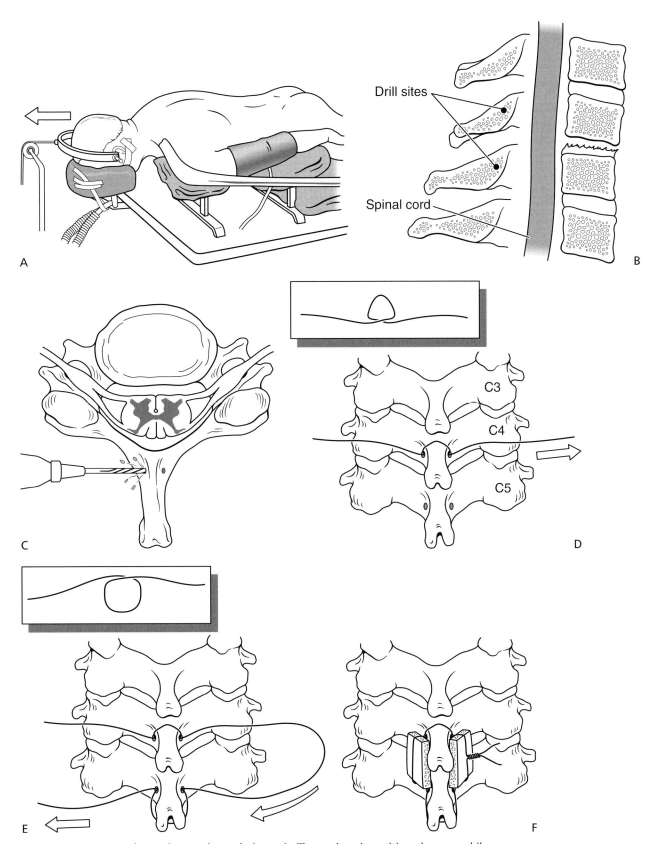

FIGURE 30.5. Rogers interspinous wire technique. **A:** The patient is positioned prone while maintaining traction on a turning frame. **B:** The location for wire placement is at the base of the spinous process, just above the spinal canal. **C:** A 3-mm drill hole is placed on each side with a high-speed burr. The hole is completed with a Levin clamp. **D:** A 20-gauge wire is passed through the drill hole, above the cranial edge of the spinous process, and back through the hole. **E:** The wire is passed through the hole in the caudal spinous process, around its caudal edge, and back through. **F:** Corticocancellous plates of bone graft are placed under the wires on each side as the wires are tightened. All slack is taken up before tightening.

the wire. Alternatively, two wires can be used, one in each spinous process. These are similarly looped around the spinous processes and back through the hole. The wires are then tightened simultaneously over the bone graft. The laminae and facets are decorticated and packed with additional cancellous bone graft.

The muscles and fascia are closed in two layers. Attempt to repair the ligamentum nuchae to the spinous processes. The subcutaneous layer and skin are closed per routine.

Bohlman Triple-Wire Technique

The Bohlman triple-wire technique involves placing a midline Rogers interspinous wire and then adding a second and third wire that rigidly hold corticocancellous plates of graft along the spinous processes (18). After placement of the interspinous wires, 22-gauge wires or cable are passed through the holes in each spinous process (Fig. 30.6A). Corticocancellous plates of bone, 1.5 cm by 3 cm by 1 cm, are harvested and contoured to lie along the spinous processes. Three-millimeter holes are placed through the grafts that align with those in the spinous processes. The wires are passed through the grafts, which are then held down onto the vertebrae. The wires are then tightened and crimped (Fig. 30.6B). A lateral radiograph is taken to assure correct placement of wire and reduction.

Facet Wire

The technique of facet wiring requires placement of a hole starting dorsally in the inferior facet that passes into the facet articulation and has sufficient bone stock to give adequate stability. A 3-mm hole is placed with a high-speed burr starting at the center of the lateral mass and directed slightly caudal into the articulation. The hole is examined to assure penetration into the joint. An elevator is placed into the facet joint to aid visualization and act as a back stop for the burr. A malleable multistrand wire or cable is passed from a dorsal to ventral direction through the hole, into the facet joint. It is grasped and pulled out through the joint. The process is repeated at as many levels as are desired.

In the Southwick stabilization technique, which is used to stabilize the cervical spine following multilevel laminectomies, multiple facet wires are placed. Struts of rib or long segments of iliac graft are placed inside the arms of each wire and then secured by wire tightening. Usually, stabilization is extended from one level above to one below the laminectomy defect or as cranially as C2. Postoperative immobilization with the halo vest is recommended.

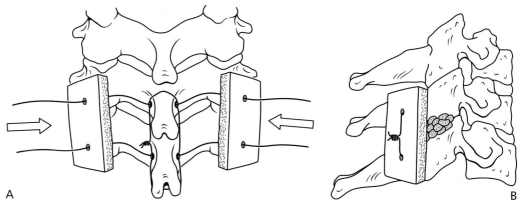

A

B

FIGURE 30.6. Bohlman triple-wire technique. **A:** A midline interspinous wire is placed, similar to the Rogers technique. The second and third wire are passed through each spinous process. Corticocancellous plates of bone graft are harvested. Appropriately spaced 3-mm drill holes are placed in the grafts. **B:** Wire tightening secures the bone graft to the spinous processes.

The oblique wire technique utilizes a facet wire placed as described previously (17). The wire on the fractured or dislocated side is looped around the next caudal spinous process and tightened. A midline interspinous wire using the Rogers technique is added. Bone graft is placed onto the decorticated laminae and facet joints.

Postoperative Care

Patients are immobilized in a cervicothoracic brace such as a Minerva brace for 6 to 8 weeks. In patients with fewer degrees of instability, a hard collar may be used. Patients with more comminuted fractures or multiple-level injuries may require a halo brace. At 6 to 9 weeks, flexion-extension radiographs are obtained to confirm fusion.

COMPLICATIONS OF WIRE FIXATION OF THE CERVICAL SPINE

Complications are infrequent using posterior wire techniques. In the atlantoaxial articulation, loss of fixation can occur secondary to unstable patterns, poor bone quality, or improper immobilization. Sublaminar wire placement requires a controlled technique to avoid spinal cord injury. Prior to wire placement, adequate space must be present as determined by preoperative imaging and intraoperative radiographs. Nonunion occurs in about 5% of cases and can be treated using a similar technique with postoperative halo vest immobilization or by C1–2 transarticular screws.

In the lower cervical spine, preexisting injury, immature bony structure, or excessive tensioning may lead to intraoperative or postoperative fracture of the spinous process. Placement of drill holes too deep in the spinous process can cause epidural wire placement and the potential for neurologic deficits. Nonunion occurs in less than 3% of cases and is usually associated with loosening of the implant. Wire breakage is seen more frequently with single-strand wire, especially when kinked during implantation. The use of cable or multistrand wire can mitigate this problem. Infections occur more frequently in patients with acute spinal cord injuries and are treated by incision and drainage and 6 weeks of antibiotics.

CONCLUSION

Wire fixation has an important role in achieving fixation and arthrodesis of the cervical spine. It is safe, effective, and low cost. The use of multistrand wire or cable is recommended. Postoperatively, patients should be immobilized in cervicothoracic orthoses until healing has occurred.

REFERENCES

1. Rogers WA. Treatment of fracture-dislocation of the cervical spine. *J Bone Joint Surg Am* 1942;24:245–258.
2. Bohlman HH. Acute fractures and dislocations of the cervical spine. An analysis of three hundred hospitalized patients and review of the literature. *J Bone Joint Surg Am* 1979;61:1119–1142.
3. Callahan RA, Margolis RM, Keggi RN, et al. Cervical facet fusion for control of instability following laminectomy. *J Bone Joint Surg Am* 1977;59:991–1002.
4. Gallie WE. Fractures and dislocations of the cervical spine. *Am J Surg* 1939;46:494–499.
5. Brooks AL, Jenkins EB. Atlanto-axial arthrodesis by the wedge compression method. *J Bone Joint Surg Am* 1978;60:279–284.
6. Songer MN, Spencer DL, Meyer PR, et al. The use of sublaminar cables to replace Luque wires. *Spine* 1991;6:S418–S421.

7. Star AM, Jones AA, Cotler JM, et al. Immediate closed reduction of cervical spine dislocations using traction. *Spine* 1990;15:1068–1072.
8. Grant GA, Mirza SK, Chapman JR, et al. Risk of early closed reduction in cervical spine subluxation injuries. *J Neurosurg* 1999;90(suppl 1):13–18.
9. Eismont FJ, Arena MJ, Green BA. Extrusion of an intervertebral disc associated with traumatic subluxation or dislocation of cervical facets. Case report. *J Bone Joint Surg Am* 1991;73:1555–1560.
10. Cotler JM, Herbison GJ, Nasuti JF, et al. Closed reduction of traumatic cervical spine dislocation using traction weights up to 140 pounds. *Spine* 1993;18:386–390.
11. Blumberg KD, Catalano JB, Cotler JM, et al. The pullout strength of titanium alloy MRI-compatible and stainless steel MRI-incompatible Gardner-Wells tongs. *Spine* 1993;18:1895–1896.
12. Rushton SA, Vaccaro AR, Levine MJ, et al. Bivector traction for unstable cervical spine fractures: a description of its application and preliminary results. *J Spinal Disord* 1997;10:436–440.
13. Hanley EN, Harvell JC. Immediate postoperative stability of the atlantoaxial articulation: a biomechanical study comparing simple midline wiring, and the Gallie and Brooks procedures. *J Spinal Disord* 1992;5:306–310.
14. Montesano PX, Juach EC, Anderson PA, et al. Biomechanics of cervical spine internal fixation. *Spine* 1991;16:S10–S16.
15. Grob D, Crisco JJ, Panjabi MM, et al. Biomechanical evaluation of four different posterior atlantoaxial fixation techniques. *Spine* 1992;17:480–490.
16. Crisco JJ, Panjabi MM, Oda T, et al. Bone graft translation of four upper cervical spine fixation techniques in a cadaveric model. *J Orthop Res* 1991;9:835–846.
17. Edwards CC, Matz SO, Levine AM. The oblique wiring technique for rotational injuries of the cervical spine. *Orthop Trans* 1986;10:455.
18. Weiland DJ, McAfee PC. Posterior cervical fusion with triple-wire strut graft technique: one hundred consecutive patients. *J Spinal Disord* 1991;4:15–21.
19. Coe JD, Warden KE, Sutterlin CE, et al. Biomechanical evaluation of cervical spinal stabilization methods in a human cadaveric model. *Spine* 1989;14:1122–1131.
20. Sutterlin CE, McAfee PC, Warden KE, et al. A biomechanical evaluation of cervical spinal stabilization methods in a bovine model. Static and cyclical loading. *Spine* 1988;13:795–802.
21. Traynelis VC, Donaher PA, Roach RM, et al. Biomechanical comparison of anterior Caspar plate and three-level posterior fixation techniques in a human cadaveric model. *J Neurosurg* 1993;79:96–103.
22. Ulrich C, Woersdoerfer O, Kalff R, et al. Biomechanics of fixation systems to the cervical spine. *Spine* 1991;16:S4–S9.
23. Weis JC, Cunningham BW, Kanayama M, et al. *In vitro* biomechanical comparison of multistrand cables with conventional cervical stabilization. *Spine* 1996;21:2108–2114.
24. Scuderi GJ, Greenberg SS, Cohen DS, et al. A biomechanical evaluation of magnetic resonance imaging-compatible wire in cervical spine fixation. *Spine* 1993;18:1991–1994.

POSTERIOR LATERAL MASS PLATING

MARSHAL D. PERIS
JAMES D. KANG

Surgical conditions requiring posterior cervical spinal surgery fall into many diagnostic categories. These include deformity and degenerative, traumatic, infectious, and neoplastic conditions. The two most common techniques for posterior fixation in the cervical spine are wiring and plating. Although either technique can provide adequate fixation to achieve a fusion, it has been shown by many authors that posterior plating is biomechanically superior (1–9). Indications for using the plating technique include nonunion of anterior fusion, trauma with intact posterior bony elements, postlaminectomy kyphosis or other deformity, or additional fixation after anterior cervical surgery. Contraindications to using the plating technique are trauma to the lateral masses, congenital anomalies, or anatomic variations of the facets, vertebral arteries, or nerve roots.

Plain radiographs, computed tomographic (CT) myelography, and magnetic resonance imaging (MRI) all have specific diagnostic roles in preoperatively evaluating patients. For example, CT scans are invaluable for assessing the bony details of the cervical spine and may be particularly helpful in planning for spinal instrumentation. MRI scans in general do not provide accurate bony detail, but they do provide good neurologic anatomy. Both studies can provide adequate localization of the vertebral arteries in relation to the lateral masses.

Several different techniques for lateral mass screw insertion have been described in the literature. The original technique described by Roy-Camille places the screw in a straight trajectory in the sagittal plane and 10 degrees lateral in the coronal plane. The Magerl technique places the screw parallel to the facet joint in the sagittal plane and 25 degrees lateral in the coronal plane. The An technique, which is a modification of the Magerl technique, is described later in this chapter.

COMPLICATIONS

Complications can include screw breakage or pullout, plate breakage, nonunion, vertebral artery injury, nerve root injury, and spinal cord impingement. Graham et al. (5) performed a prospective study of 21 consecutive patients with posterior lateral mass plating using a total of 164 screws. They found no vertebral artery or spinal cord injury, but did find 1.8% risk of radiculopathy per screw placed. Wellman et al. (10) retrospectively reviewed 43 patients with 281 screws placed and found no root injury or vertebral artery injuries, but did report one hardware failure requiring additional surgery.

BIOMECHANICS

Biomechanical testing comparing posterior cervical fixation has been ongoing for at least two decades. In 1988, Gill et al. (11) concluded that plates with bicortical screws provided the most stiffness when compared with plates with unicortical screws and intraspinous wiring, but this was not a statistically significant result. In 1991, Montesano et al. (8) tested the strengths of the constructs with two different screw placement techniques. They found that angulating the screws both cephalad and lateral was superior to no cephalo-caudad angulation in terms of load to failure.

In reference to reconstruction of the cervical spine, two studies have been performed to address the biomechanics of additional posterior cervical fixation. The first, by Kirkpatrick et al. (12), tested flexibility after corpectomy and strut grafting alone compared with the addition of anterior or posterior plates. They found the stiffness and load to failure to be greatest after anterior strut and posterior plating. Swank et al. (13) retrospectively reviewed 17 patients after anterior multilevel decompression and strut grafting with posterior plating. They found no nonunions and one radiculopathy associated with a malplaced screw.

AUTHORS' PREFERRED METHOD

The technique in using lateral mass plating has evolved over many years. For procedures involving lateral mass plating, we recommend prone positioning because it gives the sur-

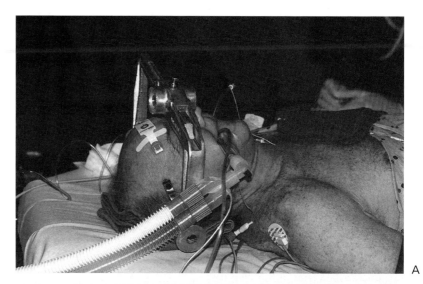

A

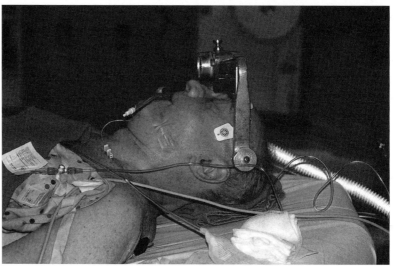

B

FIGURE 31.1. Application of Mayfield tongs prior to placing the patient in the prone position.

geon a counterforce for the use of the drill and insertion of the screws. The prone position also allows for easy retraction of both sides of the spinal musculature, and gravity allows the plates and bone graft to remain in the wound. Prior to positioning the patient in the prone position, we recommend using Mayfield tongs for head positioning and stabilization (Fig. 31.1). The Mayfield tongs provide excellent stability to the head and neck area during the dissection as well as during the instrumentation. In addition, the risk to the eyes is minimized compared with those devices (such as a horseshoe headrest) that have been associated with blindness from retinal artery thrombosis (14). Once the body and neck are positioned and the head is stabilized, the arms should be tucked at the patient's side and the shoulders taped down (Fig. 31.2). The benefit of taping is to provide easier visualization for your intraoperative radiograph and to remove the skin creases from the posterior cervical skin.

Once a lateral radiograph is taken to verify spinal level, only the levels to be fused should be exposed laterally in order to preserve the facet joints of unfused levels. A time-saving hint is to harvest the iliac crest bone graft while your radiograph is being developed. Depending on the number of levels being fused, the amount of bone graft necessary may be minimal. After the exposure is completed, the surgeon may at this time consider decompressing the neural elements if the diagnostic condition requires it. If a decompression is not necessary, the surgeon may proceed with the spinal fusion and instrumentation. A postoperative lateral radiograph should be taken prior to wound closure to ensure good placement and angulation of the screws and good position of the spine (Fig. 31.3). After instrumentation is complete, we use a 4-mm burr to decorticate the levels to be fused, including the facet, lamina, and spinous process. The bone graft is then placed over these levels to achieve a biological arthrodesis. After closure and sterile dressing, we use a rigid collar for 6 weeks followed by a soft collar for the ensuing 6 weeks as needed.

Currently, we recommend using titanium plates to allow ease of imaging postoperatively. We recommend using a system that allows freedom of screw direction and also has multiple options for hole diameter. The plate should be contoured to the desired lordosis prior to fixation. In a multilevel fusion, we drill and place a screw in our most proximal hole first, and then the most distal hole. This leaves the plate flush with the spine if contoured correctly and allows easy placement of the remaining intermediate screws. We also use a drill stop (at 14 mm) with a drill guide to control the depth of drilling. The screws should be 3.5 mm in diameter, with the possibility of using a 4.0-mm screw as a rescue screw. All holes should be tapped prior to screw insertion, and a depth gauge should be

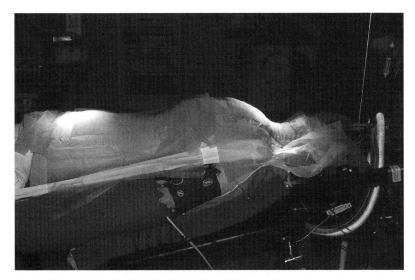

FIGURE 31.2. Patient in prone position with arms tucked and taped prior to draping.

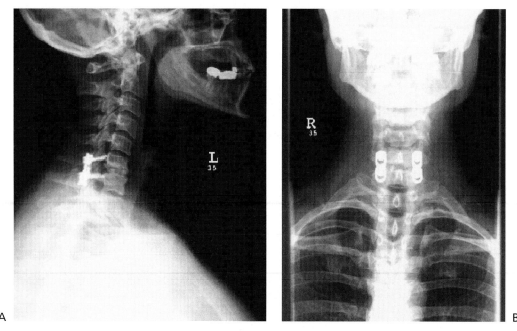

FIGURE 31.3. Postoperative anteroposterior and lateral radiographs.

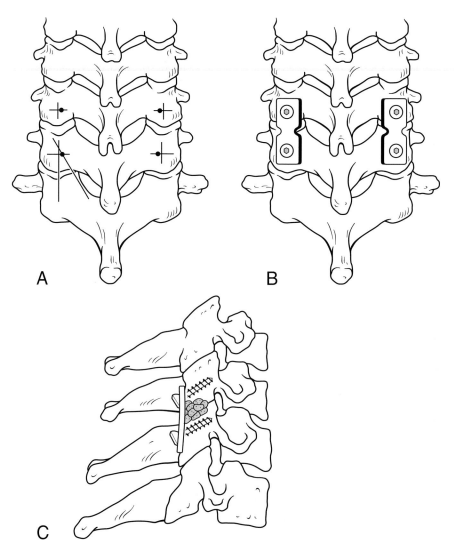

FIGURE 31.4. Diagram showing appropriate starting point and angulation of screw in relation to the lateral mass and facet joint. (Redrawn from An HS, Cotler JM, eds. *Spinal instrumentation,* 2nd ed. Philadelphia: Lippincott Williams & Wilkins, 1999, with permission.)

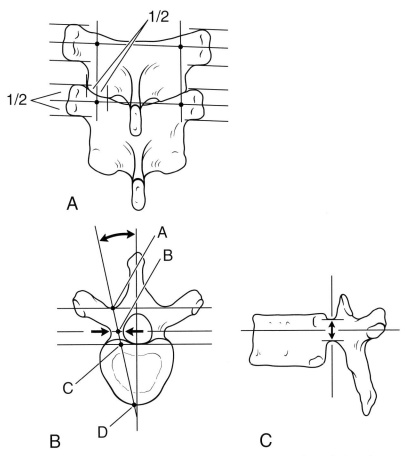

FIGURE 31.5. Diagram showing appropriate starting point and angulation of screw for pedicle insertion. (Redrawn from An HS, Cotler JM, eds. *Spinal instrumentation,* 2nd ed. Philadelphia: Lippincott Williams & Wilkins, 1999, with permission.)

used to make accurate screw length measurements. Most patients can accommodate a 14-mm screw in their lateral masses as a unicortical screw. Although some authors have advocated bicortical screw purchase to achieve optimal stabilization, we believe that this is usually not necessary. Unicortical screws have shown equally successful clinical results, and they minimize the risk to the vertebral artery and the nerve roots (15).

The optimal direction for the drill and screw has been researched extensively. We currently utilize the technique recommended by An et al. (16), which uses an entry point 1 mm medial to the center of the lateral mass and angled 30 degrees lateral and 15 degrees cephalad (Fig. 31.4). We recommend using the intraoperative radiograph to assess cephalad angulation at each level. Often, to achieve good fixation at the cervicothoracic junction, pedicle screws must be used. If these screws are needed, a laminoforaminotomy should be performed to palpate the pedicle prior to drilling and screw insertion (Fig. 31.5). Another option, if necessary, is to place transfacet screws. Klekamp et al. (17) performed an *in vitro* assessment of screw pullout strength that compared the standard lateral mass fixation to transfacet fixation. They found the pullout strength of the transfacet screw placement to be comparable to, if not greater than, lateral mass placement.

CONCLUSION

Posterior lateral mass plating is an excellent technique for posterior cervical fusion. It has shown biomechanical superiority over other techniques, with improved fusion rates and higher rigidity. As with any surgical technique, there is a learning curve associated with lateral mass plating, but close attention to anatomic details and precise placement of the screws will limit potential disastrous complications. Unless anatomy dictates otherwise, posterior lateral mass plating should be used for most posterior cervical fusions in the subaxial spine, with expected excellent results.

REFERENCES

1. Anderson PA, Henley MB, Grady MS, et al. Posterior cervical arthrodesis with AO reconstruction plates and bone graft. *Spine* 1991;16S:S72–S79.
2. Cooper PR, Cohen A, Rosiello A, et al. Posterior stabilization of cervical spine fractures and subluxations using plates and screws. *Neurosurgery* 1988;23:300–306.
3. Ebraheim NA, An HS, Jackson WT, et al. Internal fixation of the unstable cervical spine using posterior Roy-Camille plates: preliminary report. *J Orthop Trauma* 1989;3:23–28.
4. Errico T, Uhl R, Cooper P, et al. Pullout strength comparison of two methods of orienting screw insertion in the lateral masses. *J Spinal Disord* 1992;7:429–438.
5. Graham AW, Swank ML, Kinard RE, et al. Posterior cervical arthrodesis and stabilization with a lateral mass plate: clinical and computed tomographic evaluation of lateral mass screw placement and associated complications. *Spine* 1996;21:323–328.
6. Grubb MR, Currier BL, Stone J, et al. Biomechanical evaluation of posterior cervical stabilization after a wide laminectomy. *Spine* 1997;22:1948–1954.
7. Montesano PX, Juach E, Jonsson H Jr. Anatomic and biomechanical study of posterior cervical spine plate arthrodesis: an evaluation of two different techniques of screw placement. *J Spinal Disord* 1992;5:301–305.
8. Montesano PX, Juach E, Anderson PA, et al. Biomechanics of cervical spine internal fixation. *Spine* 1991;16(suppl):S10–S16.
9. Sutterlin CE III, McAfee PC, Warden KE, et al. A biomechanical evaluation of cervical spinal stabilization methods in a bovine model. *Spine* 1988;13:795–802.
10. Wellman BJ, Follett KA, Traynelis VC. Complications of posterior articular mass plate fixation of the subaxial cervical spine in 43 consecutive patients. *Spine* 1998;23:193–200.
11. Gill K, Paschal S, Corin J, et al. Posterior plating of the cervical spine: a biomechanical comparison of different posterior fusion techniques. *Spine* 1988;13:813–816.
12. Kirkpatrick JS, Levy JA, Carillo J, et al. Reconstruction after multilevel corpectomy in the cervical spine: a sagittal plane biomechanical study. *Spine* 1999;24:1186–1191.
13. Swank ML, Sutterlin CE III, Bossons CR, et al. Rigid internal fixation with lateral mass plates in multilevel anterior and posterior reconstruction of the cervical spine. *Spine* 1997;22:274–282.
14. Wolfe SW, Lospinuso MF, Burke SW. Unilateral blindness as a complication of patient positioning for spinal surgery. A case report. *Spine* 1992;17(5):600–605.
15. Seybold EA et al. Characteristics of unicortical and bicortical lateral mass screws in the cervical spine. *Spine* 1999;24(22):2397–2403.
16. An HS, Gordin R, Renner K. Anatomic considerations for plate screw fixation to the cervical spine. *Spine* 1988;13:813–816.
17. Klekamp JW, Ugbo JL, Heller JG, et al. Cervical transfacet versus lateral mass screws: a biomechanical comparison. *J Spinal Disord* 2000;13:515–518.

32

OCCIPITOCERVICAL FUSION

CHRISTOPHER M. BONO
CHRISTOPHER P. KAUFFMAN
FRANK EISMONT
STEVEN R. GARFIN

Numerous processes can lead to instability between the cranium and the cervical spine, including infection, trauma, neoplasm, and inflammatory disorders (1–4). Frequently, instability is manifest as gradual compression of the cranium onto the cervical spine. This is known as basilar invagination. Rarely, these are distractive lesions, such as traumatic occipitoatlantal dislocations (5). Despite the etiology, instability can lead to significant neurologic complications secondary to spinal cord, cerebrovascular, cerebellar, or brainstem injury. A high index of suspicion and prompt diagnosis are critical to minimize these sequelae. In most cases, early stabilization in the form of occipitocervical fusion is indicated to treat instability.

Several methods of posterior occipitocervical fusion have been described (6–20). They vary from simple on-lay bone grafting without hardware (20) to techniques of rigid plate and screw fixation (8). Fusions can be limited, including only C1 or C2, or can extend as far caudad as T5 (1,5). Postoperative immobilization with a cervical collar or halo vest can be used. Though not universally agreed upon, the choice of halo versus cervical orthosis is influenced by the quality of intraoperative fixation.

Successful craniocervical fusion is dependent on a detailed knowledge of operative anatomy and relevant biomechanical principles. Awareness of the available surgical techniques, their relative stability, and their advantages and disadvantages is helpful in choosing the optimal method of arthrodesis. It is the authors' goal to augment the reader's understanding of these issues.

ANATOMY AND BIOMECHANICS

Occipital Region

The occipital bone is the diploic posterior-inferior aspect of the cranium that cradles the cerebellum and brainstem. At its anterior and inferior aspect, it forms the posterior part of the foramen magnum, which transmits the spinal cord into the spinal canal. The occiput has several bony structures that are useful surgical landmarks. At its topographical center, the external occipital protuberance (EOP) is a dense uprising that marks the thickest portion of the bone. The superior nuchal line is a ridge that extends medial and lateral from the EOP. The inferior nuchal line is a similar condensation running parallel and below its superior counterpart. Though not a useful surgical landmark, the lambdoidal suture denotes the borders of the occipital bone at its fused junctions with the temporal and maxillary bones. The occiput curves sharply anterior from the superior nuchal line to the foramen magnum. This feature makes plate or rod fixation challenging, necessitating accurate contouring of the implant to match the skeletal geometry.

The occiput is a two-tabled structure, with dense inner and outer cortices separated by a spongy layer of bone. Bony dimensions vary with location. Zipnick et al. (21) found the bone at the EOP to be the thickest, measuring an average of 18 mm. Bone cephalad to the superior nuchal line is thicker than that caudad to it (21) and is progressively thinner at increased distances lateral from the midline, measuring as little as 3.0 mm (22). These variations in thickness have an influence on the optimal location for occipital fixation. In a cadaveric biomechanical investigation, Haher et al. (23) demonstrated the highest pull-out strengths for wires and screws at the EOP. As the bone thickness diminished laterally, pull-out strengths also decreased. Interestingly, unicortical fixation at the external protuberance was comparable to bicortical fixation at other locations. Though bicortical screw fixation was strongest in all regions, no significant difference was detectable between unicortical screws compared with wires.

The occiput interacts with the cervical spine through bilateral articular condyles on either side of the foramen magnum. Together with the posterior and anterior ligaments, the occipitoatlantal joints stabilize the head on the neck. Motion at this junction is minimal, allowing 13 degrees of flexion/extension, 8 degrees of lateral bending, and no rotation (24).

Atlantoaxial Region

The upper cervical vertebrae are unique compared to the subaxial spine. The atlas has large broad-based articular processes to interface with the occipital condyles superiorly and the axis inferiorly. An articular surface on the posterior aspect of the anterior arch faces the odontoid process of the axis. The posterior ring of C1 is quite thin, with no discrete spinous process. The vertebral artery exits the posterior occipitoatlantal membrane approximately 1.5 cm lateral to the midline before entering the foramen in the transverse processes of C1. Together with the constrained bony dimensions, it substantially limits the safety of screw insertion into the lateral masses of the atlas.

The axis articulates with C1 at three points: broad bilateral superior articular surfaces and the odontoid process. By its morphology, it allows approximately 47 degrees of rotation (50% of axial rotation of the entire cervical spine), while limiting flexion/extension to 10 degrees (24). Virtually no lateral bending is permitted at the atlantoaxial articulation (24). The axis marks the transition between the upper and lower cervical spine. In so doing, the inferior articular processes of C2 are offset posteriorly. Because of this offset, the pars interarticularis sustains high shear forces with axial loading, predisposing it to the classic hangman's fracture pattern. A foramen in the transverse processes transmits the ascending vertebral artery. The cervical nerve roots exit through foramina formed by adjacent superior and inferior pedicle walls.

Placement of a C2 pedicle screw endangers the neural elements (spinal cord) medially, the vertebral artery laterally, and the nerve roots superiorly and inferiorly. The bony anatomy of C2 displays substantial variation. Panjabi et al. (25) reported C2 pedicle heights ranging from 9 to 11 mm, while width varied from 7 to 9 mm. Madawi et al. (26) observed asymmetry of the groove for the vertebral artery and noted its influence on the effective pedicle dimensions. In some cases, it decreased the available space for screws to less than 2.1 mm. This is not likely to be appreciated from intraoperative visualization of the posterior surfaces of the lateral masses. Thin-section computed tomography (CT) angling the gantry along the line of screw insertion is recommended to accurately assess whether pedicle screws can be placed.

OPERATIVE SETUP AND SURGICAL APPROACH

A detailed preoperative neurologic examination should be performed just before surgery. In the unstable upper cervical spine, an awake fiberoptic intubation is recommended. The excessive extension of the neck required for standard intubation maneuvers can lead to acute neurologic deficit. In the supine position, baseline evoked potentials can be obtained. Before induction of general anesthesia, the patient is then rolled prone onto a spine table with well-padded bolsters. The face, nipples, abdomen, and genitals must be freed of any undue pressure. After prone positioning, a cursory neurologic exam or evoked potentials or both can be repeated. With confirmation of the neurologic status, general anesthesia is then initiated. If head-holding devices are used, preoperative imaging (that will be used intraoperatively) should be checked to ensure that the critical anatomy can be visualized. Because access to the occiput with drills and screw drivers is often limited, we often use a soft sponge head holder on the end of a radiolucent table to avoid radiographic influence.

The posterior scalp and neck are shaved clean. After standard surgical scrub and prep, the neck and occiput are draped from 2 cm above the occipital protuberance to the spinous process of C7. The posterior iliac crest is also prepared for bone graft harvesting. A midline incision is created extending from the EOP to the spinous process of C4. If fusion is to be extended to the lower cervical spine, the incision may be carried caudad. Sharp dissection is carried to the level of the trapezius muscle fascia. Palpation of the spinous processes and visualization of the decussation of tendon fibers confirm the midline. The fascia is incised down to the bone. Periosteal dissection is carried laterally, elevating the paraspinal muscles off the posterior arches of C1 and C2 as well as exposing the surface of the occiput. This must be visualized from the level of the EOP down to the occipitoatlantal articulation. Care must be taken to avoid lateral dissection of more than 1.5 cm at the level of C1 for fear of injuring the traversing vertebral arteries. The surgeon must also be attentive to the underlying spinal canal.

If decompression is indicated, it may be performed at this stage. Using sharp, curved curettes, the ligamentum flavum and tectorial membranes are meticulously elevated from the inferior and superior borders of the C1 posterior arch, respectively. Using up-biting Kerrison rongeurs, the lamina is removed and can be saved as subsequent bone graft. If necessary, partial resection of the posterior foramen magnum can also be performed at this time.

SPECIFIC TECHNIQUES FOR OCCIPITOCERVICAL FUSION

On-Lay Bone Grafting

This technique is discussed for historical perspective rather than for current application. Before using wires for internal fixation in the cervical spine became popular, surgeons placed bone graft over a decorticated spinal segment to induce arthrodesis. Though this seems simplistic by contemporary standards, it is still a common and effective practice in the lumbar spine and has occasional utility at the occipitocervical junction. The disadvantage of this method is that it offers no immediate stability. Perry and Nickel (27) documented good results using this method supplemented by halo immobilization until solid fusion. Likewise, Newman and Sweetnam (20) reported satisfactory outcomes using a similar procedure and maintaining their patients in cervical traction for 6 weeks postoperatively. Fundamentally, the main difference between this technique and more modern methods is the manner in which the spine, and the graft, is stabilized.

Wire and Bone Graft Fixation

Numerous variations of wiring techniques have been reported (4,28,29). Fixation relies on the use of wires to rigidly fix a large piece of bicortical or tricortical iliac crest bone graft that spans the occipitocervical junction. In this manner, the bone graft acts as both a fusion medium and a structural support. Techniques vary in their pattern of wire looping and graft placement.

Technique

A large corticocancellous piece of iliac bone autograft is harvested. The dimensions can vary, because some surgeons fashion bilateral strips and others use one wider central piece of bone. The cancellous portion is placed over the posterior aspect of the occiput and the posterior arches of C1 and C2 and fixed with sublaminar and transosseous occipital wires. Cancellous bone graft can then be used to supplement the fusion. To supplement the graft, the outer table of the occiput below the EOP can be cut using an osteotome and flapped down over the occipitocervical junction prior to wiring the graft. The patient is usually then placed in a halo fixator.

Carlson and Bohlman (30) have described a similar method using bilateral strips of corticocancellous iliac bone. The surgeons recommend passing a wire through drill holes in the EOP and the spinous process of C2 (Fig. 32.1). In addition, they pass sublaminar wires around the posterior arch of C1 (Fig. 32.1). Wires are then passed through the two strips of iliac graft (Fig. 32.2). The occipital wire is tensioned transversely to itself, while the two cervical wires are paired longitudinally and tensioned (Fig. 32.3). Additional bone graft is implanted around the construct. A halo vest is fitted postoperatively.

McAfee et al. (28) reported successful fusions in 33 of 37 patients with myelopathy associated with basilar invagination using this method. Their technique involved creation of unicortical troughs on either side of the EOP (Fig. 32.4). Using a drill to connect these bony burrows, a 22-gauge wire was then passed. Similarly, a wire was passed through a drill hole in the spinous process of C2. After harvesting two long specimens of corticocancellous iliac bone, holes were predrilled at either end to accept the occiput and axis wires. The upper and lower tails of the wires were then twisted together to tension the graft in place. Additional cancellous graft was then packed to further enhance fusion. Patients remained in a halo vest for 3 months, at which time they were converted to a hard cervical collar for an additional month.

In addition to neurologic injury during wire passage intraoperatively, wire migration within the spinal canal has been reported. Fraser et al. (31) described this complication 5 years after craniocervical fusion with a sublaminar wire technique. The patient presented with progressive neurologic deficit and radiographic evidence of continued cranial settling and atlantoaxial subluxation. The bone graft had completely resorbed, and

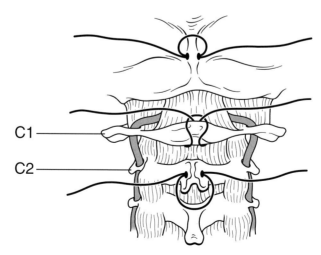

FIGURE 32.1. A burr is used to create unicortical holes on either side of the external occipital protuberance. This is then connected using a sharp towel clip or pointed bone clamp. A wire is then passed and looped to cinch down to the occiput. A sublaminar wire is then carefully passed around the posterior ring of C1. A third wire is inserted through the spinous process of C2.

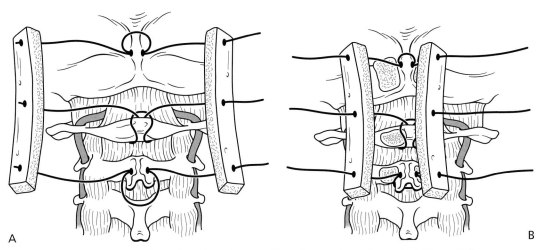

A   B

FIGURE 32.2. Two rectangular strips of corticocancellous iliac crest are harvested. Three drill holes are created in each specimen. The wire tips are passed through the holes in the graft so that the grafts are oriented longitudinally across the craniocervical junction.

the wire fixation had failed. The patient was effectively treated with stabilization by a posterior plate and lateral mass screws and was found to have a solid fusion at 9 months.

Biomechanics

Though the stability of several methods for occipitocervical fusion has been biomechanically compared, the present authors could find no *in vitro* investigation evaluating the stability of a wire and bone graft construct. It is likely that it offers some stability to flexion; minimal resistance to axial compressive, torsional, or lateral bending loads; and limited resistance to extension.

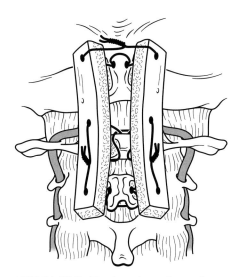

FIGURE 32.3. The two top wire ends are tightened to each other. This is one continuous wire and can be tensioned independently. The bottom two wire tips on either side are tensioned to each other. This must be performed on both sides simultaneously, since tightening on either side represents two distinct wires. Multiaxial cable can also be used, though overtightening and cracking of the graft can more easily occur.

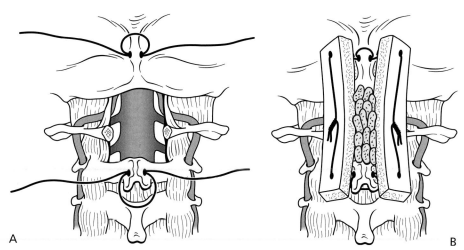

FIGURE 32.4. An alternative technique avoids passing wires at C1. Wires passed through the external occipital protuberance and spinous process of C2 are passed through two drill holes in the graft. Tensioning is performed on both sides simultaneously.

Advantages and Disadvantages

The advantages to this technique are its simplicity, relative safety, and acceptable fusion rate (89%) (28). A decompression of the spinal canal at C1 can be concurrently performed, while still allowing fixation of the graft to C2. However, if C2 must be decompressed, the fusion must be extended caudally. Among other disadvantages are the necessity of rigid external postoperative stabilization (often a halo vest) and the morbidity associated with harvesting large cortical samples from the iliac crest. Passage of wires incurs some risk of neural and vascular injury. Additionally, there is limited ability to correct sagittal or axial deformities. Although wires are considered "rigid" by some, cranial settling is not well controlled with this method (4,28,29). McAfee et al. (28) felt this to be a contributing factor for the poor rate (40%) of neurologic recovery in patients with basilar invagination, despite preoperative traction and postoperative halo immobilization. Lordotic (or, less typically, kyphotic) deformities are better controlled with more rigid segmental stabilization such as lateral mass screw-rod or plate constructs.

Rigid Loops or Rectangles

As techniques in spinal stabilization advanced to more stable constructs, methods of occipitocervical fusion followed. With documented success in the thoracolumbar spine, Luque rectangles were modified for the craniocervical region (10,14). The use of rigid wires to fix metal loops or rectangles improved immediate fixation strength and offered greater facility to reduce and maintain deformity correction. However, these systems are bulky and often prominent to the patient. Several variations on this theme have been documented, which employ a variety of materials and types of metal devices. Common to these techniques are segmental fixation of the occiput and cervical vertebrae by way of rigid wires tensioned to metal rods or loops (7,10,13,14,18).

Technique

Using the standard posterior approach, the occiput and upper cervical spine are exposed. A single rod or rectangle is contoured to simultaneously contact the EOP and rings of C1 and C2. Alternatively, two rods can be used but should be cross-linked cranially or caudally or both to recreate the "loop" configuration. Longer implants can be used if more segments are to be included in the fusion. After satisfactory shaping of the rod or rods, they are laid on the back table. Wires are then carefully placed through drill holes in the occiput. In the cervical vertebrae, wires can be passed around the laminae or through drill holes in the spinous processes of C2 and the more caudal elements. Sublaminar wires provide more rigid fixation at each level but increase the neurologic risk to the patient. The contoured rods are then laid over the wires. The wires are carefully tensioned to the rods at each level. Autogenous bone grafting is then performed, often in an on-lay manner, but grafts can be fixed to the spinous processes with wires passed through them and through or around the graft.

Ransford et al. (7) were one of the first groups to describe the use of a Luque rod to achieve arthrodesis of the occipitocervical junction. In a series of three patients, contoured steel loops were applied to the posterior aspects of the occiput and cervical spine (Fig. 32.5). Cranially, the loop was fixed to the occiput through bilateral wires passed from the decompressed foramen magnum to drill holes in the upper occiput. Cervical stabilization included bilateral segmental sublaminar wires. Patients were placed in a cervical collar for early mobilization. Solid fusion was documented in all three cases. Similarly, Ellis and Findlay (14) and MacKenzie et al. (10) reported good results using an identical technique in six and twenty patients, respectively. All patients were maintained in a cervical collar only, while one required halo stabilization.

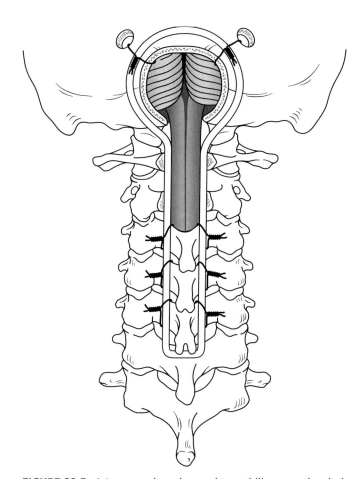

FIGURE 32.5. A Luque rod can be used to stabilize an arthrodesis at the occipitocervical junction. In this technique, the loop is fixed to the occiput through bilateral wires passed from the decompressed foramen magnum and exiting via drill holes in the lower occiput. Caudally, the rod is stabilized to the cervical vertebrae with bilateral segmental sublaminar wires.

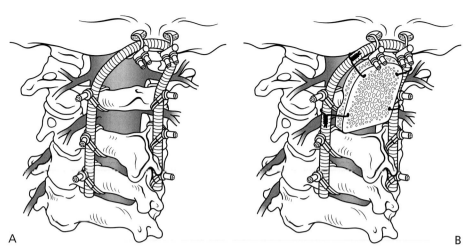

A   B

FIGURE 32.6. A threaded Steinmann pin bent into a upside-down **U** shape can also be used instead of a Luque rod to stabilize the occipitocervical junction. The pin is fixed to the bone using wires. A large piece of corticocancellous graft can be wedged between the occiput and C2 and wired to the pin along its periphery.

More recently, Apostolides et al. (18) reported use of a threaded Steinmann pin bent into an upside-down **U** shape instead of a Luque rod in 37 patients with a variety of diagnoses (Fig. 32.6). Fusion was documented in 95% of patients. Hardware failure occurred in 3 patients, including breakage of the Steinmann pin in 2 cases and wire breakage in another. Fortunately, solid fusion was achieved in each. The majority of patients were maintained in a halo vest until radiographic union. Importantly, axial correction was maintained in all patients, and none developed progressive cranial settling. The authors did not report on sagittal alignment.

Fehlings et al. (13) reported on the use of two Cotrel-Dubousset rods linked at the caudal end by a device for transverse traction (cross-link), forming a **U**-type device. Fixation to the occiput was similar to that described by Ellis and Findlay (14), MacKenzie et al. (10), and Ransford et al. (7). However, wires were passed transversely across drill holes in the spinous processes and tensioned to both rods on either side (Fig. 32.7). Fusion was reported in 93% of cases, with only 3 of 16 patients requiring halo immobilization.

Biomechanics

In vitro biomechanical comparisons suggest inferior rigidity with metal loop and wire constructs versus screw-fixed methods (32,33). Oda et al. (32) found Luque rod and wire fixation significantly weaker than most screw-rod constructs. These included both plate and rod techniques. Wire techniques offered stability against flexion/extension and axial rotation forces, while resistance to anterior-posterior translation and lateral bending moments was not significantly different than intact specimens. Hurlbert et al. (33) found that wire constructs permitted more motion than screw-plate fixators did.

Advantages and Disadvantages

Perhaps the clearest advantage of loop-wire methods is the nearly universal availability of the implants. They are inexpensive and have proven effectiveness with high fusion rates. Still, they have the potential complications associated with intracanal hardware and the dangers of wire passage. In addition, wire fixation to the rod requires an intact posterior arch. This is a clear disadvantage when decompression of the upper two cervical vertebrae must be performed, because the construct must be extended caudally to at least two intact vertebral levels. Although some surgeons report the ability to correct and maintain

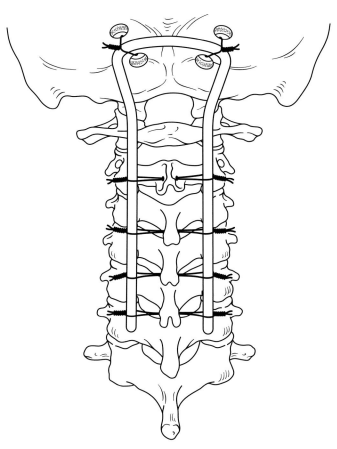

FIGURE 32.7. In this technique, fixation to the occiput was similar to that described in Figures 32.5 and 32.6. Cervical fixation was achieved using wires passed transversely across drill holes in the spinous processes and tensioned to both rods on either side.

deformities, there is little clinical evidence to support these claims. Another limitation is that halo vest immobilization is often necessary.

Screw-Fixed Rod and Plate Constructs

The latest technical developments for occipitocervical fusion have been the application of screw-rod or screw-plate constructs (8,9,11,19,34). This development corresponds with the rising use of lateral mass screw devices in the cervical spine. Initial fixation strength is substantial with the use of screws placed in both the occiput and cervical vertebrae (32,33). C2 screws are analogous to pedicle screws and offer a rigid fixation point in this vertebra. Screws in the occiput have greater *in vitro* pull-out strength than wires (23). Controversy exists on the necessity of bicortical versus unicortical occipital fixators. Screws can be fixed to plates or rods, with a variety of designs available.

Techniques

The posterior occiput and cervical spine are exposed as described previously. Currently available plate and rod systems are precontoured by the manufacturer, although adjustments are usually required for proper seating. Some surgeons describe use of 3.5-mm reconstruction plates that necessitate careful templating to match the anatomy and avoid notching the plates, which can increase the likelihood of fatigue failure (Fig. 32.8).

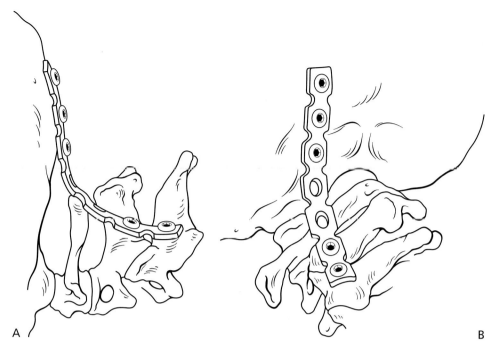

FIGURE 32.8. The popularity of lateral mass plating has helped develop methods of occipito-cervical plate fixation. Plates are contoured carefully, as implants left too proud in the region of the occiput can be easily palpable and troublesome to the patient postoperatively. Unicortical screws are used to fix the plate to the occiput. Pull-out strength is proportional to the number of screws used. Cervical fixation is provided by lateral mass screws placed into C2.

Lateral mass (pedicle) screws are first inserted into the cervical vertebrae. Screw fixation in C1 is difficult and risky. The pedicle is thin and intimately associated with the vertebral artery as it exits the tectorial membrane approximately 1.5 cm from the midline. Most surgeons avoid placement of implants at this level. Limited fixation in C1 can be achieved using a transarticular Magerl-type screw from C1 to C2. However, C1 lateral mass pedicle screws are being placed (35). Screws can be more safely implanted into C2 (Fig. 32.9). The pedicle is larger than at C1, although considerable anatomic variation and asymmetry can exist (25,26,36). Medial notching of the groove

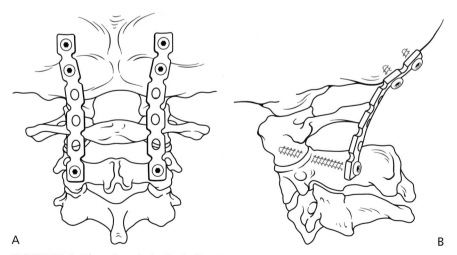

FIGURE 32.9. Though technically challenging, transarticular lateral mass screws (pedicle screws) can be inserted into C1 to provide an additional fixation point.

for the vertebral arteries reduces the effective pedicle diameter (26). Implants can be placed just in C2 as a pedicle screw or across the C1–2 facet joint, affording two-level fixation.

The insertion point lies over the posterior border of the inferior articular facet of C2. The entry point should be about 7 mm lateral to the lateral border of the spinal canal and 5 mm below the superior border of the C2 lamina (36). Safe placement into C2 requires the proper insertion angle. For C2 pedicle screws, the drill or awl should be angled medially about 30 degrees and cranially about 20 degrees. The pedicle can and should be visualized on lateral and anteroposterior (open-mouth) fluoroscopic views intraoperatively. For transarticular screws, the drill or awl must be directed more cephalad, approximately 45 degrees. In the lower cervical spine, purely lateral mass screws are inserted without entering the pedicle proper. Thus, screw direction is different from that used for C2. With a starting point along the lateral aspect of the inferior articular process, the drill or awl is directed 30 degrees laterally and 20 degrees cranially (37).

The surgeon must ensure that the head and neck are in the desired alignment. In most cases, a neutral orientation is desirable. This can be reliably determined on an intraoperative lateral radiograph (38). The plates or rods are then fitted and fixed to cervical screws. Proper seating of the longitudinal member is confirmed prior to connection to the screws. If the plate or rod is contoured in too much lordosis, for example, the plate will lift off the posterior cranium during cervical screw-rod tightening. Even in rod constructs, the rod is continuous with a plate-type device for occipital fixation (Fig. 32.10). Occipital screws are drilled through the plate, as their position is determined by the implant. Depending on the system's design, either lateral or midline occipital screws can be inserted. Biomechanical pull-out strength of midline fixtures, especially in the EOP, is superior to laterally placed implants (23). Bicortical screws placed lateral to the midline

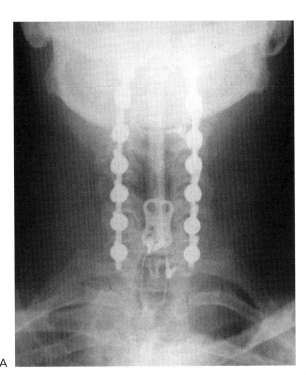
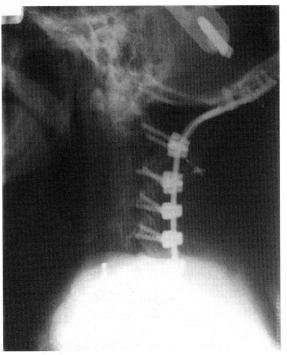

A   B

FIGURE 32.10. After anterior corpectomy and strut grafting from C2 to C7, posterior occipitocervicothoracic fusion was achieved. A continuous plate-rod was used to stabilize the construct. Polyaxial lateral mass screws were inserted into C2 through C7. The plate portion of the plate-rod was secured with unicortical occipital screws. T1 was stabilized with spinous process wiring to C7.

are mechanically comparable to unicortical EOP fixation (23). Although bicortical implants have greater *in vitro* pull-out strength, the risk of cerebellar injury during drilling and insertion detracts from their attractiveness.

Numerous variations of these constructs have been developed. Grob et al. (11) used a Y plate and transarticular C1/C2 screws in 14 patients with varying etiologies of craniocervical instability. In addition to good clinical results, in no case did either sagittal or axial deformity recur. All patients fused, with 12 of 14 demonstrating bony bridging by the sixth postoperative week. Only a soft cervical collar was used for a period of 6 to 8 weeks. Vale et al. (34) used a three-plate construct to fuse the cranium to the cervical spine in 24 patients. Two bilateral plates spanned the craniocervical junction, while an additional T plate was connected transversely over the superior nuchal line to facilitate screw fixation to the EOP. Fusion was observed in all cases.

Some authors advocate use of two reconstruction rods for stabilization (8,30). Two 3.5-mm reconstruction plates are contoured to fit the convex curve of the inferior occiput and the concave valley of the occipitocervical junction. These are placed in line with the lateral masses of the cervical vertebrae. Placement should ensure three-screw purchase into the occiput on each side. The plate extends as caudad as fusion is desired.

Abumi et al. (19) utilized a plate-rod construct in 26 patients. The implant had a plate region for occipital fixation confluent with a rod region for cervical stabilization. Notably, both C2 pedicle screws and lateral mass screws were placed into the same vertebra. C2 was the caudal extent of the construct. Fusion was achieved in 92% of spines, with maintenance of intraoperative alignment. Importantly, no complications related to pedicle screw insertion were reported.

Biomechanics

Screw-fixed constructs have demonstrated greater rigidity in all planes of motion compared with wire techniques. In a biomechanical cadaveric investigation, Hurlbert et al. (33) tested four different U-shaped constructs fixed with combinations of wires and cervical and/or occipital screws. The two most rigid techniques were a Mayfield loop or the authors' custom-designed OCTA system, which consisted of a plate-rod implant that enabled multiple-screw insertion into the EOP and superior nuchal line. Wire constructs allowed more motion than screw-fixed constructs. In a similar investigation, Oda et al. (32) demonstrated the biomechanical superiority of bilateral plate-rods fixed to C2 by pedicle and lateral mass screws. The plate was fixed to the occiput with six para-midline screws. Interestingly, three constructs with two midline screws were weaker, although this may be accounted for by the thinner rod dimensions and the lower absolute number of screws inserted into the occiput.

Advantages and Disadvantages

The advantages of screw-fixed methods are numerous. They enable laminectomy and decompression at the fused levels. This is not possible with wire-rod or wire–bone graft techniques. The immediate multiplanar stability decreases the need for rigid postoperative immobilization, enables deformity correction that can be effectively maintained, and leads to high rates of fusion. However, these systems are expensive and not universally available. The surgeon must have an in-depth familiarity with the surgical anatomy and instrumentation. Screw insertion into the cervical spine is associated with a learning curve. Screw misplacement can endanger the spinal cord, vertebral artery, and nerve cervical roots. In the occiput, the dura is often violated because it is opposed to the thin inner table. Covering the screw tip with bone wax before insertion is helpful in stopping cerebrospinal fluid leak.

SUMMARY

Occipitocervical fusion is a useful technique in the treatment of craniocervical instability. Many methods of stabilization exist. Wire and bone grafting procedures can lead to high fusion rates but often require prolonged halo use postoperatively. Metal loop constructs offer better postoperative stability and may maintain axial correction of cranial settling. However, their utility in correcting sagittal deformities is unclear. Although screw-fixed systems appear to have clear mechanical advantages, there are no available surgical series demonstrating their clinical superiority to other methods.

REFERENCES

1. Jackson R, Gokaslan Z. Occipitocervicothoracic fixation for spinal instability in patients with neoplastic processes. *J Neurosurg* 1999;91:81–89.
2. McGuire R, Harkey H. Primary treatment of unstable Jefferson's fractures. *J Spinal Disord* 1995;8: 233–236.
3. Tseng S, Cheng Y. Occiput-cervical fusion for symptomatic atlantoaxial subluxation in a 32-month old child with Down syndrome: a case report. *Spinal Cord* 1998;36:520–522.
4. Ranawat C, O'Leary P, Pellicci P, et al. Cervical spine fusion in rheumatoid arthritis. *J Bone Joint Surg Am* 1979;61:1003–1010.
5. Zigler J, Waters R, Nelson R, et al. Occipito-cervico-thoracic spine fusion in a patient with occipito-cervical dislocation and survival. *Spine* 1986;11:645–646.
6. Weiland D, McAfee P. Posterior cervical fusion with triple-wire strut graft technique: one hundred consecutive patients. *J Spinal Disord* 1991;4:15–21.
7. Ransford A, Crockard H, Pozo J, et al. Craniocervical instability treated by contoured loop fixation. *J Bone Joint Surg Br* 1986;68:173–177.
8. Pait T, Al-Mefty O, Boop F, et al. Inside-outside technique for posterior occipitocervical spine instrumentation and stabilization: preliminary results. *J Neurosurg* 1999;90:1–7.
9. Olerud C, Lind B, Sahlstedt B. The Olerud cervical fixation system: a study of safety and efficacy. *Ups J Med Sci* 1999;104:131–143.
10. MacKenzie A, Uttley D, Marsh H, et al. Craniocervical stabilization using Luque/Hartshill rectangles. *Neurosurgery* 1990;26:32–36.
11. Grob D, Dvorak J, Panjabi M, et al. Posterior occipitocervical fusion. A preliminary report of new technique. *Spine* 1991;16:S17–S24.
12. Grob D, Dvorak J, Geschwend N, et al. Posterior occipito-cervical fusion in rheumatoid arthritis. *Arch Orthop Trauma Surg* 1990;110:38–44.
13. Fehlings M, Errico T, Cooper P, et al. Occipitocervical fusion with a five-millimeter malleable rod and segmental fixation. *Neurosurgery* 1993;32:198–207.
14. Ellis P, Findlay J. Craniocervical fusion with contoured Luque rod and autogeneic bone graft. *Can J Surg* 1994;37:50–54.
15. Dormans J, Drummond D, Sutton L, et al. Occipitocervical arthrodesis in children. A new technique and analysis of results. *J Bone Joint Surg Am* 1995;77:1234–1240.
16. Bryan W, Inglis A, Sculco T, et al. Methylmethacrylate stabilization for enhancement of posterior cervical arthrodesis in rheumatoid arthritis. *J Bone Joint Surg Am* 1982;64:1045–1050.
17. Berghe AV, Ackerman C, Veys E, et al. Occipito-cervical fusion in rheumatoid arthritis. *Acta Orthop Belg* 1991;57:94–98.
18. Apostolides P, Dickman C, Golfinos J, et al. Threaded Steinmann pin fusion of the craniovertebral junction. *Spine* 1996;21:1630–1637.
19. Abumi K, Takada T, Shono Y, et al. Posterior occipitocervical reconstruction using cervical pedicle screws and plate-rod systems. *Spine* 1999;24:1425–1434.
20. Newman P, Sweetnam R. Occipital cervical fusion. *J Bone Joint Surg Br* 1969;51:423–431.
21. Zipnick R, Merola A, Gorup J, et al. Occipital morphology: an anatomic guide to internal fixation. *Spine* 1996;21:1719–1724.
22. Ebraheim N, Lu J, Biyani A, et al. An anatomic study of the thickness of the occipital bone. Implications for occipitocervical instrumentation. *Spine* 1996;21:1725–1729.
23. Haher T, Yeung A, Caruso S, et al. Occipital screw pullout strength. *Spine* 1999;24:5–9.
24. White A, Panjabi M. The clinical biomechanics of the occipitoatlantoaxial complex. *Orthop Clin North Am* 1978;9:867–878.
25. Panjabi M, Duranceau J, Goel V, et al. Cervical human vertebrae. Quantitative three dimensional anatomy of the middle and lower regions. *Spine* 1991;16:861–869.
26. Madawi AA, Solanki G, Casey A, et al. Variation of the groove in the axis vertebra for the vertebral artery. Implications for instrumentation. *J Bone Joint Surg Br* 1997;79:820–823.

27. Perry J, Nickel V. Total cervical spine fusion for neck paralysis. *J Bone Joint Surg Am* 1959;41:37–60.
28. McAfee P, Cassidy J, Davis R, et al. Fusion of the occiput to the upper cervical spine. A review of 37 cases. *Spine* 1991;16:S490–S494.
29. Chan D, Ngian K, Cohen L. Posterior upper cervical fusion in rheumatoid arthritis. *Spine* 1992;17:268–272.
30. Carlson G, Bohlman H. Surgical techniques for occiput to C2 arthrodesis. In: Dillian W, Simeone F, eds. *Posterior cervical spine surgery.* Philadelphia: Lippincott–Raven Publishers, 1998:41–52.
31. Fraser A, Sen C, Casden A, et al. Cervical transdural intramedullary migration of a sublaminar wire. A complication of cervical fixation. *Spine* 1994;19:456–459.
32. Oda I, Abumi K, Sell L, et al. Biomechanical evaluation of five different occipito-atlanto-axial fixation techniques. *Spine* 1999;24:2377–2382.
33. Hurlbert R, Crawford N, Choi W, et al. A biomechanical evaluation of occipitocervical instrumentation: screw compared with wire fixation. *J Neurosurg* 1999;90:84–90.
34. Vale F, Oliver M, Cahill D. Rigid occipitocervical fusion. *J Neurosurg* 1999;91:144–150.
35. Floyd T, Grob D. Translaminar screws in the atlas. *Spine* 2000;25:2913–2915.
36. Ebraheim N, Rollins J, Jackson W. Anatomic consideration of C2 pedicle screw placement. *Spine* 1996;21:691–695.
37. Magerl F, Grob D. Dorsal fusion of the cervical spine with the hook plate. In: Kehr P, Weidner A, eds. *Cervical spine I.* Vienna: Springer-Verlag, 1985:217–221.
38. Phillips F, Phillips C, Wetzel F, et al. Occipitocervical neutral position. Possible surgical implications. *Spine* 1999;24:775–778.

CERVICOTHORACIC FIXATION

JEFFREY S. FISCHGRUND

Posterior instrumentation of the lower cervical and upper thoracic spine has changed dramatically over the past decade. Although traditional methods of interspinous and occasionally sublaminar wiring remain viable options, more rigid fixation is often required, especially in the face of marked instability. Surgical procedures for degenerative conditions leading to neural compression often require the use of decompressive procedures, such as laminectomy, which greatly hinder the use of most forms of wire fixation. Neoplasms and traumatic deformities often require more rigid forms of fixation in order to support anterior or posterior column insufficiency. The acceptance of lateral mass screws in the lower cervical spine and the recent introduction of pedicle screws in the lower cervical spine as well as upper thoracic spine has spawned a new generation of surgical implants that can be used to reconstruct even the most difficult cervicothoracic deformity.

Posterior spinal instrumentation can assist in correcting spinal alignment, as well as preventing further malalignment from occurring. Spinal fixation devices have also been shown to enhance fusion rates and allow early immobilization of patients. Specific to the cervical spine, spinal instrumentation has made it possible to perform spinal reconstruction without the need for postoperative rigid immobilization, such as a halo brace (1).

ANATOMY

The bony architecture of the midcervical spine from C3 to C6 is similar, with a minimal increase in size proceeding from C3 to C6. C7 is a transitional vertebra and has characteristics common to both the cervical and thoracic spines. Important anatomic landmarks for posterior plate and screw instrumentation include the superior and inferior facet joints, the medial and lateral margins of the lateral mass, and the inclination of the facet joints. The junction between the lamina and lateral mass is generally quite distinct from C3 to C6, with the lateral edge of the lateral mass forming a ridge running down toward the transverse process. However, the lateral mass of C7 is more elongated in a superior-inferior direction, and thinner in an anterior-posterior direction (2). The articulating facet joint between C7 and T1 is more similar to a typical thoracic facet joint than to the cervical facet joints.

The vertebral artery is the major blood supply of the cervical cord and cervical spine. The artery originates from the subclavian artery and generally enters the transverse foramen at the C6 level. However, studies have shown that the foramen transversarium at C7 will contain the vertebral artery vein and associated nerve fibers in approximately 5% of patients. Therefore, careful review of preoperative computed tomography (CT), magnetic resonance imaging (MRI), or magnetic resonance angiography is mandatory to determine the course of the vertebral arteries prior to posterior fixation at this level (3).

Morphometric analysis of the pedicles has been completed by both An and Simpson (1) (Table 33.1) and Jones et al. (4). These studies indicate that the inner diameter of the C7 pedicle ranges from 4 to 6 mm, with a slight increase in size at T1 and T2. A discrepancy in the medial angulation of the C7 pedicles was noted by the two groups, with An

TABLE 33.1 MORPHOMETRIC ANALYSIS OF THE PEDICLES

	Diameter$_0$ (mm)	Diameter$_1$ (mm)	Angulation$_m$ (degrees)
C7			
Average	5.2	6.9	34
Range	4–6	6–8	27–40
T1			
Average	6.3	8.5	31.8
Range	5–9	7–12	27–37
T2			
Average	5–5	7.5	26.5
Range	5–7	6–9	20–35

From An HS, Simpson JM. Spinal instrumentation of the cervical spine. In: An HS, Simpson JM, eds. *Surgery of the cervical spine.* London: Martin-Dunitz, 1994:379–400, with permission.

and Simpson reporting medial angulation averaging 34 degrees and Jones et al. reporting a mean of 45 degrees. This angle can easily be measured on preoperative MRI or CT scan, and ranges from 27 to 59 degrees. This angulation does not vary greatly as one proceeds from the lower cervical to upper thoracic spine. Generally, the direction of the pedicles at the cervicothoracic junction is perpendicular to the sagittal plane; however, this angle can vary widely, depending on preexisting deformity, and is greatly influenced by the patient position on the operating room table.

BIOMECHANICAL CONSIDERATIONS

Biomechanical comparisons of the pullout strengths of lateral mass and pedicle screws have been performed at the cervicothoracic junction. Jones et al. (4) noted a mean load to failure of 608 N for pedicle screws at C7, compared with 295 N for lateral mass screws placed at the C7 level. They noted no significant correlation between pullout values and bone density, screw length, or vertebral level for either screw insertion location.

In the series of Jones et al. (4), 3.5-mm cortical screws were used, except when the pedicle diameter was less than 5.0 mm, in which case a 2.7-mm cortical screw was used. No significant difference was noted in the pullout values between the 2.7- and 3.5-mm pedicle screws. The authors felt that this was most likely due to the amount of cortical purchase in the pedicle canal. Obviously, the 2.7-mm screws have a small diameter, but they can engage a similar amount of cortical bone within the pedicle compared with the larger 3.5-mm screws (which were placed in correspondingly wider pedicles). The predominant cortical purchase of the screws also explains why screw length did not affect pullout values, since the cortical purchase in the pedicles has a greater effect on the pullout values than any purchase in the cancellous vertebral body.

INDICATIONS

Posterior stabilization of the cervicothoracic spine can be performed for numerous indications. An anterior pseudarthrosis at the C7-T1 level, following either corpectomy or discectomy, can often be treated by posterior fusion alone. Frequently, successful posterior fusion and instrumentation at this level posteriorly will lead to eventual arthrodesis anteriorly as well. Traumatic injuries, such as facet fracture and dislocations at the cervicothoracic junction, can often be treated posteriorly alone, following either a closed or open reduction. Extensive anterior decompressions for cervical spondylitic myelopathies often require posterior stabilization, and if the decompression includes the lower cervical spine, posterior fixation is often extended distally to include the cervicothoracic junction. Posterior cervical osteotomies for deformities due to ankylosing spondylitis are generally performed at the C7-T1 level. Although these procedures can be performed without instrumentation, posterior instrumentation systems may increase the chance of successful fusion and, in selected cases, obviate the need for a halo brace. Finally, post-laminectomy kyphosis reconstruction of the cervical spine often involves both posterior and anterior procedures. Because of the extensive nature of this surgery, anterior and posterior fixation methods are often used, with the posterior instrumentation extending into the upper thoracic spine.

CONTRAINDICATIONS

There are no true contraindications to the use of posterior cervicothoracic fixation; however, the specific diagnosis and surgical procedure will often dictate the type of fixation required. Additional anatomic considerations, as previously mentioned, may also limit the hardware choices. Following cervical laminectomy, interspinous wiring procedures cannot be performed unless additional levels are incorporated in the fusion. Although facet wiring is an option following decompressive procedures, the more rigid fixation systems, such as plates and rods, afford better means of stabilization. Decompression for an epidural abscess is a relative contraindication for immediate surgical fixation. Most surgeons avoid placing hardware in the posterior spine in the face of active infection. However, if instability is noted following the decompression, the posterior procedure can be staged, with the instrumentation occurring at a later date, after the active infection has been treated.

SURGICAL TECHNIQUE

Posterior cervicothoracic fixation is usually performed with the patient in the prone position. The patient may occasionally be positioned in the upright position, although care should be taken to reduce the risk of air embolism. Extreme care should be taken when positioning the patient, especially around the face. There should be no pressure on the eyes, because prolonged pressure can lead to either unilateral or bilateral blindness. Although horseshoe headrests are an option, they must be well padded, and the anesthesiologist must frequently check the eyes to make sure the head is not rotated, with resultant pressure on one or both of the eyes. To significantly decrease the risk of pressure on the eyes with this positioning, the patient can be placed in a Mayfield headrest (Fig. 33.1). This is usually accomplished by placing three pins in the skull and then tightening to a pressure of 40 to 60 pounds. The multiple articulations between the Mayfield headrest and the operating table allow great variability in positioning of the head and the neck.

The exact indications for the surgical procedure must be take into account when considering what position to place the head and neck during the surgery. Patients with significant stenosis and cervical myelopathy should not be placed in a hyperextended position because this could worsen cord pressure, leading to neurologic deterioration even before the actual surgical procedure begins. If the spine is unstable due to fracture or tumor, extreme care must be taken when turning the patient from the supine to prone position and then locking the headrest with the head and neck in a neutral position.

If there are significant concerns about cord compression during positioning the patient, spinal cord monitoring can be utilized. Baseline signals can be obtained with the patient in the supine position on the hospital gurney. After the patient has been positioned, responses can again be checked to make sure there has been no change from the

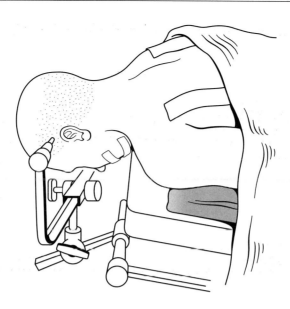

FIGURE 33.1. Patient is positioned in a Mayfield headrest. Tape is used to depress the shoulders to facilitate surgical exposure and improve x-ray quality.

baseline status. Frequently, the arms are placed along the side, since if the arms are placed above the head, they can get in the way of surgeon positioning and usually block any attempts at radiographic evaluation. Even with the arms placed at the sides and tape on the shoulders to depress the shoulders, it is often difficult to visualize the cervicothoracic junction on plain x-rays. Occasionally, fluoroscopic visualization of the lateral cervicothoracic junction can be feasible if the patient is relatively thin.

WIRING PROCEDURES

If a posterior decompression has not been performed and there is no fracture of the spinous processes or lamina, various wiring procedures are available for cervicothoracic fixation. Wiring techniques are generally effective in preventing flexion, but their effectiveness decreases in preventing rotation or extension. Generally, a 2- or 3-mm burr can be used to drill a hole at the base of the spinous processes, bilaterally, at the level to be instrumented. The drill hole site should be at the proximal aspect of the cephalad spinous process. Typically, the wire can pass underneath the caudad spinous process, since the downward sloping spinous processes will not allow the wire to disengage. After the hole is burred, a towel clip can be used to complete the tunnel through the spinous process, and then either an 18- or 20-gauge wire can be passed through the spinous process. Other options for wire fixation are braiding a smaller gauge wire or passing a braided titanium cable. The simplest technique of interspinous wiring involves a single wire going through the base of the superior spinous process and then around the inferior border of the caudal spinous process. The wire is then tightened. If more than one level is to be fused, the middle spinous process can be incorporated in a figure-of-eight fashion.

Additional stability for the wire construct can be created using a triple-wire technique, with interspinous process wires. A wire is passed through the cephalad part of the superior spinous process and then under the inferior part of the caudad spinous process. A second and third wire are then passed in similar fashion through and around the spinous processes and then through a cortical cancellous bone graft. After decortication of the lamina and facets, the wires are tightened down, thereby compressing the cortical cancellous grafts against the decorticated lamina.

Other wiring techniques include the passage of Kirschner wires through the base of the spinous process (Fig. 33.2), as well as the use of Wisconsin buttons and Luque rings.

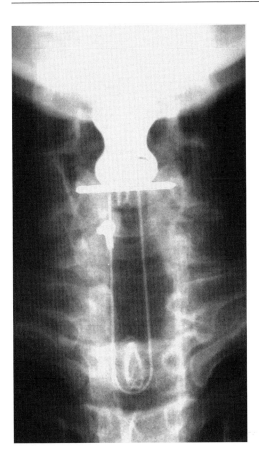

FIGURE 33.2. Posterior spinous wiring at the cervicothoracic junction. A Kirschner wire has been placed through the base of the spinous process at C6, with the wire passing underneath the spinous process of T2.

Sublaminar fixation of the cervicothoracic spine is generally not recommended, because this poses an increased risk of neurologic injury.

SCREW FIXATION

Placement of pedicle screws at the cervicothoracic junction can be performed either with the pedicles under direct visualization or through standard anatomic landmarks. With either technique, the preoperative imaging studies should be carefully examined to determine the medial angulation of the pedicle. Frequently, evaluation of the CT scan can also be very helpful in defining superficial landmarks. The relationships of the transverse processes to the pedicles can be noted and can occasionally be useful when determining the starting point for the pedicles.

There are several considerations when determining the appropriate time in the operative procedure to place posterior cervicothoracic hardware. Obviously, it would be safer to place all hardware prior to any laminectomies or decompressions because the neural elements will be protected by the lamina should there be an inadvertent handling of the instrumentation required to insert the screws, hooks, or rods. However, since the surface anatomy of the cervicothoracic spine is very variable from patient to patient, it is often difficult to find the correct starting points based on topographic features alone. Therefore, it is generally recommended that pedicle screws in this region should be placed with the pedicles under direct visualization.

If a laminotomy at C6–7 or a laminectomy at this level has already been performed, the C7 pedicle can easily be visualized and probed with a hockey-stick type of retractor. After determining the superior, medial, and inferior borders of the pedicle, the starting point is located, and a 2- or 3-mm burr is used to penetrate the posterior cortex. The

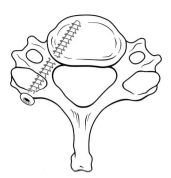

FIGURE 33.3. Axial schematic view of the correct starting point and placement of a cervical pedicle screw.

pedicle can generally then be sounded with a variety of devices. A small straight curette can be used to go within the confines of the pedicle, unless the bone is of such density that excessive force is needed to advance the curette. A power drill with an automatic stop on the guide can also be used (5). Minimal force should be used when advancing the drill, because the drill bit should be allowed to find its way in the confines of the pedicle. After drilling within the pedicle and just into the intervertebral body, the drill bit is removed and the walls of the pedicle can be probed with a small, flexible ball-tip probe. Frequently, a portion of the pedicle will need to be tapped, due to the dense cortical bone. The screw can then be placed, with palpation of the borders of the pedicle, again with the right-angle probe, to confirm there has been no breach of the cortical walls of the pedicle (Fig. 33.3).

As the complexity of the cervicothoracic deformity increases, it can become increasingly difficult to perform instrumentation procedures. It is generally not difficult to correctly place lateral mass screws in the cervical spine. Even with a greatly distorted anatomy, the landmarks for lateral screw placement in the mid to lower cervical spine can usually be found, as well as the entry points for pedicle screws at the cervicothoracic junction. Finally, even in the face of severe deformity, thoracic hooks, sometimes in pediatric sizes, can be placed in either sublaminar, subpedicular, or transverse processes in the thoracic spine. One of the great difficulties in severe deformities is connecting these various hooks to a single fixation device. Previous attempts used longer lateral mass plates that were designed for use in the lateral masses of the cervical spine, alone. Increase in the length of these plates does allow points of fixation for screws in the lateral masses of the cervical spine, down to the upper thoracic spine. However, with increasing deformity, as well as variations in anatomy, the starting points for screws often will not line up along a straight line. The surgeon is then faced with the difficult choice of attempting to fit the implant to the patient, with resultant placement of screws in a nonideal position.

As these difficulties became encountered more frequently, various modifications were made to existing hardware. One of the earliest modifications was a plate-rod device, described by Vaccaro et al. (6). This device provides a means of instrumenting the cervicothoracic junction by using a lateral mass or pedicle screw plating device that is transformed into a hook or wire attachment device in the thoracic spine (Fig. 33.4). Through the use of various connectors in the thoracic spine, there is sufficient offset so that screws can be placed in their correct starting points, thereby fitting the rod to the patient rather than compromising correct starting points due to hardware constraints. This device greatly increased the feasibility of posterior cervicothoracic fixation. Placement of lateral mass or pedicle screws in the cervical spine through the holes in the plate allowed for a semiconstrained fixation, whereas placement of hooks or screws in the lower portion of the rod allowed for rigid fixation at this level.

As the hardware continues to evolve, posterior cervicothoracic rodding designs that allow for greater variability and flexibility of screw placement have been introduced. Many newer devices allow placement of lateral mass screws in the cervical spine or pedicle screws in the cervical and thoracic spine. These constrained devices can also allow offset between the screws and rods, thereby allowing the surgeon to place all screws at the correct anatomic starting points. The use of dual-diameter rods (Fig. 33.5) allows larger

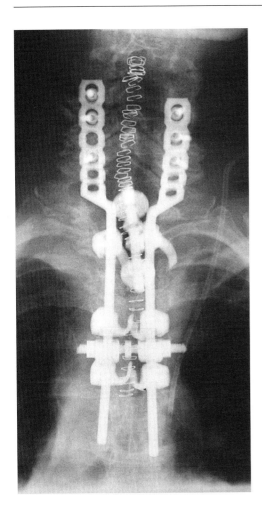

FIGURE 33.4. Posterior cervicothoracic fixation using a custom plate/rod device. The patient previously had anterior instrumentation placed at the level of a thoracic corpectomy defect.

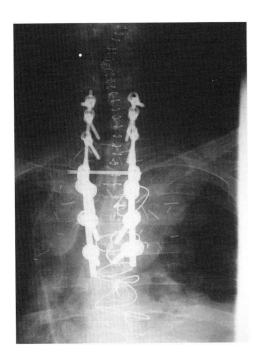

FIGURE 33.5. Dual diameter rod fixation of the cervicothoracic spine. Lateral mass screws are placed at C6, while pedicle screws are placed at C7 and T1, and larger-diameter pedicle screws are placed at T3, T4, and T5.

screws or hooks to be placed in the thoracic spine, while also allowing the smaller screws to be placed in the cervical spine. Because this technology is relatively new, long-term outcomes have not yet been recorded. Care should be used, especially in complex reconstructions in which excessive forces may be imposed on the fixation device.

REFERENCES

1. An HS, Simpson JM. Spinal instrumentation of the cervical spine. In: An HS, Simpson JM, eds. *Surgery of the cervical spine.* London: Martin-Dunitz, 1994:379–400.
2. An HS. Anatomy of the cervical spine. In: An HS, Simpson JM, eds. *Surgery of the cervical spine.* London: Martin-Dunitz, 1994:1–39.
3. Jovanovic MMS. A comparative study of the foramen transversarium of the sixth and seventh cervical vertebrae. *Surg Radiol Anat* 1990;12:167–172.
4. Jones EL, Heller JG, Silcox DH, et al. Cervical pedicle screws versus lateral mass screws. *Spine* 1997;22:977–982.
5. Albert TJ, Klein GR, Joffe D, et al. Use of cervicothoracic junction pedicle screws for reconstruction of complex cervical spinc pathology. *Spine* 1998;23:1596–1599.
6. Vaccaro AR, Conant RF, Hilibrand HS, et al. A plate-rod device for treatment of cervicothoracic disorders: comparison of mechanical testing with established cervical spine *in vitro* load testing data. *J Spinal Disord* 2000;13:350–355.

34

CERVICAL PEDICLE SCREW FIXATION

KUNIYOSHI ABUMI
MANABU ITO
YOSHIHISA KOTANI

Pedicle screws provide a number of advantages over other spinal fixation methods in treating a variety of conditions. Despite increasing acceptance among spine surgeons of the use of pedicle screws in the lumbar spine, many surgeons have been reluctant to extend their indication beyond the distal thoracic spine. As for the cervical pedicle, screw insertion has been considered too risky for the neurovascular structures, except at the C2 and C7 levels (1). However, biomechanical studies revealed the superior stabilizing effect of pedicle screw fixation over that of other internal fixation procedures in the cervical spine (2–4). This procedure allows rigid fixation to provide the high correction capability to restore physiologic sagittal alignment of the cervical spine, as well as sufficient correction of malalignment in the occipitoatlantoaxial region (5–8). In addition, the pedicle screw fixation procedure, which does not require use of the lamina as a stabilizing anchor, is quite valuable in patients who undergo one-stage posterior cervical decompression and stabilization and in patients who undergo posterior reconstruction after previous cervical spine laminectomy (9,10). On the other hand, the risks of neurovascular complications caused by inadequate screw placement into the cervical pedicle cannot be completely obviated (11,12). Thorough knowledge of local anatomy and the application of established surgical techniques are essential for this procedure.

INDICATIONS AND BENEFITS

A pedicle screw fixation procedure can be indicated for almost all of the pathological conditions requiring posterior stabilization or reconstruction or both of the occipitocervical spine, cervical spine, or cervicothoracic junction:

- Injuries with posterior disruption or anterior and posterior disruption without severely disrupted vertebral bodies
- Cervical spinal instability caused by nontraumatic lesions, including metastatic tumor, rheumatoid arthritis, and destructive spondyloarthropathy
- Correction of cervical malalignment in the sagittal plane, including postlaminectomy and posttraumatic kyphosis
- Stabilization of the unstable motion segment caused by decompression of the nerve root or spinal cord
- Posterior reduction and stabilization at the cervicothoracic junction
- Salvage of previous anterior surgeries

In addition, screws inserted into the cervical pedicles can be the rigid stabilizing anchors of craniocervical fixation.

CONTRAINDICATIONS AND LIMITATIONS

Patients with infectious disorders at the posterior portion of the cervical spine are contraindicated for pedicle screw fixation. Pedicles with the following conditions are inadequate for screw insertion:

- Pedicles destroyed by injuries, tumors, or marked osteoporosis
- Extremely small pedicles
- Pedicles of the vertebrae associated with major anomalies of the vertebral artery

SPECIFIC PREOPERATIVE CONSIDERATIONS

The pedicles in some patients are too small in diameter to allow screw insertion (13,14) (Fig. 34.1). Preoperative oblique projection plain x-ray films are valuable for evaluation of the pedicle size. In oblique projection plain films, the contralateral pedicle is seen as

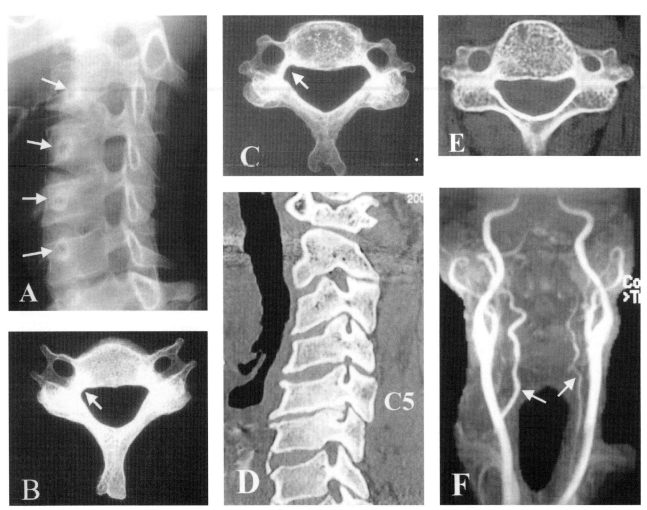

FIGURE 34.1. Preoperative radiological evaluation. **A:** Oblique projection plain film: Contralateral pedicle is seen as an oval (*arrows*) projected onto the vertebral body. **B:** Normal size of the cervical pedicle. **C:** Pedicles with small diameter. **D:** Narrowed intervertebral foramen demonstrated by reconstructive computed tomography (CT). **E:** CT showing dominance of the right vertebral artery. **F:** Domination of the right side of the vertebral artery in magnetic resonance angiography.

an oval projected onto the vertebral body, showing the outer and inner diameter of the pedicle (Fig. 34.1A). Computed tomography (CT) evaluations (adjusted to the bone windows) are essential to assess the pedicle morphometry and determine pedicle size, which allows surgeons to choose the appropriate pedicle screw diameter, length, and direction in the coronal plane. Figures 34.1B and C demonstrate different diameters of the pedicles. Reconstructive CT in the oblique plane provides useful information on the size of the neural foramen. Figure 34.1D shows intervertebral foramina narrowed by spondylosis.

Preoperative evaluation of the morphology of the vertebral artery is important in preventing serious complications involving the artery. The incidence of ischemic brain complication caused by unilateral obstruction of the vertebral artery is low (15). However, if the dominant vertebral artery is injured, serious neurologic complications can occur. CT (see Fig. 34.1E) and magnetic resonance imaging (MRI) provide information regarding the right-left domination and anatomic variations of the vertebral artery. Magnetic resonance angiography must be conducted for patients with evidence of abnormalities or in whom these abnormalities are suspected. Figure 34.1F (same patient as in Fig. 34.1E) shows domination of the right side of the vertebral artery.

OPERATION ROOM SETUP AND POSITIONING

The surgeon is recommended to stand at the head of the patient, to assure symmetrical insertion of the right and left screws, while the assistant surgeon usually stands on the left side of the patient (Fig. 34.2). The radiograph display is placed at the left side of the patient near the patient's pelvis for easy viewing by the surgeon (Fig. 34.2A). The patient is placed prone on a Relton-Hall frame using a horseshoe-type headrest or Mayfield head holder. The shoulders are pulled caudally by a heavy bandage for intraoperative lateral radiograph imaging of the lower cervical spine (Fig. 34.2B).

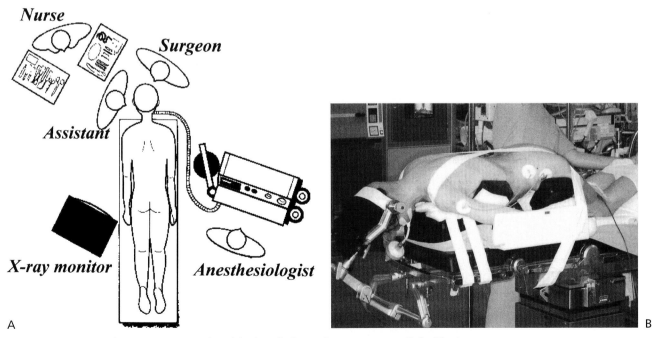

A   B

FIGURE 34.2. Operating room setup and positioning. **A:** Operating room setup. **B:** Positioning of the patient using a Relton-Hall frame and Mayfield head holder.

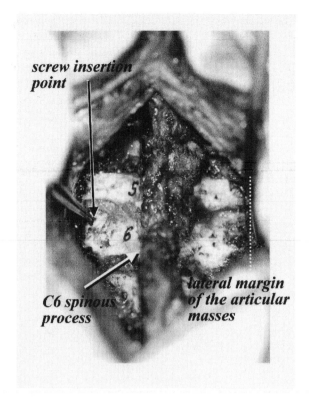

FIGURE 34.3. Exposure of the lower cervical spine. The paravertebral muscles are dissected laterally to expose the lateral margins of the articular masses.

EXPOSURE

A skin incision, usually longer than required for a standard spinous process wiring, is made (Fig. 34.3). The cephalad adjacent lamina of the uppermost fixed vertebra should be exposed entirely, with care taken to protect the surrounding facet joint capsule. The paravertebral muscles are dissected laterally to expose the lateral margins of the articular masses.

INSTRUMENTS

Screws with diameters of 3.5, 4.0, and 4.5 mm, according to pedicle diameter, are recommended for cervical pedicle screw fixation. The length of the screw is 20 or 22 mm for C3 to C7. A 24-mm-long screw is required to penetrate the anterior cortex of the vertebral body to increase the C2 screw stability. A constrained type of locking mechanism connecting the screws and plates or rods is essential to obtain the rigid stabilizing effect of this procedure.

PEDICLE SCREW PLACEMENT

Pedicle Screw Insertion Points and Directions

C3 to C7 Screws

The points of screw penetration for the C3 through C7 pedicles are slightly lateral to the center of the articular mass and close to the inferior margin of the inferior articular process of the cranially adjacent vertebra (Fig. 34.4). The insertion angle of the pedicle screw from C3 to C7 is intended to be 25 to 45 degrees medial to the midline in the transverse plane (Fig. 34.4A). The lateral margin of the articular mass of the cervical spine has a notch approximately at the level of the pedicle. The pedicles are located approximately below the lateral vertebral notch at C2, at the notch at C3 to C6 (Fig. 34.4B), and at or slightly above the notch at C7 (16).

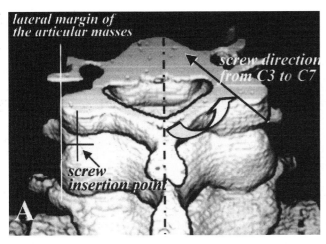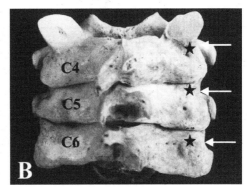

FIGURE 34.4. A: Pedicle screw insertion point and screw direction for C3 through C7. **B:** Screw insertion points (*asterisk*) and the lateral vertebral notch (*white arrows*)

C2 Screw

The craniad margin of the lamina of C2 is the landmark for the point of screw penetration for C2 (Fig. 34.5). To confirm the screw insertion points in C2, a slightly curved small spatula can be inserted into the spinal canal along the cranial margin of the C2 lamina to the superomedial surface of the pedicle of C2 (Fig. 34.5A). The angle for the C2 pedicle should be 15 to 25 degrees medial to the midline in the transverse plane (Fig. 34.5B).

Screw Insertion

The cortex at the point of insertion is penetrated with a high-speed burr (Fig. 34.6A). The surgeon can see the pedicle cavity directly in many cases by enlarging the insertion hole with a curette. After creating the insertion hole, a small pedicle probe, tap, and

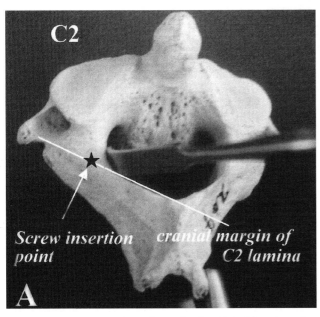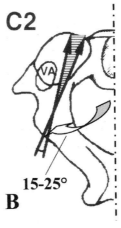

FIGURE 34.5. A: Screw insertion point for C2. **B:** Direction of screw for C2.

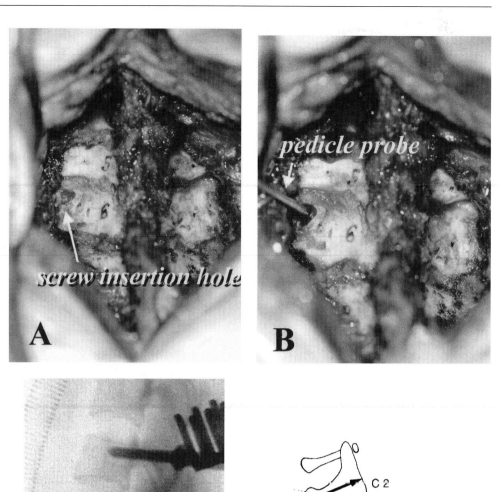

FIGURE 34.6. A: Screw insertion hole (*arrow*). **B:** Pedicle probe insertion into the pedicle. **C:** Intraoperative x-ray image shows a pedicle probe inserted into the vertebral body through the pedicle. **D:** Screw direction in the sagittal plane.

screws are inserted into the pedicle with the help of a lateral image intensifier to confirm the direction and insertion depth (Fig. 34.6B,C) The cortex of the cervical pedicles is always thinnest laterally toward the vertebral artery (13,14). Therefore, the surgeon should keep this in mind during probing and tapping of the pedicle and while placing the screws. A drill bit must never be used to penetrate the cortex of the lateral mass or to make a hole for screw advancement. The intended angle of screw insertion in the sagittal plane is parallel to the superior endplate for the pedicles of C5 through C7, and is in a slightly cephalad direction in C2 through C4 (Fig. 34.6D), according to its angulation in the sagittal plane. The neurocentral junction in the cervical spine, which is near the base of the pedicle in the vertebral body, is sometimes hard to pass with the pedicle probe. In such cases, the junction can be perforated with a Kirschner wire to make a path for the pedicle probe into the vertebral body (17).

PLATE OR ROD FIXATION IN THE CERVICAL SPINE

The neural foramina in patients with degenerative disorders or rheumatoid arthritis are sometimes stenotic preoperatively. There is a risk of iatrogenic nerve root lesion due to foraminal stenosis caused by reduction of anterior translation or correction of kyphosis. Use of a washer under the plate or rod for the cranial vertebral screws is helpful in situations where excessive reduction would occur during screw tightening. During correction of kyphosis, surgeons must also avoid applying excessive compression force at the spinal segment with neural foraminal stenosis due to degenerative changes. A prophylactic foraminotomy is recommended for patients with marked stenosis of the neural foramen.

The vertebral artery is sometimes obstructed unilaterally in patients with severe deformity at the craniocervical junction. In such patients, marked change of the vertebral alignment exposes the viable contralateral artery to injury. Confirmation of the arterial flow during reduction by using arterial ultrasonic Doppler provides for a safe reduction.

Prior to plate or rod application, the cortex of the lateral masses and laminae must be decorticated, and bone chips obtained from spinous processes and laminae are placed (Fig. 34.7A). In the final stage of instrumentation, inserted screws are connected by

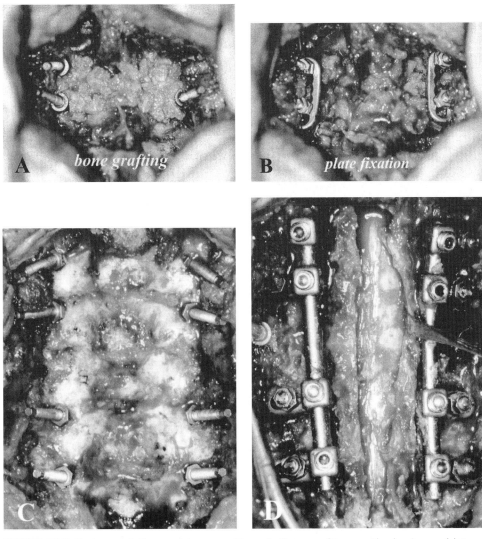

FIGURE 34.7. Instrumentation and bone grafting. **A:** Bone grafting on the lamina and lateral mass. **B:** Plate fixation. **C:** Screw insertion prior to decompression. **D:** Rod fixation after decompression.

plates or rods (Fig. 34.7B). Simple plate fixation is preferred for one- or two-segment fixation. However, the direction of inserted screws in the coronal plane may be varied randomly in multilevel fixation. Therefore, a rod with large freedom of connection with a screw rather than a plate is recommended for multilevel fixation of over three segments (Figs. 34.7C,D). Posterior decompression by laminectomy or laminoplasty must be performed prior to plate or rod application for patients with spinal canal stenosis because of the risk of neurologic deterioration by changing vertebral alignment after longitudinal connection of the screws.

CASE PRESENTATION

For patients with traumatic dislocation, reduction of anterior translation by nut tightening must be performed by applying distraction force between the inserted screws, avoiding deterioration of spinal cord lesions by traumatic herniated discs (17) (Fig. 34.8). The patient shown in Figure 34.8 with distractive flexion injury of C5–6 had incomplete spinal cord lesion. Preoperative lateral x-ray film shows local kyphosis and narrowed disc space (Fig. 34.8A). Preoperative MRIs revealed extruded disc herniation compressing the spinal cord (Fig. 34.8B). Single posterior reduction and fixation using a cervical pedicle screw-and-plate system was conducted. Distraction force was applied during reduction by nut tightening. Postoperative radiograph shows that distraction force opened the injured disc space (Fig. 34.8C). The postoperative MRI demonstrates reduction and reversal of the disc herniation (Fig. 34.8D). Spinal cord compression disappeared after posterior indirect decompression was achieved by placement of the cervical pedicle screw system.

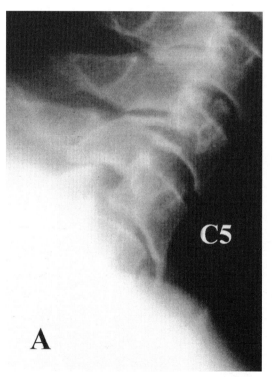 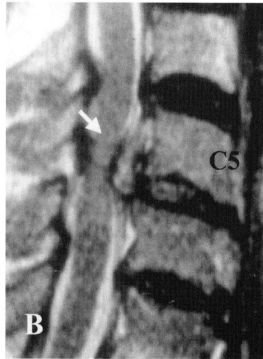

FIGURE 34.8. Distractive flexion injury at C5–6 with traumatic disc herniation. **A:** Lateral film shows subluxation of C5 and narrowed disc space. **B:** Magnetic resonance image shows spinal cord compression by herniated disc. *Continued.*

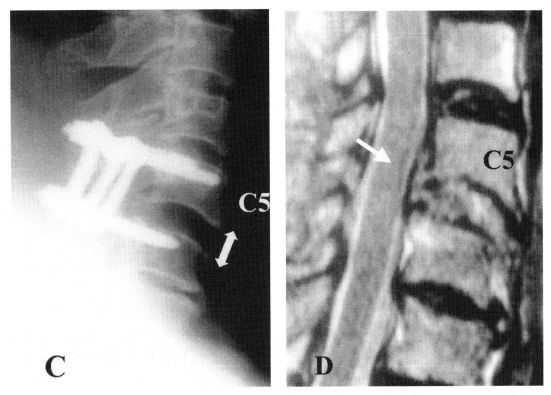

FIGURE 34.8. *(continued)* **C:** Postoperative radiograph shows the opened disc space. **D:** Postoperative magnetic resonance image demonstrates reduction and reversal of the disc herniation.

OCCIPITOCERVICAL FIXATION

Many patients who require occipitocervical fixation possess combined deformities in the sagittal plane. These consist of anterior translation of the atlas on the axis, vertical subluxation of the odontoid process, and flexion deformity caused by anterior subluxation or dislocation of the occipitoatlantal complex on the axis. If atlantoaxial dislocation is irreducible and the dislocation is a causative factor of neurologic deficits, anterior decompression and fusion by a transoral or mandibular splitting approach will be required. However, these procedures involve complicated perioperative management and the risks of infection, and it will be difficult to obtain solid fusion with these procedures without support by rigid external fixation using a halo vest or cast. The combined use of cervical pedicle screws and occipitocervical rods for reconstruction of occipitocervical lesions provides sufficient correction of malalignment of the craniocervical junction by application of the combined force of extension and distraction. As a result of the reduction, indirect decompression of the anterior portion of the medulla oblongata is obtained by decrease of the mechanical stress (6).

Surgical Technique of Occipitocervical Fixation

After insertion of the pedicle screws, decortication of the posterior cortex of the lateral masses and residual laminae is performed with a burr. Washers, 2.5 or 5.0 mm in height, are placed on the C2 pedicle screws to reduce anterior translation of the atlas on the axis and to allow a space for monocortical on-lay bone graft between the rod and the lateral mass. The occipitocervical rods are contoured at the plate-rod junction to reduce hyperflexion at the occipitocervical junction. The plate portion of the rod is fixed by self-tapping

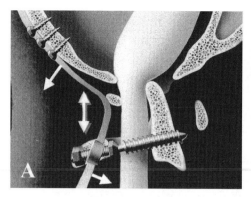
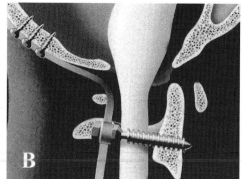
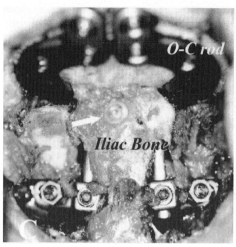

FIGURE 34.9. Occipitocervical fixation. **A:** Application of extension and distraction force for reduction of atlantoaxial subluxation and vertical subluxation of the odontoid process. **B:** Indirect decompression achieved by reduction. **C:** Iliac bone grafting between the occiput and the axis (an *arrow* indicates an absorbable screw to stabilize the grafted iliac bone).

screws onto the occiput. The caudal end of the rod is cut to the proper length, leaving adequate length to allow distraction force to correct upward migration of the odontoid process. Figure 34.9 shows reduction and fixation of anterior subluxation and vertical subluxation of C2.

Hyperflexion alignment of the occipitoatlantoaxial complex is corrected by application of extensional force created by tightening the nut to the pedicle screws. Distraction force is applied with a spreader between the plate portion of each rod and the head of each screw inserted into the pedicle of C2 or C3 to reduce the upward migration of the odontoid process (Figs. 34.9A,B). These reduction maneuvers work by application of the combined force of extension and distraction and are conducted alternately on each side to avoid excessive force applied on one side. After reduction by application of proper force, rods and screws are fixed by tightening the set screws of the connectors. The massive monocortical iliac bone for bridging a graft between the occiput and the axis is trimmed and packed between the two rods. Chipped cancellous and cortical bones are grafted on the remaining exposed laminae and lateral masses at all the fusion levels (Fig. 34.9C). In Figure 34.9C, a white arrow indicates an absorbable screw to stabilize the grafted iliac bone.

CASE PRESENTATION

A patient with rheumatoid arthritis had suffered from quadriparesis and respiratory problems (Fig. 34.10). The patient could not remain in a sitting position without halo vest stabilization because of respiratory disturbance. The neurologic disturbance was caused by compression of the medulla oblongata by massive flexion deformity at the occipitocervical

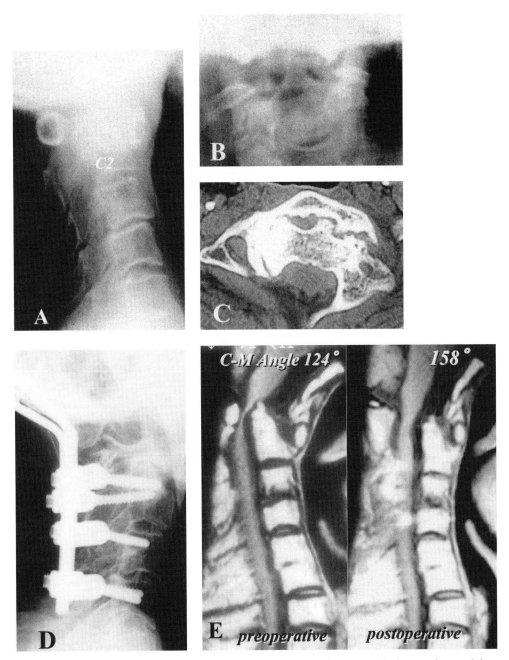

FIGURE 34.10. A patient with rheumatoid arthritis. **A:** Lateral laminograph shows atlantoaxial subluxation and vertical subluxation of the odontoid process. **B:** Anteroposterior laminograph shows tilting of the occipitoatlantoaxial complex. **C:** Computed tomography (CT) scan demonstrates rotatory fixation of the atlantoaxial joint. **D:** Postoperative CT scan shows reduction of atlantoaxial subluxation and vertical subluxation of the odontoid process. **E:** Preoperative and postoperative magnetic resonance images demonstrate the decrease in anterior compression of the medulla oblongata and improvement of the cervicomedullary angle from 124 degrees to 158 degrees.

junction and upward migration of the odontoid process (Figs. 34.10A–C). This patient underwent correction of flexion deformity and vertical subluxation by using cervical pedicle screws and occipitocervical rods (Fig. 34.10D). Preoperative and postoperative MRIs demonstrate the decrease of anterior compression of the medulla oblongata and improvement of the cervicomedullary angle from 124 degrees to 158 degrees. In this patient, screws were inserted into the pedicles of C2, C3, and C4 to correct the rigid flexion deformity.

CONCLUSION

Pedicle screw fixation is a useful procedure for reconstruction of the cervical spine in various kinds of disorders. Complications associated with cervical pedicle screw fixation cannot be completely obviated; however, they can be minimized by sufficient preoperative imaging studies of the pedicles, thorough knowledge of local anatomy, and strict control of screw placement.

REFERENCES

1. Roy-Camille R, Salient G, Mazel C. Internal fixation of the unstable cervical spine by a posterior osteosynthesis with plates and screws. In: The Cervical Spine Research Society, eds. *The cervical spine,* 2nd ed. Philadelphia: JB Lippincott Co, 1989:390–403.
2. Jones EL, Heller JG, Silcox DH, et al. Cervical pedicle screw versus lateral mass screws: anatomic feasibility and biomechanical comparison. *Spine* 1997;22:977–982.
3. Kotani Y, Cunningham BW, Abumi K, et al. Biomechanical analysis of cervical stabilization systems: an assessment of transpedicular screw fixation in the cervical spine. *Spine* 1994;19:2529–2539.
4. Oda I, Abumi K, Haggerty CJ, et al. Biomechanical evaluation of five different occipito-atlanto-axial fixation techniques. *Spine* 1999;24:2377–2382.
5. Abumi K, Ito H, Taneichi H, et al. Transpedicular screw fixation for traumatic lesions of the middle and lower cervical spine. Description of the techniques and preliminary report. *J Spinal Disord* 1994;7:19–28.
6. Abumi K, Takada T, Shono Y, et al. Posterior occipitocervical reconstruction using cervical pedicle screws and plate-rod systems. *Spine* 1999;24:1425–1434.
7. Abumi K, Shono Y, Taneichi T, et al. Correction of cervical kyphosis using pedicle screw fixation systems. *Spine* 1999;24:2389–2396.
8. Abumi K, Ito M, Kaneda K. Surgical treatment of cervical spine disorders associated with long-term hemodialysis. *Spine* 2000;25:2906–2912.
9. Abumi K, Kaneda K. Pedicle screw fixation for non-traumatic lesions of the cervical spine. *Spine* 1997;22:1853–1863.
10. Abumi K, Kaneda K, Shono Y, et al. One-stage posterior decompression and reconstruction of the cervical spine by using pedicle screw fixation systems. *J Neurosurg (Spine 1)* 1999;90:19–26.
11. Abumi K, Shono Y, Ito M, et al. Complication of pedicle screw fixation in reconstructive surgery of the cervical spine. *Spine* 2000;25:962–969.
12. Abumi K, Ito M, Kotani Y. Complications of cervical pedicle screw placement. *Semin Spine Surg* 2002;14:112–124.
13. Karaikovic EE, Daubs MD, Madsen RW, et al. Morphologic characteristics of human cervical pedicles. *Spine* 1997;22:493–550.
14. Panjabi MM, Shin EK, Chen NC, et al. Internal morphology of human cervical pedicle. *Spine* 2000;25:1197–1205.
15. Smith MD, Emery SE, Dudley A, et al. Vertebral artery injury during anterior decompression of the cervical spine. *J Bone Joint Surg Br* 1993;75:410–415.
16. Karaikovic EE, Kunakornsawat S, Daubs MD, et al. Surgical anatomy of the cervical pedicles: landmarks for posterior cervical pedicle entrance localization. *J Spinal Disord* 2000;13:63–72.
17. Abumi K, Shono Y, Kotani Y, et al. Indirect posterior reduction and fusion of the traumatic herniated disc by using a cervical pedicle screw system. *J Neurosurg (Spine 1)* 2000;92:30–37.

INDEX

Page numbers followed by *f* indicate figures; page numbers followed by *t* indicate tables.